CANCER ETIOLOGY, DIAGNOSIS AND TREATMENTS

Additional books in this series can be found on Nova's website under the Series tab.

Additional e-books in this series can be found on Nova's website under the e-book tab.

DERMATOLOGY - LABORATORY AND CLINICAL RESEARCH

Additional books in this series can be found on Nova's website under the Series tab.

Additional e-books in this series can be found on Nova's website under the e-book tab.

CANCER ETIOLOGY, DIAGNOSIS AND TREATMENTS

MELANOMA

MOLECULAR BIOLOGY, RISK FACTORS AND TREATMENT OPTIONS

CANCER ETIOLOGY, DIAGNOSIS AND TREATMENTS

MELANOMA

MOLECULAR BIOLOGY, RISK FACTORS AND TREATMENT OPTIONS

ALEXANDER C. JONES
EDITOR

New York

For permission to use material from this book please contact us:
Telephone 631-231-7269; Fax 631-231-8175
Web Site: http://www.novapublishers.com

Additional color graphics may be available in the e-book version of this book.

Library of Congress Cataloging-in-Publication Data

ISBN: 978-1-62808-608-9

LCCN: 2013945019

Published by Nova Science Publishers, Inc. † New York

CONTENTS

PREFACE

Melanoma accounts for only 4% of all skin cancer cases but most of skin cancer-related death. The rising incidence of melanoma makes this tumor an important public health problem. In this book, the authors present current research in the study of the molecular biology, risk factors and treatment options for melanoma. Topics include the role of P13K/AKT and Wnt/β-Catenin pathways in melanoma's progression to metastatic disease; cutaneous melanoma; molecular determinants of melanoma vasculogenic mimicry; new aspects of the molecular biology of melanoma metastasis; the surgical extent of regional lymph node dissection for cutaneous melanoma and its novel techniques and modifications; the epidemiology of melanoma in young individuals; cardiac involvement in malignant melanoma; poor Karnofsky performance status and high serum lactate dehydrogenase level identifies patients with brain metastases from malignant melanoma who do not benefit from palliative whole brain radiotherapy; interferon-beta therapy; and boron neutron capture therapy.

Chapter 1 - Worldwide, melanoma has the most rapidly rising incidence rate of any human cancer. It arises from the malignant transformation of the melanocyte cells of the skin. Due to the inefficacy of present chemotherapeutic regimens and the resistance of melanocyte cells to radiotherapy, 95% of stage IV metastatic melanoma patients die within five years of diagnosis. Metastasis, the spread of a cancer from the site of the primary tumour to distant sites of the body, makes melanoma very hard to treat. Risk factors associated with malignant melanoma include excessive sun exposure and associated mutations in specific genes and deregulation of signal transduction pathways.

Malignant melanoma is characterized by frequent metastasis; however, specific changes that cause this malignancy are yet to be characterized. Several oncogenes, tumour suppressor genes, and pathways are implicated in melanoma; for example, NRAS, which activates RAF kinases in response to growth factors is overactive in 15–20% of melanomas. P16 (INK4A) tumour suppressor expression is lost by mutation, deletion, or transcriptional silencing of the CDKN2A locus in many melanomas. BRAF mutations are often found alongside P16 mutations. Phosphatase and tensin homolog (PTEN) mutations and deletions are also present in a significant number of melanomas, coinciding with BRAF mutations. Since these two mutations often occur together PTEN loss reflects the importance of two RAS-effector pathways in melanoma. Another genomic aberration associated with melanoma is the amplification of microphthalmia-associated transcription factor (MITF).

The occurrence of several different mutations implies that several signal transduction pathways are perturbed in melanoma. Of particular interest to this review are mutations in the Wnt/β-catenin pathway as well as the PI3K pathway. Elevated levels of nuclear β-catenin are observed in ~30% of human melanomas. In fact, melanoma is one of the first cancer types associated with β-catenin/Wnt signaling mutations. Mutations in the Wnt signaling pathway that result in over-activation of β-catenin signaling are readily observed in melanomas, but the functional implications of these mutations in melanoma progression remain unclear.

The PI3K pathway is likely the most frequently deregulated pathway in melanoma, although the mechanism underlying the over-activation in most cases remains largely elusive. Growth factor stimulation of receptor tyrosine kinases (RTK) and/or non-RTKs results in the activation of PI3K and the conversion of phosphatidylinositol-bis-phosphate (PIP2) to phosphatidylinositol-tri- phosphate (PIP3). The presence of PIP3 mediates the phosphorylation and activation of Akt/PKB by PDK1/PDK2 at Threonine 308 (T308) and Serine 473 (S473). Activated Akt (phosphorylated Akt [P-Akt]) is the central effector of many downstream signaling pathways regulating protein synthesis, cell cycle, cell death, cell growth, and cell survival. In Melanoma, the loss of the tumour suppressor protein and negative regulator of the PI3K/Akt pathway, PTEN, is a common event leading to the constitutive activation of PI3K/Akt signaling. The consitutive activation of this pathway with PTEN loss and the resulting elevation of the P-AKT signaling axis may be a method for promoting/sustaining melanoma progression. This includes modes of regulation between PI3K/Akt and other pathways such as 1) cross-talk with the Wnt/GSK3β/β- catenin pathway, 2) cross-talk with FOXO family of transcription factors and 3) mammalian target of rapamycin (mTOR).

This review will discuss the current evidence available for PI3K/PTEN/Akt and Wnt- β-catenin mediated signaling in melanoma progression.

Chapter 2 - Cutaneous Melanoma is the neoplasia with the fastest growing incidence worldwide. Early diagnosed tumors are mostly curable by surgery. However, when it metastasizes, only a minority of patients can be cured; treatment options are still limited, in part due to its refractory nature to conventional therapies. In this section the authors will revisit the main risk factors associated to this disease and will perform an integral analysis of its biology, taking into consideration key signatures and signaling pathways. In light of the increasing knowledge about Cutaneous Melanoma biology and its immunogenic nature, the authors will go through new therapies that focus on targeted therapies and immunotherapy, including vaccines.

Chapter 3 - The rising incidence of melanoma makes this tumor an important public health problem. Standard systemic therapies have not been adequately effective in the management of melanoma. Moreover, melanoma is resistant to antiangiogenesis therapy suggesting the existence of alternative blood circulation system. For years sprouting angiogenesis has been considered as exclusive mechanism of tumor vascularization. However, in recent years another mechanism of tumor vascularization has been identified that does not involve endothelial cells, a process called vasculogenic mimicry (VM).VM describes the unique ability of highly aggressive tumor cells to express a multipotent, stem cell-like phenotype, and form capillary-like structures (CLS) and matrix-rich patterned network in three-dimentional culture that mimic embryonic vasculogenic network. VM occurrence is tumors strongly associated with poor prognosis.

This review will focus on molecular determinants and signaling pathways involved in melanoma VM. The authors will discuss the mechanisms that operate at the initial phase of CLS formation by melanoma cells. The authors will provide the experimental evidence that CLS formation requires apoptotic cell death through activation of caspase-dependent mechanism. In addition, the authors will describe the status of VM under the condition of angiogenesis blockage.

Chapter 4 - Metastatic melanoma is a highly aggressive tumor and compared to other types of skin cancer, it has recently shown the highest increase in incidence and studies in several countries indicate that this increase is expected to continue over the next two decades. If this type of cancer has of good prognosis when diagnosed during the early stages of development (5-year survival estimated at 88-98%), the metastatic 5-year survival is less than 20%, the currently used chemotherapy protocols having a poor efficiency. It is therefore necessary to better understand the process of metastatic spread of this type of cancer in order to identify new targets and to gain better insight into potentially efficient therapies. The metastatic dissemination of tumor cells can be divided in four main steps intravasation, adhesion, extravasation and secondary tissue colonization. Many attempts have been made to identify molecules involved in the three first steps and some mechanisms are now beginning to be better understood. The interactions with the endothelium have notably been described by different groups, and seem to involve several immune molecules.

To colonize secondary tissue, the last step but not the least, cells must adapt to their new microenvironment before proliferating. This is a critical step for the spread of metastases and melanoma particularly succeeds in it. Among the several models that have been suggested to explain these properties one is particularly of interest suggesting that melanoma progression may be driven by phenotype-switching. This would be triggered by cell adaptation to changes in tumor microenvironment, made possible by an important plasticity of melanoma cells. Therefore, melanoma would regularly shift between aggressive/proliferative phases and invasive phases. All this progress in the understanding of melanoma biology highlights different aspects of the development of metastatic melanoma (i.e. plasticity and immune mimetic mechanisms) and might hopefully help to develop new therapeutic strategies.

Chapter 5 - With the advent of the sentinel lymph node biopsy technique, the rate of patients with melanoma who have microscopic nodal metastases has increased. However, patients with clinical nodal disease are still encountered despite the development of sentinel lymph node biopsy. Although surgery is still the most important staging tool and treatment option for patients with microscopic or clinical nodal metastases and because surgery offers the chance for regional control and cure, the therapeutic value and the appropriate surgical extent of lymph node dissection and the appropriate selection of patients for lymph node dissection remain unclear. There are few specific recommendations available in the published guidelines, and there are reports with only low levels of evidence supporting the appropriate surgical extent of lymph node dissection of the cervical, axillary, and ilioinguinal regions. Ultimately, the individual surgeon decides the extent of lymph node dissection that is appropriate for each patient.

The indications for regional lymph node dissection for patients with melanoma continue to evolve. Several studies regarding the extent of dissection, its novel techniques, and modifications of the procedure to reduce postoperative morbidity have been reported. In this chapter, the authors will review the currently available information on regional lymph node dissection for cutaneous melanoma, assess the current strategies of lymph node dissection, discuss relevant controversial issues, and examine future steps required to improve the regional control of metastasis.

Chapter 6 - Cutaneous melanoma arises in the skin from melanocytes and is one of the most deadly forms of skin cancer. Worldwide incidence of cutaneous melanoma has been increasing dramatically, particularly among young adults[1]. Fortunately, the skin is easily examined and biopsied, leading to early diagnosis, effective surgical treatment and positive clinical outcomes in most cases. However, the most important prognostic indicator of a primary tumor is the depth of invasion into the skin, and once the primary tumor has invaded lower layers of the skin and/or spread to lymph nodes or distant sites, mortality rates increase exponentially. This mortality rate is primarily due to the lack of effective treatment, particularly for metastatic melanoma, although recent advances have generated more effective therapy. Research into the molecular mechanisms that initiate and drive melanoma has improved the author's understanding of melanoma biology and may lead to new treatment options in the future.

Chapter 7 - Skin cancer is the most common type of cancer affecting patients today. Cutaneous melanoma is one of the more serious forms of skin cancer, which originates from melanocytes usually in the dermal-epidermal junction. The rates of cutaneous melanoma have been steadily increasing; 1/500 in 1935, 1/600 in 1960, and 1/75 in 2000 with a projected steady increase in incidence in the future; current estimates suggest that the rates are 1/50. Particularly, melanoma rates continue to grow, especially in younger individuals.

There are a variety of different epidemiological studies which have shown that younger individuals are at an ever increasing risk for developing melanoma. Childhood and adolescence are considered to be "critical periods of vulnerability" when individuals are vulnerable to the effects ultraviolet radiation. 25% of sun exposure occurs before the age of 18 and sun exposure during those years is often more intense than those in later years due to the behavior of the younger individuals. In addition to being at a much higher risk for sunlight exposure young individuals are also less likely to practice proper sun-protection. Studies have shown that there is an increased risk of melanoma after receiving a sunburn during the adolescent and childhood periods. This is hypothesized to occur because exposure may lead to alteration in the DNA of melanocytes which increases the risk of malignant degeneration as the individual ages.

Many younger individuals also spend time tanning in indoor tanning machines which exposes them to increased levels of UV radiation which can lead to DNA damage and skin cancer in the long term. Many studies have shown strong associations between UV exposure via tanning beds and risk of melanoma.

In young individuals, social pressures have contributed to increased desire to achieve greater skin pigmentation, often through use of tanning beds. Tanning bed use leads to a great deal of negative health effects, including melanoma. In young adults, cutaneous melanomas from 1975-2000 were the most common cancers in the 25-29 year old population of females and was 12% of cancers in 20-40 year old females. In the past few years there has been a sharp uptick in the number of patients with cutaneous malignancies; from 1970 to 2009, the incidence of melanoma has skyrocketed in males aged 18 to 39 (4-fold increase) and females in the same age range (8-fold increase).

Younger individuals may be at a greater risk for developing melanoma due to tanning bed use and greater exposure to the ultraviolet radiation. Education programs targeted at highlighting risky behaviors and leading to increased protection from UV radiation and other toxic exposures can limit the incidence of melanoma as the individual progresses from childhood to adulthood.

Chapter 8 - Skin is a complex tissue, whose outer layer, epidermis, protects against ultraviolet radiation and several pathogens. Thus, epidermal cells have a high risk of acquiring gene mutations leading to cancer. Malignant melanoma is a tumor derived from genetically altered epidermal melanocytes; it is highly aggressive, often associated with rapid progression. Familial melanomas represent about 10% of all melanoma cases. The study of familiar cases led to the identification of several melanoma susceptibility genes in chromosomes 1, 6, 7, 9, and 10. Some of the molecular pathways altered in malignant melanoma regard tyrosine kinase receptors pathways, cell cycle regulation pathways, epigenetic gene expression regulation, apoptosis pathways, common apoptosis effectors, and protein chaperoning and degradation.

The presence of lymph-node metastases decreases the 5-year survival rate by approximately 40%. However, 25% of patients free of lymphatic metastasis have disease recurrence and die.

Malignant melanoma has a high rate of cardiac metastases. It is rarely detected ante mortem, and can involve almost any cardiac structure. Heart involvement is usually silent, or the patient complains of nonspecific symptoms. Right or left heart failure, cardiac tamponade and atrioventricular block can also occur. Echocardiography is a first-line imaging technique for heart evaluation. Disease staging is performed by means of tomographic scanning of chest, abdomen, and brain, magnetic resonance imaging of and whole-body 18 Fluorodeoxyglucose. Prognosis is poor, as therapeutic options are usually limited to palliative treatments. However, patients with metastases in the form of single intra-cardiac masses can undergo excision, at least for symptoms relief.

Chapter 9 - Malignant melanoma has a high propensity for intracranial seeding. By the time brain metastases are diagnosed, the majority of patients also suffer from uncontrolled extracranial disease.

For this prognostically unfavorable group, and especially for patients with multiple or progressive intracranial metastases, there are no existing scores that are able to reliably predict whether the patients can benefit from palliative whole brain radiotherapy (WBRT) or best supportive care.

In a previous analysis, Karnofsky Performance Status (KPS) and lactate dehydrogenase level (LDH) independently predicted overall survival. The present study was undertaken to test these parameters in a larger patient cohort.

The authors present a retrospective analysis of 107 patients with initial multiple intracranial lesions or with progression of brain metastases after resection and/or radiosurgery, who were treated with palliative WBRT between 1988 and 2012. Uni- and multivariate analyses were used to analyze the impact of the following patient-, tumor- and treatment-related parameters on overall survival: age, sex, KPS, neurologic symptoms, serum LDH, number of intracranial metastases, prior neurosurgical resection or stereotactic radiosurgery as well as the number and site of extracranial metastases prior to WBRT.

In accordance with the author's previous findings, low KPS (defined as <70) and high serum LDH (defined as >240 U/L) were identified as the only independent prognostic factors for overall survival with a hazard ratio of 4.8 [95% CI 2.8–8.1] and 2.5 [95% CI 1.6–4.1] The combination of these two parameters (KPS/LDH Index) classified the patients into 4 distinct survival groups.

The median overall survival was 175 days for patients with high KPS and low LDH; 111 days for patients with high KPS and high LDH; 47 days for patients with low KPS and low LDH; and 34 days for patients with low KPS and high LDH. 76 patients presented with neurological symptoms at the time of WBRT. At the end of therapy no improvement or even a deterioration of neurological symptoms had been recorded in 64.2% of these patients.

The authors' updated analysis confirmed that the KPS/LDH Index was highly predictive in identifying patients with a more favorable or a very unfavorable prognosis. Patients of the latter group did not benefit from WBRT in terms of improved survival. Disappointing results were also obtained in terms of improving quality of life in patients with neurological symptoms.

Chapter 10 - Interferon (IFN)-β is a naturally occurring secretary glycoprotein. At present two subtypes of IFN-β, "natural" IFN-β (nIFN-β) and "recombinant" IFN-β (rIFN-β), are being used clinically. According to *in vitro* studies examining the anti-tumor activity of IFN-β, both nIFN-β and rIFN-β inhibited the proliferation of, and showed apoptotic effects on, melanoma cells. Moreover, some *in vivo* studies have demonstrated that the local administration of nIFN-β and rIFN-β leads to anti-tumor activity on human melanoma xenograft models. Despite such experimental outcomes, the results of phase II clinical trials involving metastatic melanoma patients indicated that systemic administration of neither nIFN-β nor rIFN-β was significantly effective. In contrast, clinical trials in Japan involving intratumoral injections of nIFN-β resulted in an efficacy rate of 50% against cutaneous metastatic melanomas. Due to this finding, nIFN-β is now approved in Japan and is frequently used, especially as a part of post-operative adjuvant chemotherapy such as "DAV-IFN-β therapy", a combination of dacarbazie, nimustine, vincristine, and local subcutaneous injections of nIFN-β. After DAV-IFN-β therapy, nIFN-β alone can be administered for maintenance therapy. While the efficacy of nIFN-β when combined with DAV therapy has not yet been fully confirmed in clinical investigations, a recent study examining single-agent maintenance therapy with sequential, local injections of nIFN-β demonstrated significant improvement of the prognosis of stage II melanoma patients. Although further randomized studies are needed, adjuvant therapy using local injections of nIFN-β may be a viable option for post-operative melanoma patients.

Chapter 11 - Recent evidence suggests that molecular targeted therapy using BRAF or MEK inhibitors on melanoma (with BRAF V600E mutation) is promising. In addition, combined BRAF and MEK inhibition is proved to be superior, because MEK inhibitors are able to prevent BRAF-inhibitor-induced side effects; that is, cutaneous squamous cell carcinoma, which is associated with paradoxical activation of MAPK pathway by BRAF inhibitors.

Although molecular targeted therapy on melanoma seems to be successful, there remains an unsolved problem; drug resistance. Increasing volumes of evidence indicate that mechanisms of drug resistance are not only cell-intrinsic but also cell-extrinsic. One of cell-intrinsic mechanisms is BRAF gene amplification, and novel driver mutations reported recently may also contribute to drug resistance. On the other hand, regarding cell-extrinsic mechanisms, tumor-microenvironment-mediated drug resistance has been demonstrated; that is, HGF-high stroma is attributable to drug resistance, and HGF-cMet axis inhibitors are useful to resolve drug resistance.

Collectively, further understanding of drug resistance mechanisms will improve outcomes of molecular targeted therapy on melanoma.

Chapter 12 - Boron Neutron Capture Therapy (BNCT) is a therapeutic tool for treatment of many types of tumors. It is based on the administration of a compound containing the element boron - isotope 10 (^{10}B), followed by thermal neutron irradiation. This results in a nuclear reaction and consequent release of high linear energy transfer, by alpha particles and lithium production. The products created by this reaction have a short range (5-9 μm) and thus reaches only cells that incorporate ^{10}B. This therapy is therefore a cellular irradiation suited to treat tumors that have infiltrated into healthy tissues. Some compounds have been studied to increase the uptake selectivity by tumor cells. The most frequently compounds with 10B used clinically are BSH ($Na_2H_{11}{}^{10}B_{12}SH$, sulfhydryl borane) and an amino acid derivative known as BPA [$(HO)_2\ {}^{10}B\text{-}C_6H_4\text{-}CH\ (NH_2)\ CO_2H$, Boronophenylalanine]. These compounds are nontoxic and may be administered in high doses. BNCT has been used clinically to treat patients with cutaneous melanomas which have a high mortality. These patients were either not candidates for, or had declined, conventional therapy. Melanoma is the most aggressive skin cancer and frequently involves distant and locoregional spread, usually with no efficient treatment. Metastatic melanoma remains a highly lethal disease, with an incidence that continues to increase faster than any other cancer. Almost all adjuvant treatments fail to control this malignancy. This therapy can potentially target tumor tissue selectively, sparing normal cells damage due to radiation. BNCT induces cell cycle arrest by cyclin D1 decrease, antiproliferative effects by Ki67 decrease and apoptosis by mitochondrial electric potential decrease and cleaved caspase 3, 7, 8 and 9 protein levels increase only in melanoma cells. As a result, BNCT acts as a localized therapy with minimal side effects for the melanoma treatment. This way, BNCT can be used as an adjunctive treatment in combination with other modalities, including surgery and chemotherapy, may lead to an improvement in patient survival.

In: Melanoma
Editor: Alexander C. Jones
ISBN: 978-1-62808-608-9

Chapter 1

MELANOMA PROGRESSION TO METASTATIC DISEASE: THE ROLE OF THE PI3K/AKT AND WNT/B-CATENIN PATHWAYS

Jaskiran Sidhu, Geetha Venkateswaran and Sujata Persad*
Department of Pediatrics, Faculty of Medicine and Dentistry, University of Alberta, Edmonton, Alberta, Canada

ABSTRACT

Worldwide, melanoma has the most rapidly rising incidence rate of any human cancer. It arises from the malignant transformation of the melanocyte cells of the skin. Due to the inefficacy of present chemotherapeutic regimens and the resistance of melanocyte cells to radiotherapy, 95% of stage IV metastatic melanoma patients die within five years of diagnosis. Metastasis, the spread of a cancer from the site of the primary tumour to distant sites of the body, makes melanoma very hard to treat. Risk factors associated with malignant melanoma include excessive sun exposure and associated mutations in specific genes and deregulation of signal transduction pathways.

Malignant melanoma is characterized by frequent metastasis; however, specific changes that cause this malignancy are yet to be characterized. Several oncogenes, tumour suppressor genes, and pathways are implicated in melanoma; for example, NRAS, which activates RAF kinases in response to growth factors is overactive in 15–20% of melanomas. P16 (INK4A) tumour suppressor expression is lost by mutation, deletion, or transcriptional silencing of the CDKN2A locus in many melanomas. BRAF mutations are often found alongside P16 mutations. Phosphatase and tensin homolog (PTEN) mutations and deletions are also present in a significant number of melanomas, coinciding with BRAF mutations. Since these two mutations often occur together PTEN loss reflects the importance of two RAS-effector pathways in melanoma. Another genomic aberration associated with melanoma is the amplification of microphthalmia-associated transcription factor (MITF).

* Correspondence to: Dr. Sujata Persad Associate Professor, Department of Pediatrics Faculty of Medicine and Dentistry University of Alberta 3020 Katz Group Centre for Pharmacy and Health Research Edmonton, Alberta, Canada T6G 2E1 TEL: 780 492 5201 E-mail: sujata.persad@ualberta.ca.

The occurrence of several different mutations implies that several signal transduction pathways are perturbed in melanoma. Of particular interest to this review are mutations in the Wnt/β-catenin pathway as well as the PI3K pathway. Elevated levels of nuclear β-catenin are observed in ~30% of human melanomas. In fact, melanoma is one of the first cancer types associated with β-catenin/Wnt signaling mutations. Mutations in the Wnt signaling pathway that result in over-activation of β-catenin signaling are readily observed in melanomas, but the functional implications of these mutations in melanoma progression remain unclear.

The PI3K pathway is likely the most frequently deregulated pathway in melanoma, although the mechanism underlying the over-activation in most cases remains largely elusive. Growth factor stimulation of receptor tyrosine kinases (RTK) and/or non-RTKs results in the activation of PI3K and the conversion of phosphatidylinositol-bis-phosphate (PIP2) to phosphatidylinositol-tri- phosphate (PIP3). The presence of PIP3 mediates the phosphorylation and activation of Akt/PKB by PDK1/PDK2 at Threonine 308 (T308) and Serine 473 (S473). Activated Akt (phosphorylated Akt [P-Akt]) is the central effector of many downstream signaling pathways regulating protein synthesis, cell cycle, cell death, cell growth, and cell survival. In Melanoma, the loss of the tumour suppressor protein and negative regulator of the PI3K/Akt pathway, PTEN, is a common event leading to the constitutive activation of PI3K/Akt signaling. The consitutive activation of this pathway with PTEN loss and the resulting elevation of the P-AKT signaling axis may be a method for promoting/sustaining melanoma progression. This includes modes of regulation between PI3K/Akt and other pathways such as 1) cross-talk with the Wnt/GSK3β/β- catenin pathway, 2) cross-talk with FOXO family of transcription factors and 3) mammalian target of rapamycin (mTOR).

This review will discuss the current evidence available for PI3K/PTEN/Akt and Wnt-β-catenin mediated signaling in melanoma progression.

1. PI3K/AKT Signaling Pathway and Its Components

1.1. Overview

The Phosphatidylinositol-3-kinase/AKT (Protein Kinase B) pathway (PI3K) serves a role in altering cellular functions in response to extracellular signals, and it is a central integrator of metabolism, survival and growth signals [1]. With respect to metabolism, various studies have shown PI3K pathway's role in insulin sensitivity [2]. Several membrane receptors, in particular receptor tyrosine kinases (RTKs), G-protein coupled receptors (GPCR) and cytokine receptors activate PI3Ks. A number of the components of the pathway have been found mutated or deregulated in a wide variety of human cancers highlighting the key role of this pathway in cellular transformation and further in tumourigenesis [3]. The PI3K pathway has been shown to be prominently involved in tumour development and also in the tumour's potential response to cancer treatment. Many of the new "targeted agents" have been specifically designed to act on PI3Krelated targets [4].

1.2. Components of the PI3K Pathway

1.2.1. PI3K Isoforms

PI3K is a member of a large family of lipid kinases that are characterized by their ability to phosphorylate the inositol ring 3'-OH group in inositol phospholipids [4]. They are sub-classified based on their structure and preferred substrates [5]. The PI3Ks are comprised of three classes, Class I, II and III. The three classes differ in structure, substrate preference, tissue distribution, mechanism of activation and, ultimately, in function [6]. Class I serves an important role in cancer development through its role in cell growth regulation. Class II and III PI3Ks, on the other hand, are less studied and are recognized for their involvement in membrane trafficking and receptor internalization, and vesicle trafficking, respectively [7, 8, 1]. In this review, we will focus mainly on Class IA PI3K as they have been shown to be most relevant in cell growth regulation and cancer development. Although frequent genetic alterations in the PI3K group of enzymes and the pathway effectors makes this pathway the most frequently deregulated pathway in cancer, only the Class IA PI3Ks have been implicated in human cancer [9]. Throughout this review we will be refer to Class IA PI3K as PI3K unless otherwise stated.

Class I PI3Ks (PI3Ks) are divided into four members based on their mechanism of activation. They present as a heterodimeric complex comprising of a regulatory subunit p85α and any of three catalytic subunits; p110α, p110β and p110δ. The p110 isoforms (α, β, δ) have the same basic structure, a p85 binding domain, a kinase domain and a C2 domain for membrane anchoring [10]. The p110α subunit additionally has a Ras-binding domain (Ras-BD) and a helical domain [11]. The regulatory subunit contains SH2 and SH3 domains, which are involved in associating with target proteins that have the appropriate binding sites [12]. In particular, the p85α subunit of PI3Ks encodes an adaptor-like protein that has two SH2 domains and an inter-SH2 domain that binds constitutively to the p110 catalytic subunit [10]. The regulatory subunits are subject to further splicing. The two splice variants (p55α and p50α) retain such regions but lacks an amino terminal SH3 domain (mediates the binding of proline rich sequences) and a breakpoint cluster region (BCR) homology domain (a protein-protein interaction motif) [10]. PI3K p110α domain isoform is the most mutated amongst cancers, causing the kinase to be more active [13, 14, 15] and perpetuating a constitutively active PI3K pathway.

1.2.2. Phosphatase and Tensin Homologue Deleted on Chromosome 10 (PTEN)

The tumour suppressor, PTEN, is a negative regulator of the PI3K pathway. PTEN is a dual phosphatase that acts on Tyr, Ser and Thr residues on lipid and protein substrates [16]. The lipid phosphatase-hydrolysing activity of PTEN occurs at position 3' from phosphoinositides [17]. PTEN can dephosphorylate the D3 position of PIP_3 thus antagonizing signaling through the PI3K pathway [18]. The lipid phosphatase role of PTEN effectively reduces the activation of Protein Kinase B (PKB/AKT) and prevents the downstream signaling events that are controlled by AKT [12]. This therefore controls the activity of the PI3K pathway in regulating cell survival and growth via signaling from growth factor receptors and components of the extracellular matrix [17].

Loss of PTEN is observed in many cancers [19] and further germline alterations are associated with a group of syndromes known as PTEN hamartoma tumour syndromes, which are characterized by the presence of developmental and neurological defects and cancer susceptibility. Along with PTEN loss, mutations in AKT and RTK amplifications, presents a class of frequent genomic aberrations that promotes tumourigenesis through upregulation of the PI3K signaling axis [9]. Loss of PTEN results in suppression of apoptosis and accelerated cell cycle progression [20].

PTEN is tightly regulated at the transcriptional level as well as by post translational modification, primarily ubiquitylation. Incidentally, the activity of PTEN is also controlled by the PI3K pathway. Transcriptionally, the levels of PTEN are controlled by PI3K through the regulation of the transcription factor NF-κB, while PPARβ/δ agonists and TNFα repress PTEN expression [1, 21]. In p85 conditional knockout mice, the loss of p85 resulted in PTEN activity, while loss of p110δ isoform regulated PTEN activity through a RhoA-ROCK-dependent signaling [1, 22]. Currently, NEDD4-1 is the first and only identified E3 ligase for PTEN [1, 23]. Similar to PTEN, NEDD4-1 is also regulated by the PI3K pathway, thus representing a positive feedback for PTEN degradation and PI3K activation [1, 24]. More often than not, heterozygous alterations of PTEN are most common in the initial steps of tumourigenesis. Surprisingly, complete PTEN deletion does not have pro-tumourigenic effect.

1.2.3. AKT

The formation of PIP_3 is the central initiating event which functions to recruit plekstrin homology (PH) domain containing proteins to the plasma membrane. Of relevance here, is AKT/PKB, as it is the critical mediator of signal transduction events downstream of the PI3K cascade. There are three members of the AKT family (AKT1, AKT2, and AKT3) with AKT1 being the major isoform implicated in cancers. AKT2 is known for its involvement in insulin signaling and glucose transport whereas AKT3 is thought to play specific roles in brain tissue [13, 25].

The AKT gene encodes a serine/threonine kinase with an amino-terminal PH domain, a central catalytic domain, and a carboxyl-terminal regulatory domain. The regulation of AKT function is two- fold, requiring its translocation to the plasma membrane and its sequential phosphorylation at Threonine 308 (T308) and Serine 473 (S473). In unstimulated cells, AKT is constitutively phosphorylated at S124 and T450. When PIP_3 is generated it interacts directly with AKT via the PH domain which recruits AKT to the plasma membrane. Here, PDK1 phosphorylates AKT on T308 which is the priming event to mediate the phosphorylation of S473 by PDK2, which is thought to be mammalian target of rapamycin complex 2 (mTORC2). This secondary phosphorylation event is necessary for maximal activation of AKT increasing the kinase activity 10-fold [13, 26, 27]. AKT has multiple substrates within the cytoplasm and nucleus and the activation of AKT regulates many cellular processes including cell proliferation and survival, cell size and glucose homeostasis, metabolism, angiogenesis, and tissue invasion [13].

Phosphorylation of AKT in response to various stimuli can lead to an anti-apoptotic response. This is affected through a series of phosphorylation/inhibition of key pro-apoptotic proteins including, BAD, MDM2 and members of the Forkhead family of proteins. AKT also phosphorylates the pro-death enzyme, caspase 9, and inhibits its catalytic activity. An indirect mechanism by which AKT regulates apoptosis is mediated by the NF-κB and p53 pathways. Specifically, phosphorylation and activation of IκB kinase (IκK) results in the degradation of the NF-κB inhibitor, IκB. This causes the nuclear translocation of NF-κB and the expression of anti-apoptotic genes. The pro-apoptotic effects of p53 tumour suppressor protein are also mediated by phosphorylation of the p53 binding protein, MDM2 by AKT. MDM2 is a negative regulator of p53 function as it targets p53 for ubiquitin mediated proteosomal degradation through its E3 ubiquitin ligase activity. The phosphorylation of MDM2 increases the efficiency by which MDM2 translocates to the nucleus and thereby enhancing p53 degradation [13].

The proliferative effects of AKT activation can also be attributed to the inhibition of the enzyme, glycogen synthase kinase (GSK) 3β at its Serine 9 phosphorylation site as well as its role in inactivating the cell cycle inhibitor p27 and p21. AKT has an important role in preventing cyclin D1 degradation by inhibiting GSK3β, which phosphorylates cyclin D1, thereby increasing cyclin D1 levels resulting in cell cycle progression. The regulation of cell cycle progression is regulated throughcyclin-dependent kinase (CDK) complexes and CDK inhibitors (CKI). p27 and p21 are CKIs that become phosphorylated by AKT and through indirect mechanisms, can modulate the expression of CKIs as well as their activities. Cyclin D1 expression is also tightly controlled by the transcription factor FOXO3A, in that FOXO3A is a transcriptional repressor of the Cyclin D1 gene. When AKT phosphorylates FOXO3A, it is removed from the nucleus resulting in decreased transcriptional repression and thus increased cyclin D1 expression [28].

1.3. PI3K Pathway Activation and Downstream Targets

The activity of PI3K is regulated within the cell by growth factor-receptor interactions [9]. In a quiescent cell, PI3K is inactive and localized in the cytoplasm, far removed from its plasma membrane substrates. Under such unstimulated conditions p85 binds to p110 resulting in the inhibition of its kinase activity. Moreover, only a small fraction of these PI3Ks become activated upon growth factor stimulation [9]. PI3K is activated upon receptor occupation by several growth factors, including fibroblast growth factor (FGF), vascular endothelial cell growth factor (VEGF), human growth factor (HGF), angiopoietin I (Ang1), insulin like growth factor 1 (IGF-1), and insulin. The growth factor activated receptors are receptor tyrosine kinase (RTK) that undergoes transphosphorylation and activation upon binding their respective growth factor ligands. Upon growth factor stimulation, the SH2 domain (Roussarcoma-oncogene homology-2 domains) of p85 binds to phosphorylated tyrosine in YxxM motifs in RTKs or their substrate adaptor proteins. This binding relieves the inhibition of p110 and mediates recruitment of the catalytic subunit of PI3K in close proximity to its lipid substrates at the plasma membrane [29].

In the simplest scenario, phosphorylated residue on receptor becomes a docking site for the p85 subunit of heterodimeric PI3K. In some cases, however, receptor phosphorylation mediates the recruitment of an adaptor protein. For example, when insulin activates the insulin receptor, the insulin receptor substrate protein (IRS) must be recruited to facilitate PI3K binding. Similarly, focal adhesion kinase (FAK) serves as an adaptor protein, docking PI3K via its p85 regulatory domain when integrins (instead of RTK) are activated. In each case, an SH2 or SH3 domain of the p85 subunit of PI3K binds to the adaptor protein at an autophosphorylated site [12].

The preferred substrates of PI3K are the non-phosphorylated phosphatidylinositol (PI), inositol monophosphate (PI(4)P), and phosphatidyl-bis-phosphate ($PI(4,5)P_2$). PI3Ks mediate the addition of a phosphate group in the D-3 position of the inositol ring to generate PI(3)P,

PIP_2, and PIP_3, respectively [30, 31]. PI-3,4-bisphosphate promotes cell proliferation (growth) and resistance to apoptosis (survival), unlike its precursor PI-4-phosphate. Finally, PIP_2 is converted to PI-3,4,5-trisphosphate (PIP_3), which modulates cell adhesion, growth, and survival [12]. PIP_3 serves to recruit proteins containing the pleckstrin homology (PH) domain. The PH domains are diverse in their structure, providing varying degrees of selectivity. This interaction controls the timing and localization of protein-membrane association and in this way regulates protein activity. The interaction of the protein with the lipid may also change protein conformation to alter protein function. The generation of PIP_3 promotes the movement of the PH domain-containing enzyme phosphoinositide-dependent kinase 1 (PDK1) to the plasma membrane [12]. AKT/Protein Kinase B (PKB), a PH domain containing protein, is a central protein involved in normal and pathological signaling. Upon recruitment to the plasma membrane, AKT is phosphorylated at two sites, specifically at Thr 308 by PDK1 and Ser 473 by PDK2. However, the exact mechanism of these phosphorylations is yet unclear [4]. Phosphorylated-AKT (pAKT) results in a cascade involving various downstream signaling proteins [32, 33, 34]. A high level of pAKT is correlated with poor prognosis of many cancers, whereas pAKT is mostly undetectable in normal tissue [35]. Along with several downstream effectors as mentioned in the previous section, activated AKT inhibits GSK3β, which normally prevents up-regulation of cell proliferation due to increased cyclin D1 degradation. Also, inhibition of GSK3β is shown to spare free β-catenin from degradation in cancer cells [35]. Further, increased β-catenin can bind and stabilize cyclin D1 mRNA, which leads to enhanced expression of the latter protein and promotion of G1-phase/S-phase progression [36]. Another key effector downstream of PI3K is mTOR [37, 38]. It has been shown that mTOR is a serine/threonine kinase that plays a central role in protein translation, cell proliferation and evasion of apoptosis [37]. Components of this pathway have been implicated in carcinogenesis and cancer progression at many levels such as excessive growth signals, insensitivity to growth inhibitory signals, evasion of apoptosis, limitless replicative potential, sustained angiogenesis, and tissue invasion and metastasis [39]. AKT, through the phosphorylation of these target proteins, fulfills a role as a key regulator of a variety of critical cell functions including glucose metabolism, cell proliferation and survival [40].

1.4. PI3K in Cancer

Activating mutations in PIK3CA, the gene encoding the p110α catalytic subunit of PI3K, were recently identified as novel mechanisms of inducing oncogenic PI3K signaling [41]. PI3K gene amplifications are frequently seen in ovarian and gastric tumours, and mutations of PI3K are common in breast and colorectal cancer [29]. The most frequent mutations of PI3K are in its kinase domain and helical domain causing different impacts on PI3K targets [42]. Deregulation of the pathway is usually caused by oncogenic activation of the RTKs upstream of PI3K. Alternatively, amplifications of genes encoding the catalytic unit of PI3K, and activating mutations in the regulatory subunit of PI3K, also cause excessive activation of the pathway [3].

2. PI3K Pathway in Melanoma

2.1. Melanoma

2.1.1. Overview

Worldwide, melanoma has the most rapidly rising incidence rate of any human cancer. It arises from the malignant transformation of melanocyte cells of the skin. Due to the inefficacy of present chemotherapeutic regimens and the resistance of melanoma cells to radiotherapy, 95% of stage IV metastatic melanoma patients die within five years of diagnosis [43, 44, 45]. Metastasis, the spread of a cancer from the site of the primary tumour to distant sites of the body, makes melanoma very hard to treat. A risk factor associated with malignant melanoma is sun exposure which can cause mutations in specific genes and deregulation of signal transduction pathways.

2.1.2. Stages of Melanoma

Malignant melanoma is characterized by the uncontrollable proliferation of melanocytes, cells originating from neural crest cells. The liver, brain, and lungs are the most common targets of melanoma metastasis, and patients with metastasized melanoma have a median survival of six months [46].

Melanocytes are located in the basal layer of the epidermis surrounded by keratinocytes. Keratinocytes maintain controlled growth of melanocytes through (1) extracellular communication through paracrine growth factors, (2) intracellular communication through second messengers and signal transduction, and (3) intercellular communication through cell–cell adhesion molecules, cell–matrix adhesion, and gap junctional intercellular communication [47]. Perturbations in the cellular environment can lead to alterations in molecules involved in cell-cell adhesion and cell communication, leading to melanoma development [48]. Uncontrolled proliferation, homeostatic balance perturbation through deregulation of signal transduction, and loss in cell adhesion can all lead to melanoma progression to metastasis.

Normal melanocytes are transformed to malignant melanocytes through distinct phenotypic changes, as they progress through the process of Epithelial to Mesenchymal Transition (EMT). This is characterized by a disruption in adherens junctions of melanocytes as a result of the down regulation of the epithelial E-cadherin and up regulation of the mesenchymal N-cadherin (the "cadherin switch") [49]. The result is a loss of cell adhesion and an increase in cell mobility. Loss of E-cadherin allows melanocytes to escape from keratinocyte growth control and allows malignant melanocytes to escape from the primary tumour focus [50]. EMT must take place for cells to progress to a metastatic stage, as cells must shed their epithelial phenotype and gain a mesenchymal phenotype. To gain metastatic potential, cells must invade the basement membrane and make their way into the bloodstream.

The American Joint Committee on Cancer (AJCC) has devised a system to categorize melanoma. This system incorporates tumour thickness, nodal status, and metastatic disease [51]. Melanoma progresses through distinct phases, clustering of cells on the skin begins with a benign nevus stage, which can be defined as a mole. This then progresses to a dysplastic nevus, and with further proliferation to a radial growth phase. As cells progress through EMT, changes in cells cause invasion into the sub-epidermal tissue in a vertical fashion, known as the vertical growth phase. The final stage of melanoma is a metastatic stage, when cells invade through the basement membrane and travel through the vascular system to distant tissues/organs and survive as single cells or colonies at these sites. The most common sites of metastasis by melanoma are lung, liver, brain and bone [52].

2.1.3. Melanoma and Common Mutations of Signaling Pathways

Several oncogenes, tumour suppressor genes, and pathways are known to be deregulated in melanoma; for example, NRAS, which activates RAF kinases in response to growth factors, is overactive in 15–20% of melanomas [53, 54]. P16 (INK4A) tumour suppressor expression is also lost by mutation, deletion, or transcriptional silencing of the CDKN2A locus in many melanomas [55]. BRAF mutations are often found with P16 mutations. PTEN mutations and deletions are also present in some melanomas, coinciding with BRAF mutations [55, 56, 57]. The frequent occurrence of these two mutations together is likely a reflection of the importance of two RAS-effector pathways (PI3K and Mitogen Activation Protein Kinase Pathway (MAPK) in melanomagenesis and progression [58]. Another genomic aberration associated with melanoma is the amplification of microphthalmia-associated transcription factor (MITF) [58]. The high incidence and low survival rate of melanoma, makes it an important area of study. Elucidation of the changes and dysregulation occurring in signal transduction pathways that leads to metastasis will allow identification of molecular targets and thus the design of efficacious therapies to treat metastatic disease [59]. Melanoma was one of the first cancer types which was associated with mutations in the β-catenin/Wnt signaling pathway [60]. However, the exact role of these mutations in melanoma has remained elusive [61]. Mutations in the Wnt signaling pathway that result in over-activation of β-catenin signaling are readily observed in melanomas, but the functional implications are still unclear [62]. Several *in vivo* and *in vitro* models have been established to study the implications of a deregulated Wnt signaling pathway in melanoma. Overactive β-catenin signaling along with a constitutively active PI3K pathway was shown to facilitate melanoma development in a mouse model [62]. Elevated levels of nuclear β-catenin are observed in ~30% of human melanomas [63]. The occurrence of multiple mutations in melanoma implies that several signal transduction pathways are likely perturbed and involved in melanoma progression. Although the PI3K pathway is one of the most frequently deregulated pathways in melanoma, the mechanism underlying the over-activation in most cases remains largely elusive [64].

2.2. PI3K and Melanoma Progression

Malignant melanoma is characterized by frequent metastasis; however, specific changes that cause this malignancy are yet to be characterized [62]. Deregulation of the PI3K pathway is used by many tumours to attain growth advantage and survival [65]. The PI3K pathway is one of the most deregulated pathways in melanoma. PTEN mutations are found in 30-40% of melanoma cell lines and 5-20% of primary melanomas [66, 67]. Loss of expression or function of PTEN is not only due to mutation and allelic loss [66, 67], but functional inactivation by epigenetic silencing [68] or altered subcellular localization [69]. Ectopic expression of PTEN has been demonstrated to suppress melanoma cell growth and melanoma tumourigenicity and metastasis [70]. Absence or inactivity of PTEN deregulates the PI3K pathway and constitutively activates the downstream effector, AKT via its phosphorylation at two critical amino acids: Serine (Ser) 473 and Threonine (Thr) 308 [71]. This results in sustained proliferative and anti-apoptotic cellular response. The importance of the PI3K pathway in malignant melanoma is underscored by the fact that over 60% of melanomas exhibit activated AKT [72] and overexpression of AKT has been shown to convert radial growth melanoma to vertical growth melanoma [73]. Further the PI3K pathway has been shown to be overactive in preclinical models of melanoma.

Upregulation of cellular processes such as cellular growth, metabolism and proliferation due to a deregulated PI3K pathway in melanoma are controlled through downstream effectors which regulate cell cycle, angiogenesis, inflammation and invasiveness [64]. A positive correlation has been determined in melanoma progression and phosphorylated/activated AKT levels. Levels of phospho-AKT correlate inversely with disease-free survival and directly with poor prognosis [70]. PI3K triggers a network that positively regulates G1/S cell cycle progression and increases cyclin D1 expression. Loss of the G1/S phase checkpoint is often seen in melanoma and allows cells to pass into the stage of cell proliferation without control [74]. In this regard, mTOR has been the target of several phase I and II trials using its inhibitor rapamycin in various cancers, including melanoma [73, 75].

3. PI3K Mediated Crosstalk in Melanoma Progression

In this section we will discuss the crosstalk between the PI3K pathway and other pathways that are altered in melanoma. There are several putative areas of crosstalk involving pathways such as the Mitogen Activated Protein Kinase (MAPK), Wnt-β catenin, Nuclear Factor kappaB (NF-κB), Transforming Growth Factor beta (TGF-β), JAK-STAT and Notch pathways. The crosstalk between the PI3K and Wnt-β catenin pathway will not be discussed in this section and will be discussed in detail in section 4.

3.1. PI3K – MAPK Crosstalk

MAPK pathway is one of the most commonly deregulated pathways in melanoma. MAPK pathway regulates important cellular processes and hence deregulation of this pathway plays a key role in cancer progression. In mammals there are 4 major isoforms of MAPK namely, the extracellular signal regulated kinase (ERK1/2), c-Jun amino (N)-terminal kinases (JNK 1/2/3), p38 isoforms (α, β, γ, δ) and ERK5. Although the signaling pathways originating from each MAPK isoform includes very specific components, the general route of the signaling occurs via a common three tier kinase cascade consisting of MAPK kinase kinase (MAP3K), MAPK kinase (MAP2K) and MAPK [76, 77, 78]. Among the four MAPK signaling pathways, the JNK and ERK modules are most frequently reported to be deregulated in melanoma and hence we will focus on these two modules in this section.

ERK 1/2 Module

ERK 1/2 is activated by several growth factors, cytokines as well as in response to stress. ERK 1/2 signaling begins with the activation of RTK or GPCR leading to transphosphorylation of Tyrosine residues in the intracellular domain. These phosphorylated residues serve as binding site for adaptor proteins like Grb2, which recruits Sos (a GEF, Guanine nucleotide exchange factor) to the plasma membrane. Sos mediates the exchange of Ras-GDP to the active Ras-GTP, resulting in the activation of MAP3K, Raf (A-Raf, B-Raf, Raf-1). Raf activation leads to the activation of the MAP2K (MEK 1/2) which in turn phosphorylates MAPK (ERK 1/2) at its Thr-Glu-Tyr motif leading to the activation ERK 1/2 [76, 77]. Once activated, ERK 1/2 translocates from cytoplasm to nucleus, where it induces transcription of its target genes [77, 78].

JNK Module

JNKs are MAPKs activated in response to stress and has three isforms JNK 1, 2, 3. The MAP2K components of JNK pathway are MKK4 and MKK7. MAP3K components are MEKK1-4, MLK-2 and 3, Tpl-2, DLK, TAO 1 and 2, TAK1 and ASK 1/2 with each MAP3K being induced specifically by different stimuli. Scaffold proteins like filamin, β-arrestin and JNK interacting protein (JIP) plays an important role in regulating the activation of JNK by optimizing the interaction of component kinases of JNK signaling module. Like ERK, JNK also requires phosphorylation of conserved Thr-Pro-Tyr motifs within its activation loop. Once activated JNK enters the nucleus where it acts on its substrates, mostly transcription factors. c-jun is the most important nuclear substrate of JNK, which when phosphorylated at Ser 63 and 73 dimerizes with c-fos to form the active AP-1 transcription factor complex. P53, ATF-2, STAT3, c-myc, Jun-B are other transcription factors that are activated by JNK [77, 78].

The PI3K and MAPK pathways are significant in cancer progression and studies have shown that treatment with PI3K inhibitor Wortmannin induced inhibiton of MAPK pathway, suggestive of potential crosstalk between these two pathways [79]. A review by Edita et al shows experimental data and computer simulations to support several points of crosstalks between these two independent parallel pathways [80]. Ras is a prominent point for crosstalk as both MAPK and PI3K are effector pathways downstream of Ras [81]. Another point of crosstalk is at Raf. PIP_3 produced from an activated PI3K pathway leads to sequential activation of GEF, Rac (small GTPase) and finally PAK (P-21 activated kinase), an effector of Rac [82, 83]. Chaudhary et al. proposed that PAK activates Raf-1 by the phosphorylation at Ser 338 [84]. However, this is contradicted by Antonio et al. who show that S338 phosphorylation of Raf-1 is independent of PI3K and PAK [85]. Raf is also activated by AKT at Ser 259 [86] and this Raf-AKT crosstalk is regulated in a concentration and ligand dependent manner [87]. AKT is also shown to inhibit the Raf/ERK pathway by phosphorylating the Ser428 and Thr439 residues in the amino terminal regulatory domain of B-Raf [88]. Alternatively, constitutive activation of Raf/MAPK has been shown to inhibit AKT and cell cycle arrest specifically through MEK-1 [89]. Another point of crosstalk between the PI3K and MAPK pathway is via PDK1, which targets MEK1 and MEK2 by phosphorylation at Ser222 and Ser226, respectively [90].

Studies have also suggested crosstalk between PI3K and JNK signaling pathway. JNK2 has been reported to convey Src/PI3K signal for growth and metastasis by enhancing GAB2 (Grb2 associated binding protein 2) expression in 4TI mammary tumour cells [91]. A study by Logan et al showed that dominant negative PI3K as well as Wortmannin blocked EGF induced JNK activation, suggesting crosstalk between PI3K/JNK pathways [92]. Studies done in nasopharyngeal cancer (NPC) has shown that activity of Matrix metalloprotease-9 (MMP9) is blocked only upon combined inhibition of PI3K and JNK, alluding to importance of JNK/PI3K crosstalk in NPC progression [93].

Hyperactivation of Ras signaling has been observed in melanoma and this attributes to alterations in both upstream and downstream components of the Ras pathway. Two important effectors of the Ras signaling are the MAPK and PI3K pathways. The significance of crosstalk between PI3K and MAPK in melanoma is supported by work of Merighi et al. in which the binding of an agonist to A3 adenosine receptor is shown to activate PLC-PI3K, which in turn reduces the pERK1/2 levels (MAPK) that is necessary for proliferation [94]. B-Raf is one of the most commonly mutated genes in melanoma. Potential mechanisms of B-Raf involvement in melanoma progression features crosstalk between AKT and ^{V600E}B-Raf. The frequently observed B-Raf mutation, ^{V600E}B-Raf results in the increased activation of MAPK that leads to senescence. On the other hand, phosphorylation at Ser^{364} and Ser^{428} of ^{V600E}B-Raf due to aberrant activity of AKT, as in case of melanoma promotes melanoma progression [95]. Brenden et al proposes that ^{V600E}B-Raf negatively regulates AKT through its interaction with mTORC2. In cells with wild type AKT signaling, ^{V600E}B-Raf interacts with mTORC2 exerting a negative effect on AKT phosphorylation which prevent cell survival. However, in cells with aberrantly activated AKT signaling (due to PTEN loss leading to PI3K activation) as in case of melanoma, the effect of the negative impact from ^{V600E}B-Raf interaction with mTORC2 on AKT is countered by strong upstream signals that activate AKT signaling and lead to cell survival and melanoma progression [96]. Crosstalk between PI3K and MAPK is also mediated via PTEN. Studies with animal model have shown that ^{V600E}B-Raf expression alone was not sufficient to cause development of melanoma. However expression of ^{V600E}B-Raf in the background of PTEN silencing resulted in melanomagenesis and progression [97].

3.2. PI3K – NF-κB Cross Talk

NFκB signaling pathway is a key player in cancer. The NFκB family proteins comprises of two subfamilies: NFκB proteins (p105, p100) and Rel proteins (RelA, RelB, c-Rel) and its activity is tightly regulated by its interaction with inhibitory proteins I-κB. NFκB remains inactive in the cytoplasm by the inhibitory effect of I-κB. When I-κ is phosphorylated by I-κB kinase (IKK), it is targeted for degradation resulting in the activation of NFκB. Once activated, NFκB enters the nucleus and activates the transcription of downstream targets that are involved in cell survival, apoptosis and cell migration and hence is implicated in tumour progression [98]. Several mechanisms of cross talk between PI3K and NFκB pathways have been reported in many cancers. NFκB was shown to be activated by AKT-induced activation of the IKK complex upon stimulation by Tumour Necrosis Factor (TNF-α) and Platelet Derived Growth Factor (PDGF) [99, 100]. Alternatively, Sizemore et al. show that AKT activates the p65/Rel A subunit of NFκB in a PI3K dependent manner in the absence ofdegradation of I-κB by IKK complex [101]. Another mechanism of crosstalk is proposed in a study by Madrid. V et al. which illustrates that the stimulation of transactivation of p65/Rel A by AKT requires IKK and p38 MAPK [102]. The PI3K-NFκB cross talk is reported to promote cell survival by suppressing apoptosis [103, 104, 105, 106, 107] and inducing EMT and metastasis [108, 109] in various cancers.

In melanoma, constitutive activation of IKK activity and enhanced degradation of I-κB was found to significantly activate NFκB compared to normal skin [110, 111, 112, 113, 114]. The nuclear levels of NFκB has been shown to increase with disease progression from dysplastic nevi to primary melanoma and metastatic melanoma, indicating that up-regulation of NFκB plays a role in enhancing melanoma progression [115]. NFκB was also shown to promote angiogenesis and metastasis in melanoma [110]. Punita et al. showed that crosstalk between the PI3K and NFκB pathways resulted in constitutive activation of AKT that resulted in up-regulation of NFκB and prevention of apoptosis in melanoma cells [72].

3.3. PI3K – TGFβ Pathway Crosstalk

TGFβ constitutes a superfamily of cytokines that regulate developmental processes and deregulation of this pathway has been shown to promote cancer genesis and progression. Binding of TGFβ to its trans-membrane Ser-Thr kinase receptor complex (TGFβR1, TGFβR2) activates intracellular mediators called Smads. There are three types of Smads; the regulatory or R-Smads (Smad – 1, 2, 3, 5, 8), co-smad (Smad-4) and inhibitory Smad (Smad 7). In the nucleus, R-Smads and co-Smad bind to various co-activators or co-repressors and regulate gene expression [116]. A comparison of the levels of different isoforms of TGFβ in normal melanocyte, nevi and melanoma showed that while TGFβ-1 is expressed in only some melanocytes, it is expressed uniformly in nevi as well as primary and metastatic melanoma. TGFβ-2 and TGFβ-3 isoforms were not expressed in melanocytes but were expressed in nevi, primary and metastatic melanoma [117]. Elevated levels of TGFβ-1 and TGFβ-2 have also been reported in patients with disseminated melanoma [118]. Inhibition of TGFβ pathway was shown to reduce bone metastasis in melanoma [119] and expression of TGFβ2 was shown to be critical for metastasis and invasiveness in melanoma [120]. Further, over-expression of Smad-7 was shown to decrease tumourigenicity and metastasis [121, 122,123]. Collectively, these reports highlight the significance of TGFβ signaling pathway in melanoma. Crosstalk between TGFβ and PI3K pathway was recently reported in a study by Fang et al, where stimulation of Nodal (member of TGFβ superfamily) was accompanied with increased levels of phospho-AKT leading to Snail-mediated EMT in melanoma [124].

3.4. PI3K – Notch Pathway Crosstalk

Notch signaling regulates the normal development of many tissues and hence perturbations in the pathway contribute to cancer development. Canonical Notch signaling involves the activation of the Notch receptor by ligands Delta and Jagged/Serate. The binding of ligands leads to the intra-membranal proteolysis of the intact receptor, releasing within the cytoplasm a soluble fragment containing intracellular domain called Notch intracellular domain (NICD). NICD has a nuclear localization sequence which allows the protein to enter the nucleus and regulates the transcription of target genes [125]. Gene expression studies support a role of Notch signaling in melanoma [126, 127]. The expression of Notch receptors and ligands are up-regulated in dysplastic nevi and melanoma compared to normal melanocytic nevi [128, 129]. Although Notch 1 signaling is elevated in melanoma, AKT and hypoxic conditions are required for melanomagenesis to occur [130]. Further, a role of Notch 1 signaling in promoting vertical growth phase of primary melanoma to aggressive phenotype was shown to be mediated by activation of AKT and MAPK pathways. This is underscored by the observation that effect of the Notch 1 signaling in melanoma progression is reversed with inhibition of either MAPK or the AKT pathways [131]. Collectively, these studies support the importance of crosstalk between PI3K and Notch signaling pathway in promoting melanomagenesis and progression.

3.5. PI3K – JAK-STAT Pathway Crosstalk

Janus kinase – signal transducer and activator of transcription (JAK-STAT) pathway conveys the information from polypeptide signals. Upon ligand binding, JAK activates the members of STAT family of proteins by phosphorylation of a single tyrosine moiety. When activated, STATs form dimers and enter the nucleus, where they bind to response elements on promoter regions of target genes and regulate their transcription [132, 133]. Reports indicate that the JAK-STAT pathway is associated with survival of melanoma cells. Different components of JAK-STAT pathway are observed to be defective in melanoma cell lines resistant to the anti-proliferative effect of interferon, highlighting a key role of this pathway in mediating the anti-proliferative signals from interferon [134]. However, this is contradicted with the study by David et al which shows presence of the components of JAK-STAT pathway in MeWo melanoma cell line that is resistant to interferon response [135]. Melanoma cells are shown to have Interleukin-29 (IL-29) receptors on the surface, which when activated by IL-29 leads to apoptosis via JAK-STAT signaling [136]. Crosstalk between the PI3K and JAK-STAT pathways was reported in a study by M Krasilnikov et al, who showed that inhibition of MAPK and PI3K pathways led to down-regulation of JAK-STAT pathway and increased sensitivity to apoptosis [137].

3.6. PI3K- mTOR Crosstalk

The mTOR signaling pathway regulates cell growth, proliferation, survival and division in response to nutrients and growth factors via the regulation of protein synthesis. mTOR is a downstream effector of many pathways but is primarily activated by the PI3K pathway. mTOR comprises of two multiprotein complexes namely mTORC1 and mTORC2. mTORC1 is sensitive to rapamycin and mediates protein translation by activating S6K1 and 4EBP1 via signaling pathways like PI3K, MAPK and AMPK. mTORC2 is insensitive to rapamycin and regulates the actin cytoskeleton by activating PKC-α and AKT [138]. mTORC1 has five components; mTOR, the catalytic domain, regulatory-associated protein of mTOR (Raptor), mammalian lethal with Sec13 protein 8 (mLST8), proline rich AKT substrate 40 (PRAS40) and DEP domain containing mTOR interacting protein (Deptor). PRAS40 and Deptor are negative regulators, whereas mLST8 positively regulates mTOR kinase activity. mTORC2 has six components; rapamycin insensitive companion of mTOR (Rictor), mammalian stress activated protein kinase interacting protein (mSIN1), protein observed with Rictor-1 (Proctor-1), mLST8 and Deptor [139]. Activation of mTOR by PI3K pathway is the prototypic mechanism. However, there are several other AKT-independent mechanisms of activation. Since this section is focussed on crosstalk with the PI3K pathway, we will selectively discuss the AKT dependent mechanism/s of activation. As previously mentioned AKT is activated upon its phosphorylation by PDK 1 and PDK 2 (mTORC2 is now accepted as a PDK2) proteins. Phosphorylated AKT further activates mTORC1 in a tuberous sclerosis protein-2 (TSC-2)-dependent or independent manner. TSC-2 suppresses the activity of Ras-related GTPase Rheb, an activator of mTORC1. Hence, inhibition of TSC-2 by AKT leads to activation of mTORC1. AKT can also bind directly to PRAS40, thereby attenuating its inhibitory effect on mTORC1 leading to mTORC1 activation independent of TSC2 [140]. Activated mTORC1 promotes translation by inhibiting 4EBP1 (inhibitor of translation) or activating the S6K1.

mTOR signaling plays a role in various facets of cancer progression such as cell motility, and apoptosis and this has been supported with several studies. Increased mRNA levels of Rictor, mTOR and Raptor has been observed in advanced stages of colorectal cancer (CRC) and CRC metastasis was shown to be reduced with inhibition of mTORC1 and mTORC2, highlighting the significance of mTOR signaling in cancer progression and metastasis [141]. An *in vivo* mouse model study showed that CRC metastasis is inhibited upon treatment with rapamycin (mTOR inhibitor) and this is mainly due to reduction of VEGF levels. This prompts a role of mTOR in angiogenesis [142]. The importance of mTOR signaling in various cancers such as prostate cancer [143], ovarian cancer [144, 145], leukemia [146], breast cancer [147], colorectal cancer [148], hematologic malignancies [149], lung cancer [150], oral cancer [151] has been reported.

Many studies support the role of PI3K/ mTOR pathway in melanoma. mTOR is shown to be activated in malignant melanoma (73%) compared to benign nevi (4%) [152] and activated mTOR pathway in melanoma was associated with poor prognosis [153]. Study by Aziz et al shows the co-expression of mTOR and PI3K, especially the p110 catalytic subunit in melanoma, signifying the role of PI3K/mTOR pathway [154]. Chemo-sensitivity of melanoma cells was shown to improve with inhibition of PI3K/ mTOR pathway [155], which highlights the importance of the PI3K/ mTOR pathway in supporting and promoting melanoma.

This section outlined the crosstalk of several signal transduction pathways with the PI3K pathway leading to melanoma progression. Section 4 will focus on the canonical Wnt signaling pathway and its crosstalk with the PI3K pathway in melanoma. The crosstalk between these two pathways is of significant interest to this review due to the role of these pathways independently and their putative crosstalk in melanoma progression.

4. Wnt/β-Catenin and PI3K Pathway

4.1. β-Catenin

4.1.1. Structure and Function

β-catenin is a 781 amino acid protein encoded by the CTNNB1 gene that is highly conserved throughout species and shares 67% homology to the Drosophila Armadillo protein [156]. β-catenin's primary structure is composed of two terminal domains; the N-terminal

(NTD) and C-terminal (CTD) domains, and a central Armadillo (ARM) domain. β-catenin's structure allows binding of specific partners at distinct sites across the terminal domains and the central domain. The ARM domain is characteristic of the Armadillo/catenin family of proteins, and is distinguished by a positively charged groove of densely packed α-helices [157] comprising of 12 imperfect repeats of 42 amino acids (total 550 amino acids) [158, 157].

The crystal structure of the ARM repeat domain shows that each repeat consists of three helices, H1, H2, and H3 [157] and the repeats pack against one another to form a positively charged superhelix. This positively charged groove is ideal for β-catenin to bind its various negatively charged partners. When these interactors are post-translationally modified by phosphorylation, effectively increasing the magnitude of the negative charge, β-catenin's binding affinity with these interactors is augmented [159]. The ARM domain folds into a single structural unit where its surface serves to bind the majority of β-catenin's partners, such as cadherins, TCF/LEF transcription factors and APC [158].

The NTD and CTD of β-catenin are less evolutionarily conserved relative to the central ARM domain. The NTD is important for the stability of the cytoplasmic levels of β-catenin while both the NTD and CTD are significant in β-catenin's role as a co-activator/transactivator of TCF/LEF transcriptional activity. The established role of the CTD in recruiting factors required for regulation of gene expression is dependent on the interaction with cellular partners at the proximal structured elements of this region, such as helix C, which directly follows the 12th arm repeat [160]. The functions for the more distal unstructured region of the CTD remain poorly defined. Furthermore, the acidic charge distribution of the NTD and CTD creates a tertiary structure that brings the NTD and CTD in close proximity to the largely basic ARM domain. Since the NTD and CTD are highly negatively charged and the structural groove of the ARM domain is highly positively charged it is likely that both the NTD and CTD tails of β-catenin interact with the groove of the ARM domain through non-specific charge interactions [158]. The NTD and CTD serve as intramolecular chaperones of the ARM repeat domain which increases the binding specificity and prevents the self-aggregation of the armadillo repeat domain region [158]. Post-translational modifications, such as phosphorylation pattern which change the charge of β-catenin may further result in conformational change or stabilization of the N and/or C tails causing a regulation in binding specific interactors [158].

The CTD also plays a role in the interaction of β-catenin with a number of nuclear factors including, TATA Binding Protein (TBP) [161] Sox 17 and 13, histone deacetylase, SMAD4, the retinoic acid receptor, the CREB binding protein and related proteins [162] as well as transcriptional inhibitors such as ICAT, and Chibby [163, 164].

At Cellular Membrane

At the cell membrane, β-catenin is an important component of the adherens junctions, where it links E-cadherin and α-catenin to the actin cytoskeleton. The adherens junction is essential in maintaining the seamless cell-cell interaction of the epithelial phenotype and provides the cell with structural integrity. The binding of E-cadherin to β-catenin spans the entire ARM region [159] although the actual sites of interaction are concentrated within ARM repeats 4-12 [165]. Tyrosine (Tyr) modification of β-catenin regulates the disassembly of adherens junctions and is regulated by phosphorylation of Tyr-654 of the final armadillo repeat which leads to decreased binding of E-cadherin and β-catenin [166]. A possible mechanism by Piedra and colleagues suggests that this may be due to decreased interaction between ARM and CTD with the phosphorylation of Tyr-654 [162]. Interestingly, this phosphorylation neither affect the association of nuclear factors such as TBP (binding site 639-729), nor TCF-4 (T-cell factor 4) at the CTD. This supports the fact that the CTD is an integral regulatory component which facilitates the interactions of β-catenin with E-cadherin [162].

In the Cytoplasm and Nucleus

While β-catenin linked to E-cadherin is deemed to be highly stable, the cytosolic and nuclear pools are quite dynamic. The subcellular localization of β-catenin is largely regulated by direct competition of β-catenin's binding to E-cadherin and TCF. The N-terminal of TCF forms extensive contacts at ARM 3-9 of β-catenin which bears structural similarities to the E-cadherin-β-catenin interaction. To this end, overexpression of cadherins has been shown to inhibit the transcriptional activity of β-catenin [167]. Furthermore, binding to cadherins can effectively sequester β-catenin within the plasma membrane/cytoplasm and inhibit its signaling efficacy [168].

4.1.2. β-Catenin/Canonical Wnt Pathway

β-catenin is a dual function protein. It plays a role in intercellular adhesion and in regulating gene expression. The latter role is associated with its oncogenic properties. Its second role is as a transcriptional co-activator of the canonical Wnt signaling pathway. The Wnt signal transduction pathway is an essential regulatory pathway that directs cell proliferation, cell polarity and cell fate determination [168]. β-catenin's fate as an adhesion molecule or a transcriptional activator is determined by its intracellular stability. The Wnt pathway largely regulates the intracellular stability of β-catenin.

In the absence of Wnt occupancy of its receptor, free cytoplasmic β-catenin levels are regulated by a multi-protein destruction complex comprising the scaffold protein Axin, the tumour suppressor Adenomatous Polyposis Coli (APC), GSK3β and Casein Kinase-1 (CK-1). Axin is a central protein of the destruction complex that functions as a scaffold that brings all the components into close proximity. APC plays a key role in the regulation of β-catenin turnover since cells containing a mutant APC have elevated β-catenin levels. GSK3β binds a central region within Axin, with a single Axin helix fitting into a hydrophobic groove in the C-terminus of GSK3β, leaving the GSK3β active site free to phosphorylate β-catenin [169]. CK1 binds Axin and phosphorylates β-catenin at Ser45 in order to prime the N-terminal for phosphorylation at residues Ser33, Ser37 and Thr41 by GSK3β [170, 171, 172]. This phosphorylation creates a site for ubiquitination of β-catenin by E3 ubiquitin ligase β-transducin repeat-containing protein (β-Trcp), resulting in β-catenin's subsequent proteosomal degradation [168].

Wnts are secreted glycoproteins that bind to frizzled (Fz) seven-transmembrane spanned receptors. There are 19 known Wnt ligands, three of which are known to stimulate the canonical Wnt pathway in humans, namely Wnt 1, 3 and Wnt8 [168]. Particular Wnt ligands are responsible for embryonic development in several different species. A complete listing of the particular Wnts is described by Dr. Roel Nusse's laboratory [173]. Wnt ligands bind to Fz receptors which are coupled with heterotrimeric G proteins. In the canonical pathway, LRP 5/6, low-density lipoprotein receptors, are co-receptors of Wnt ligands. Upon binding of Wnt ligands, the activated Fz recruits the intracellular protein dishevelled (Dvl), which in recruits the GSK3β-Axin complex. Following recruitment of this complex to the plasma membrane LRP6 is phosphorylated [174]. Wnt-induced LRP6 phosphorylation is a key event in receptor activation [175]. These phosphorylated sites serve as docking sites for Axin complex [176, 175] thereby recruiting Axin to LRP6 upon Wnt stimulation [177]. Further phosphorylation of LRP6 by CK-1 (Davidson et al. 2005; Zeng et al. 2008) results in the clustering of various proteins—including LRP6, Dvl, and Axin—to form what has been referred to as the LRP6 signalosome [178]. Formation of this complex from the phosphorylation of LRP5/6 leads to inhibition of the "destruction complex". Deactivation of the destruction complex results in stabilization of β-catenin within the cytoplasm and its targeted entry into the nucleus, where it binds to the T-cell factor (TCF)/Lymphoid Enhancer Factor (LEF) family of transcription factors leading to transcriptional activation of Wnt target genes [179].

Within the nucleus, the CTD of β-catenin interacts with the TCF family of proteins, which anchor β-catenin to specific promoters for the transcription of Wnt target genes [180]. Many of these target genes, such as cMyc, Cyclin D1, vascular endothelial growth factor A (VEGFA) and matrix metalloproteases (MMPs) have implications in cell survival, cell proliferation, growth, cell cycle progression and invasion along with several others that can be found on the following page: http://www.stanford.edu/group/nusselab/cgi-bin/wnt/target_genes [173]. Since the canonical Wnt pathway regulates transcription of genes involved in cell cycle, growth and survival, uncontrolled activation of the pathway is highly significant in disease pathophysiology. Constitutive activation of the canonical Wnt pathway results in positive regulation of cell survival and negative regulation on cell death/apoptosis. These changes in cellular properties associated with elevated cellular β-catenin are associated with poor prognosis in many human cancers including adenocarcinoma of the prostate and breast as well as melanoma [168].

4.1.3. Active β-Catenin

Upon Canonical Wnt pathway activation, GSK3β associated with the axin scaffold is inhibited allowing β-catenin to evade degradation. The cytoplasmic accumulation of β-catenin is thought to ultimately result in its translocation to the nucleus. However, this translocation alone is not sufficient for β-catenin/TCF transcriptional activity [181, 182]. Staal and colleagues demonstrated that the increased half-life of β-catenin upon Wnt signaling was not a direct consequence of its stability [182]. The phosphorylation status of the NTD of β-catenin upon Wnt signaling independently affected the signaling properties and half-life of β-catenin. In fact, it is not so much the accumulation of β-catenin per se but the dephosphorylation of specific amino acids at the NTD of β-catenin that is important in generating a transcriptionally active form of β-catenin [182, 160]. Maher and colleagues demonstrated that the cadherin free form of β-catenin unphosphorylated at S37 and T41 (transcriptionally active- β-catenin (ABC)) is largely monomeric and located mainly within the nucleus. Active-β-catenin is found to be intrinsically more transcriptionally active than the non-phosphorylated β-catenin [160]. The predominant nuclear accumulation of the active-β-catenin is due to its low concentration within the cell, which renders it less likely to be bound by the cadherins and α-catenin [160]. Furthermore, β-catenin phosphorylated at three sites; S33, S37 and T41 is found to be more retained within the cytosol, as well as subject to increased nuclear export. Maher and colleagues also established that β-catenin phosphorylated at T41/S45 strongly co-localizes with active-β-catenin within the nucleus and is largely a cadherin-free form of β-catenin. This suggests that the nuclear form of β-catenin phosphorylated at Ser45 may also be a signaling/active form of β-catenin. Referring back to the Wnt pathway, β-catenin is phosphorylated at Ser45 by CK1 in a priming mechanism, allowing subsequent phosphorylation by GSK3β at Ser 33, 37 and T41 [171]. Therefore, it is possible that the priming of β-catenin at S45 by CK1 may be a temporal regulatory mechanism that couples β-catenin phosphorylation and degradation to β-catenin nuclear signaling. The fact that β-catenin phosphorylated at the three sites of phosphorylation by GSK3β does not completely overlap with β-catenin phosphorylated at serine 45 and threonine 41, suggests a possible spatial separation of the two kinase activities of GSK3β and CK1 [160]. In addition to serving as a priming site for phosphorylation, the phosphorylation at Serine 45 may facilitate the phosphorylation pattern of β-catenin making it transcriptionally active. However, this has to be investigated further as this idea is yet primitive [160]. High levels of nuclear phospho-β-catenin are associated with significantly worse overall survival [70]. Using a phosphorylation specific antibody Kielhorn and colleagues determined that nuclear β-catenin staining was more prevalent in advanced melanomas [183]. This may be due to the specific phosphorylation pattern of β-catenin having specificity for TCF thereby allowing transcription of cancer causing genes.

4.1.4. Localization

β-catenin is present in the cytoplasmic compartment as well as the nucleus. A well-defined feature of active-β-catenin is that it is located exclusively in the nucleus [182]. However, the mechanism of the nuclear localization of β-catenin is currently unknown. β-catenin does not contain a nuclear localization sequence (NLS) nor utilize the importin transport machinery [184]. However, nuclear export of β-catenin is established to be mediated by an intrinsic export signal and its interaction with APC. The retention of β-catenin within the nucleus is thought to be due to its interaction within the nucleus with TCF, BCL-9 and pygopous [184]. However, these interactions are not a prerequisite for β-catenin's localization into the nucleus as it has been demonstrated that the protein can successfully localize to the nucleus in the absence of these interactions. Overexpression of LEF/TCF has been shown to lead to β-catenin's accumulation in the nucleus [185, 186]. It has been suggested that the nuclear import of the β-catenin/LEFcomplex is mediated by the NLS provided by LEF/TCF proteins. However, elevations in nuclear levels of β-catenin are observed even when the levels of LEF/TCF are low [186, 187]. Therefore, mechanisms independent of LEF/TCF are likely to be important for regulating the nuclear import of β-catenin *in vivo* [188]. Two groups have independently demonstrated a direct importin-independent nuclear import of β-catenin in a semi-permeabilized cell model [189, 190]. However, to date no mandatory chaperone essential to the nuclear transport of β-catenin has been identified. In summary, within the nucleus, β-catenin specifically active-β-catenin, has an oncogenic role as it serves as a transcriptional co-activator of cancer promoting target genes.

4.1.5. β-Catenin in Cancer

In carcinomas, the loss of β-catenin-E-cadherin complexes is an important step in disease progression. Loss of organization by disruption of epithelial complexes at adherens junctions is a common feature of invasiveness. Furthermore, deregulation of the Wnt signaling pathway at various levels, often leads to metastasis and cancer progression as Wnt target genes are responsible for controlling the regulation of cell cycle, proliferation and inhibition of apoptosis. A common effect of deregulated/activated Wnt pathway components is an overexpression of β-catenin. Many common cancers including, colorectal cancer (CRC) [191], hepatocellular carcinoma [192], adrenal cancers [193, 194], breast cancer [195], Wilm's tumour [196], several hematological malignancies [197] and melanomas [63] have been found to have a deregulated Wnt pathway. Some of the causative factors of this deregulation are the loss of function mutations in APC or Axin [197], or mutations in the amino acids at the NTD of β-catenin which interfere with its phosphorylation and proteosomal degradation [191]. Truncating mutations in Axin cause nuclear accumulation of β-catenin in hepatocellular carcinomas [198]. Furthermore, APC is mutated in 85% of familial and sporadic CRCs [199]. Mutations have also been found to occur in exon 3 of the β-catenin gene, affecting sites of phosphorylation by GSK3β, making β-catenin refractory to degradation [200]. The result of mutations in the Wnt pathway is an elevation of total cellular levels of β-catenin and the activation of β-catenin dependent TCF/LEF transcription which mediates its oncogenic effect in various tissues. Over activation of the canonical Wnt signaling pathway results in up regulation of several cell growth regulatory proteins and processes, consequently resulting in cancer progression.

4.1.6. β-Catenin in Melanoma

Wnt-β-catenin signaling is up regulated in melanoma, and approximately 30% of melanoma exhibit increased nuclear β-catenin [63]. The high frequency of nuclear accumulation is not all attributable to mutations in the Wnt pathway. The discrepancy between these datasets prompts the investigation of putative mechanisms responsible for the excessive accumulation of nuclear β-catenin. The mechanism that regulates β-catenin's transcriptional activity of Wnt target genes needs further investigation. Determining how this nuclear pool of β-catenin is regulated by the Wnt pathway alongside other pathways to orchestrate the transcription of target genes is an area of study that needs much anticipated investigation. This would be a leap into the study of melanoma formation and tumour progression [63]. A thorough understanding of the pathway will provide a look into cell specific molecular mechanisms involved in initiation and progression of melanoma. β-catenin expression in melanoma has been shown to be different than many other cancers. Several studies using melanoma cell lines show a decrease in nuclear and cytoplasmic staining in malignant cell lines compared to a benign nevus stage [201]. This creates contradiction of β-catenin's expression pattern in other cancers where β-catenin levels are elevated as the cancer progresses, such as hepatoma, gastric and bladder cancers [201]. Little is known specifically about changes in active-β-catenin in melanoma progression, the pool of β-catenin relevant in the transcription of genes for the proteins that promote metastasis. Demunter and colleagues showed that post-translational modifications of β-catenin rather than mutations in the CTNNB1 gene itself are responsible for the altered distribution of β-catenin in the cell (Demunter et al., 2002). The fact that β-catenin serves many roles in the cell and has variability in its phosphorylation pattern may be an explanation as to why many studies measuring overall levels of β-catenin show an inverse relationship in melanoma progression and β-catenin levels. The fact that phospho-β-catenin is more prevalent in metastatic melanomas is consistent with the fact that β-catenin serves different roles and functions in a cell [202]. Kiehlhorn and colleagues suggests that phosphorylation specific antigen of β-catenin is correlated with a better marker of disease progression than overall levels, which are masked with different pools of β-catenin. However, high transcriptional activity of β-catenin in certain disease conditions cannot be attributed to mutations in β-catenin or components of the Wnt pathway. In support of this, β-catenin, recently identified as a candidate gene for melanoma progression, was found to be mutated in 5% of melanomas but constitutively active (nuclear expression and transcriptional activity) in 40-50% of melanomas [63]. This suggests that alternate regulatory mechanisms/pathways in controlling the oncogenic/transcriptional properties of β-catenin are involved. Although the canonical Wnt pathway is well characterized in the regulation of cellular β-catenin levels, several investigations suggest that β-catenin may also be regulated by other signal transduction pathways via potential cross talk. In particular, the phosphotidylinositol-3 kinase (PI3K) pathway has been significantly implicated in the regulation of β-catenin [203].

4.2. Crosstalk between the PI3K and Canonical Wnt Pathways in Melanoma Progression

There are divergent views on the role of the PI3K pathway in the regulation of β-catenin. There are several different hypotheses around how these two pathways may be linked. The regulation of β-catenin by the two pathways may be through direct crosstalk via a common component. Since GSK3β is a common component of both pathways, several studies suggest that the inactivation of GSK3β by AKT links the PI3K pathway to the Wnt pathway in a bipartite mechanism which subsequently regulates the cytoplasmic levels of β-catenin [204]. However, other studies propose that the Wnt and PI3K pathways remain distinct and variably regulate alternate pools of GSK3β [205]. Other components such as AKT, TGFβ1, mTOR and PI3K have also been suggested as linkers between the Wnt and PI3K pathways.

4.2.1. GSK3β As a Potential Candidate to Mediate Crosstalk between Wnt/β-Catenin and PI3K Pathways

There are two schools of thought regarding PI3K/Wnt crosstalk. One hypothesis states that both pathways signal through a common pool of GSK3β while an alternative hypothesis suggests two segregated pools of GSK3β. There is evidence supporting both hypotheses: Sharma et al. [206] saw that increased levels of PI3K signaling correspond to nuclear accumulation of β-catenin in what was assumed to be a GSK3β dependent mechanism since GSK3β is deactivated via AKT phosphorylation. They noted that inhibition of PI3K reduces AKT and GSK3β phosphorylation and subsequently decreases nuclear accumulation of β-catenin. However, many other studies suggest a more segregated pool of GSK3β linking the PI3K and Wnt systems.

The PI3K pathway, via AKT, elicits cellular responses through an array of downstream effectors, one of which is GSK3β. In this pathway GSK3β serves various roles such as protein synthesis, glycogen metabolism and cell cycle regulation [207, 208]. Insulin stimulation of the PI3K pathway results in downstream phosphorylation by AKT at Ser 9 of GSK3β and Ser 21 of GSK3α, resulting in the inactivation of GSK3β [209]. This inactivation further dephosphorylates and activates glycogen synthase (GS), which promotes the synthesis of glycogen (Nature 378, 785-789). By this mechanism, the phosphorylation of GSK3β turns off its catalytic activity thereby deregulating GSK3β and activating downstream targets that are normally repressed by GSK3β.

It has been suggested that interactions of GSK3β with a specific pathway may effectively shield GSK3β from the influences from other alternate pathways resulting in its specificity of effects to any one particular pathway at any one time. Ding et al. saw that the effect of each signaling pathway is highly specific, and changes to GSK3β activity in one pathway may not affect the downstream events of the components of the other pathway [210]. Another reason that may cause differential regulation may be a difference in post-translational modification of the GSK3β. The serine 9 phosphorylation of GSK3β is specific to PI3K signaling, and is not affected by the Wnt pathway activity. As Ding and colleagues showed Wnt stimulation does not cause phosphorylation of AKT at Thr-308 or Ser-473, nor phosphorylation of GSK3β on Ser-9 [210], therefore AKT is not the mediator of endogenous Wnt signals disrupting the destruction complex. Patel and colleagues also looked at the effect on β-catenin levels following activation of the PI3K pathway via insulin stimulation, which resulted in a decrease in overall GSK3β activity. Although there was a change in GSK3β activity they saw no change in β-catenin levels and therefore concluded that β-catenin regulation is "insulated from other signaling pathways" [211]. Further support comes from Ng and colleagues who reported that the Axin bound pool of GSK3β, which comprises 3-5% of total cellular GSK3β, compartmentalizes the pools involved in the wnt pathway [205]. This sequestration of the GSK3β prevents the Wnt pathway associated GSK3 and the subsequent Wnt-induced transcriptional activity from being affected by PI3K pathway [205]. It is possible that, although GSK3β downstream of PI3K and Wnt may be segregated, activation of AKT can affect both pools of GSK3β. The resulting reduction in activity of both pools of GSK3β may then contribute synergistically to the cellular accumulation β-catenin. However, this decrease must be in the order of 75-80% to have significant effect on Wnt signaling [212], as AKT would more easily alter the activity of GSK3β not sequestered by Axin due to quantity and availability within the cytoplasm.

4.2.2. Other Potential Candidates That Mediate Crosstalk between Wnt/β-Catenin and PI3K Pathways

4.2.2.1. AKT

There may be other components of the PI3K pathway which may be involved in changes in β-catenin and the Wnt pathway such as, AKT. AKT is a key effector of the PI3K system, canonically being phosphorylated in a PI3K-dependent fashion by PDK1 and PDK2. By phosphorylating GSK3β, AKT may induce inactivation of the destruction complex and thereby allowing β-catenin to accumulate in an AKT-dependent manner. Sharma et al suggest an AKT-dependent increase in nuclear localization of β-catenin, which may operate through this type of direct mechanism [206]. Fukumoto et al suggest that while AKT activity might not be sufficient to mimic a Wnt signal, it might prolong the duration of the signal to enhance the effect of the signal [213]. Thus increased phosphorylation of AKT by deregulated PI3K pathway might lead to longer periods of destruction complex inactivation and therein induce an increased accumulation of β-catenin. AKT has also been shown to directly modulate β-catenin interaction with E-cadherin, which comprises a central portion of the adherens junction [214]. He et al [215] has shown that by phosphorylating Ser552 of β-catenin, AKT induces separation of β-catenin from E-cadherin and thereby frees it to accumulate unbound in the cell and subsequently promotes nuclear localization of β-catenin. AKT phosphorylation at additional sites of β-catenin increases its interaction with 14-3-3ζ, an oncogenic chaperone with implicated roles in signaling, cell cycle control and regulation of apoptosis [216]. Binding with 14-3-3ζ causes β-catenin to accumulate in the cytoplasm, sequestered away from E-cadherin. More importantly, this interaction inhibits β-catenin's binding with β-Trcp, inhibiting the proteosomal degradation of β-catenin and in turn increasing its stability. While binding to 14-3-3ζ reduces β-catenin's binding to B-Trcp, it actually increases β-catenin's affinity for its nuclear interactor Lef4. This may implicate 14-3-3ζ as playing a vital role as a chaperone in regulating β-catenin activity.

Dihlmann et al. show that β-catenin transcriptionally regulates AKT1, and Zhang et al. (2011) found similar regulation of AKT2 [217]. Additionally, Fukumoto et al showed that Wnt signaling induces phosphorylation of AKT in the presence of Dvl [213]. This Dvl-dependent p-AKT binds the Axin destruction complex in the presence of Dvl, phosphorylating GSK3β and inducing accumulation of β-catenin. In this manner, AKT acts in a Dvl-dependent manner to transduce the canonical Wnt signal. The mechanism by which AKT is phosphorylated is not discussed, but its phosphorylation is measured at Thr308 and Ser473, its canonical PI3K dependent phosphorylation sites. If its phosphorylation is PI3K-dependent but is induced by Wnt signaling, a cyclic interaction between the PI3K and Wnt pathways may exist. To this end, Wnt signals would increase canonical AKT phosphorylation through PI3K, and newly phosphorylated AKT may bind in a Dvl-dependent manner to the axin destruction complex, wherein it phosphorylates and subsequently deactivates GSK3β. This deactivation of GSK3β would lead to increased stability of β-catenin, which would transcriptionally activate AKT and perpetuate the cycle. If this sort of system exists, deregulation of the PI3K pathway would lead to hypersensitivity of the destruction complex to regular Wnt signaling due to an abundance of activated AKT, thus inducing increased levels of β-catenin accumulation and subsequent translocation to the nucleus.

4.2.2.2. PI3K

PI3K itself is a candidate for crosstalk between PI3K and Wnt pathways. Espada et al. found that β-catenin binds to PI3Ks regulatory subunit p85α with a higher affinity than to its transcriptional partner Lef1 [218]. β-catenin binding to p85α sequesters it away from the destruction complex by inhibiting its interaction with APC [218]. Since β-catenin is shielded from APC by p85α, binding to the catalytic domain of PI3K would inhibit its regular degradation pathway and thereby increase its stability. With sequestration from the destruction complex, β-catenin would be allowed to accumulate in the cytoplasm and translocate to the nucleus, where it can act transcriptionally. This may suggest an additional role for PI3K within the cell: its regulatory domain, p85α, may act as a chaperone for β-catenin, sequestering it from the destruction complex and thus inducting its stability. This could be accomplished by either solely sequestration or by inducing a conformational change that promotes some post-secondary modification of β-catenin.

4.2.2.3. mTOR

Some downstream targets of AKT could induce effects that become evident by alterations of AKT activity. One such target is mTOR. As discussed earlier, mTORC1 plays many roles in cellular regulation, translation and autophagy. On the other hand, mTORC2 acts as a PDK2 molecule, capable of phosphorylating molecules such as AKT, though its kinase functionality is not necessarily limited to AKT. As such, mTORC2 may play a role in transducing a signal to components of the Wnt cascade.

mTOR has been identified by Tanwar et al. as a therapeutic target for cancers characterized by deregulated PI3K activity and increased transcriptional activity of β-catenin [219]. Since this targeting is achieved via rapamycin treatment, mTORC1 is implicated. The mTORC1 complex plays roles in increasing protein synthesis through inhibition of 4EBP1, the negative regulator of elongation factor elF4E [220]. When stimulated by insulin, mTORC1 is activated through PI3K, which downregulates its negative regulator, PRAS40, which specifically inhibits Raptor, a component of mTORC1 [220]. Along with promoting protein synthesis, mTORC1 differentially regulates phosphatase activity [221], which may be required to generate hypophosphorylated active β-catenin phosphorylated at Ser37/Thr41. In the study by Harwood et al., mTORC1 inhibited the phosphatase involved in maintaining the hypophosphorylataion of Thr202 on p44/42, while at the same time promoting the activity of the phosphatase involved in dephosphorylating Tyr204. Both sites require phosphorylation in order to activate p44/42, a key member of the MEK cascade. This suggests a complex role for mTORC1 in the regulation of phosphatase activity. Okadaic acid inhibited the activity of the phosphatase involved in Thr202 in the presence of rapamycin, suggesting that the phosphatase involved is PP2A. If mTORC1 is differentially promoting and inhibiting the activity of certain phosphatases, it may be involved in the generation of selectively hypophosphorylated active β-catenin. In support of this, a study by Liu et al. indicates that nuclear translocation of β-catenin occurs in a rapamycin-sensitive mTOR-dependent manner [222]. These effects may be as a result of mTORC1-induced generation of active β-catenin.

4.2.2.4. TGFβ1

Another downstream target of AKT is TGFβ. Walsh et al. showed that TGFβ1, an isoform of the known oncoprotein TGFB, regulates β-catenin localization in an insulin/PI3K-dependent manner [223]. Upon stimulation of insulin receptors, PI3K is stimulated and production of certain matrix metalloproteinases (MMPs) is promoted downstream. These MMPs cleave latent TGFβ1, activating it so that it can subsequently bind TGFβ1 receptors. This binding results in increased stabilization and nuclear translocation of β-catenin, according to results by Welsh et al. The mechanism for this is currently unknown. However, the binding of TGFβ to TGFβR is known to activate Smad proteins. Smad activates the Snail transcription factor, inhibiting production of E-cadherin [224]. In the absence of E-cadherin, β-catenin has no major interactor at the adherens junction and is allowed to accumulate in the cytoplasm, subsequently translocating to the nucleus. Interestingly, Snail is also modified by O-GlcNAcylation [225]. Since Snail has its transcriptional activity reduced by O-GlcNAcylation in a manner similar to β-catenin, the enzyme beta-N-acetlyglucosaminidase may be downstream of TGFβR, allowing the binding of its ligand to reduce the inhibition of Snail activity through removal of the sugar modification.

Current Therapeutics of Melanoma and Concluding Remarks

Currently there are five different types of therapies for melanoma, depending on the stage of the cancer. Surgery, chemotherapy, radiation therapy, targeted therapy and biologic therapy are the treatments presented by the National Cancer Institute.

Surgery is the primary form of treatment as it excises the primary tumour or the lymph nodes to which the tumour cells have metastasized. Chemotherapy with Decarbazine or DTIC [5-(3,3-Dimethyl-1-triazenyl)imidazole-4-carboxamide] and radiation therapy are two other commonly used conventional cancer treatment regimens. Treating melanoma using chemotherapy has poor response rate and the effect is short lived. Biologic therapy targets the patient's immune system to fight the cancer. This therapy boosts the immune system by restoring the body's natural defences. An example is Interleukin -2 (IL-2), which promotes the growth and activity of lymphocytes, a group of cells used by the immune system in its defence against cancer cells. The adverse effects of such treatment are severe side effects at higher doses of these reagents. In light of this these drugs are used in low doses usually in combination with another form of therapy. Targeted therapy is focussed on signal transduction pathway components that are deregulated in melanoma [226]. This form of treatment is very specific compared to other conventional therapies. Some of the drugs that are commonly used in targeted therapy for melanoma are Vemurafenib, Sorafnib and Ipilimumab. Vemurafenib is a commonly used BRAF inhibiting drug which specifically targets BRAF substitution mutations. Sorafnib is a multikinase inhibitor that targets VEGF and Raf/MEK pathways at the level of RAF kinase. Ipilimumab, an antibody against cytotoxic T-lymphocyte (CTL) antigen, is a commonly used drug for stage IV melanoma. This drug removes inhibition of CTLs so they can target and destroy cancer cells [227]. Signaling pathways like the MAPK, PI3K, c-KIT and NFκB which are deregulated in melanoma are also targeted for treating melanoma progression. In this section we will discuss targeting of the components of the PI3K pathway, which is of primary focus in this review.

Perifosine is a novel alkyl phospholipid compound that inhibits AKT. It was shown to have cytotoxic effects in-vitro and in-vivo in human multiple myeloma cells [228]. Vyomesh Patel et al showed Perifosine to cause cell cycle arrest in-vitro in squamous carcinoma cells by inducing $p21^{WAF1}$ in a p53 independent manner [229]. Sudhir et al proposed the mechanism for induction of $p21^{WAF1}$ to be via PI3K pathway [230]. BI-69A11 is another inhibitor of AKT. Treatment of melanoma cells in-vitro with BI-69A11 led to reduced levels of AKT and intra-peritoneal injection of BI-69A11 caused primary tumour size regression in melanoma xenografts [231]. Isothiocyanates are naturally occurring compounds with anti-cancerous property. This compound targets AKT and lead to increased apoptosis in melanoma cells with low toxic effects [232]. Apart from these compounds which target AKT, some of the compounds that target mTOR are also found to be significant for melanoma therapy. Phase II study of Everolimus, an mTOR inhibitor in combination with Bevacizumab, an angiogenesis inhibitor has shown moderate efficacy in patients with metastatic melanoma. This combination treatment was also well tolerated by patients [233]. H. Niessner et al tested the effect of Lonafarnib, an m-TOR inhibitor to cause apoptosis in melanoma cells. Lonafarnib significantly decreased cell growth in combination with sorafnib, a p-Raf inhibitor, whereas it had insufficient effect when used for treatment alone or in combination with other inhibitors of AKT. Hence suggests that lonafarnib inhibits mTOR signaling and potentiates sorafnib mediated apoptosis in melanoma cells [234].

Overall, co-targeting of pathways has proven to be more effective in treating melanoma compared to targeting a single pathway and hence an understanding of crosstalks among signal transduction pathways would be invaluable in increasing and improving the scope for melanoma therapy. Crosstalk between the PI3K and Wnt/β-Catenin pathways is a novel area of study, which will provide several targets of value in melanoma therapies, possibly intervening with metastasis.

REFERENCES

[1] Carracedo, A., & Pandolfi, P. P. (2008). The PTEN-PI3K pathway: of feedbacks and cross-talks. *Oncogene,* 27, 5527-5541.

[2] Katso, R., Okkenhaug, K. et al. (2001). Cellular function of phosphoinositide 3-kinases: implications for development, homeostasis, and cancer. *Annu Rev Cell Dev Biol,* 17, 615–675.

[3] Petrocelli, T., & Slingerland, J. M. (2001). PTEN deficiency: a role in a mammary carcinogenesis. *Breast Cancer Res,* 3, 356-360.

[4] Fresno Vara, J. A., Casado, E. et. al. (2004). PI3K/Akt signaling pathway and cancer. *Cancer Treat Reviews,* 30(2), 193-204.

[5] Paez, J., & Sellers, W. R. (2003). PI3K/PTEN/AKT Pathway. A critical mediator of oncogenic signaling. *Cancer Treat Res.,* 115, 145-67.

[6] Bader, A. G., Kang, S. et. al. (2005). Oncogenic PI3K deregulates transcription and translation. *Nat Rev Cancer,* 5, 921–929.

[7] Engelman, J. A., Luo, J. et al. (2006). The evolution of phosphatidylinositol 3-kinases as regulators of growth and metabolism. *Nat Rev Genet,* 7, 606-619.

[8] Backer, J. M. (2008). The regulation and function of class II PI3Ks: novel roles for Vps34. *Biochem J,* 410, 1-17.

[9] Yuan, T. L., & Cantley, L. C. (2008). PI3K pathway alterations in cancer: variations on a theme. *Oncogene,* 27(41), 5497-510.

[10] Vivanco, I. & Sawyers, C. L. (2002). The phosphatidylinositol 3-kinase-akt pathway in human cancer. *Nature Review,* 2, 489-501.

[11] Chalhoub, N., & Baker, S. J. (2009). PTEN and the PI3-kinase pathway in cancer. *Annu Rev Pathol,* 4, 127-50.

[12] Brock,T. (2013). The PI3K Pathway: Fast Forward for Cancer. *Experimental Biology.*

[13] McCall, P. (2010). *The interaction between the PI3K/Akt cascade and the androgen receptor in the development and progression of castrate resistant prostate cancer.* PhD thesis. University of Glasgow.

[14] Ikenoue, T., Kanai, F., et al. (2005). Functional analysis of PIK3CA gene mutations in human colorectal cancer. *Cancer Res,* 65(11), 4562-4567.

[15] Samuels, Y. & Ericson, K. (2006). Oncogenic PI3K and its role in cancer. *Curr Opin Oncol,* 18(1), 77-82.

[16] Myers, M. P., & Tonk, N. K. (1997). PTEN: sometimes taking it off can be better than putting it on. *Am J Hum Genet,* 61(6), 1234-1238.

[17] Stambolic, V., Suzuki, A., et. al. (1998). Negative regulation of PKB/Akt-dependent cell survival by the tumour suppressor PTEN. *Cell,* 95, 29–39.

[18] Maehama, T., Taylor, G. S., et al. (2001). PTEN and myotubularin: novel phosphoinositide phosphatases. *Annu Rev Biochem.* 70, 247-279.

[19] Li, D. M., & Sun, H. (1997). TEP1, encoded by a candidate tumour suppressor locus, is a novel protein tyrosine phosphatase regulated by transforming growth factor beta. *Cancer Res,* 57, 2124–2129.

[20] Ramaswamy, S., N. Nakamura., et. al. (1999). Regulation of G1 progression by the PTEN suppressor protein is linked to inhibition of the phosphatidylinositol-3 kinase/Akt pathway. *Proc. Natl. Acad. Sci. USA,* 96, 2110–2115.

[21] Vasudvan, K. M., Guruurthy, S., et. al. (2007). Suppression of PTEN expression by NF-kappa B prevents apoptosis. *Mol Cell Biol,* 24, 1007-1021.

[22] Papakonstanti, E. A., Ridley, A. J., et. al. (2007). The p110delta isoform of PI 3-kinase negatively controls RhoA and PTEN. *EMBO J,* 26, 3050-3061.

[23] Wang, W., Trotman, L. C., et. al. (2007). NEDD4-1 is a proto-oncogenic ubiquitin ligase for PTEN. *Cell,* 128, 129-139.

[24] Ahn, Y., Hwang, C. Y., et. al. (2008). Tumour suppressor PTEN mediates a negative regulation of E3 ubiquitin-protein ligase Nedd4. *Biochem J,* 412, 331-338.

[25] Yang, Z. Z., Tschopp, O., et. al. (2004). Physiological functions of protein kinase B/Akt. *Biochem Soc Trans,* 32(Pt 2), 350-354.

[26] Sarbassov, D. D., Guertin, D. A., et. al. (2005). Phosphorylation and regulation of Akt/PKB by the Rictor-mTOR complex. *Science,* 307 (5712), 1098-1101.

[27] Stephens, L., Anderson, K., et al. (1998). Protein Kinase B kinases that mediate phosphatidylinositol 3,4,5-trisphosphate-dependent activation of protein kinase B. *Science,* 279 (5351), 710-714.

[28] Cully, M., You, H., et. al. (2006). Beyond PTEN mutations: the PI3K pathway as an integrator of multiple inputs during tumourigenesis. *Nature Reviews,* 6, 184-192.

[29] Bader, A. G., Kang, S., et. al. (2005). Oncogenic PI3K deregulates transcription and translation. *Nat Rev Cancer,* 5(12), 921–929.

[30] Vogt, P. K., Hart, J. R., et. al. (2010). Phosphatidylinositol 3-Kinase: the oncoprotein. *Current Topics in Microbiology and Immunology,* 347, 79-104.

[31] Carpenter, C. L., Duckworth, B. C., et. al. (1990). Purification and characterization of phosphoinositide 3-kinase from rat liver. *J Biol Chem,* 265, 19704-19711.

[32] Carnero, A., Blanco-Aparicio, C., et. al. (2008). The PTEN/PI3K/Akt signaling pathway in cancer, therapeutic implications. *Curr. Cancer Drug Targets,* 8, 187–198.

[33] Cheng, G. Z., Park, S., et. al. (2008). Advances of Akt pathway in human oncogenesis and as a target for anti-cancer drug discovery. *Curr. Cancer Drug Targets,* 8, 2–6.

[34] Gao, N., Zhang, Z., et. al. (2003). Role of PI3K/Akt/mTOR signaling in the cell cycle progression of human prostate cancer. *Biochem. Biophys. Res. Commun,* 310, 1124–1132.

[35] de la Taille, A., Rubin, M. A., et al. (2003). β-Catenin-related anomalies in apoptosis-resistant and hormone-refractory prostate cancer cells. *Clin. Cancer Res,* 9, 1801–1807.

[36] Lee, H. K., Kwak, H. Y., et. al. (2007). β-Catenin regulates multiple steps of RNA metabolism as revealed by the RNA aptamer in colon cancer cells. *Cancer Res,* 67, 9315–9321.

[37] Vignot, S., Faivre, S., et. al. (2005). mTOR-targeted therapy of cancer with rapamycin derivatives. *Ann. Oncol,* 16, 525–537.

[38] Toker, A. (2008). mTOR and Akt signaling in cancer: SGK cycles in. Mol. *Cell,* 31, 6–8.

[39] Hanahan, D. & Weinberg, R. A. (2000). The hallmarks of cancer. The hallmarks of cancer. *Cell,* 100, 57-70.

[40] Manning, B. D. & Cantley, L. C. (2007). AKT/PKB signaling: navigating downstream. *Cell* 129, 1261–1274.

[41] Samuels, Y., Wang, Z., et al. (2004). High frequency of mutations of the PIK3CA gene in human cancers. *Science,* 304, 554.

[42] Zhao L. & Vogt P. K. (2008). Class I P13K in oncogenic cellular transformation. *Oncogene,* 27(41), 5486-96.

[43] Grossman, D. & Altieri, D. C. (2001). Drug resistance in melanoma: mechanisms, apoptosis, and new potential therapeutic targets. *Cancer Metastasis Rev,* 20, 3-11.

[44] Helmbach, H., Rossmann, E., et. al. (2001). Drug-resistance in human melanoma. *Int J Cancer,* 93, 617-22.

[45] Soengas, M. S. & Lowe, S. W. (2003). Apoptosis and melanoma chemoresistance. *Oncogene,* 22, 3138-51.

[46] Kim, I. K., Lane, A. M., et. al. (2010). Survival in patients with presymptomatic diagnosis of metastaic uveal melanoma. *Arch Ophtalmol,* 128, 871-5.

[47] Haass, N. K., Smalley, K. S., et, al. (2004). The role of altered cell-cell communication in melanoma progression. *J. Mol. Histol,* 35, 309-18.

[48] Haass, N. K., Smalley, K. S., et. al. (2005). Adhesion, migration and communication in melanocytes and melanoma. *Pigment Cell Res,* 18(3), 150-9.

[49] Hao, L., Ha, J. R., et. al. (2012). Cadherin switch from E- to N- cadherin in melanoma progression is regulated by the PI3K/PTEN pathway through Twist and Snail. *Br J Dermatol,* 166(6), 1184-97.

[50] Hirohashi. S. (1998). Inactivation of the E-cadherin-mediated cell adhesion system in human cancers. *Am J Pathol,* 153, 333–9.

[51] Piris, A., Mihm, M. C Jr. et. al. (2011). AJCC melanoma staging update: impact on dermatopathology practice and patient management. *J Cutan Pathol,* 38, 394-400.

[52] Sosman, J. A. (2013). *Patient Information: Melanoma treatment; advanced or metastatic melanoma* (Beyond the Basics). Upto Date.

[53] Padua, R. A., Barrass, N., et. al. (1984). A novel transforming gene in a human malignant melanoma cell line. *Nature,* 311, 671–673.

[54] van't Veer, L. J., B, B. M. et. al. (1989). N.-ras mutations in human cutaneous melanoma from sun-exposed body sites. *Mol. Cell. Biol,* 9, 3114–3116.

[55] Yang, G., Rajadurai, A., et. al. (2005). Recurrent patterns of dual RB and p53 pathway inactivation in melanoma. *J. Invest. Dermatol,* 125, 1242–1251.

[56] Daniotti, M., Oggionni, M., et al. (2004). BRAF alterations are associated with complex mutational profiles in malignant melanoma. *Oncogene,* 23, 5968–5977.

[57] Curtin, J. A., Fridlyand, J. et. al. (2005). Distinct sets of genetic alterations in melanoma. N. *Engl. J. Med,* 353, 2135–2147.

[58] Flaherty, K. T., Hodi, F. S., et. al. (2012). From genes to drugs: targeted strategies for melanoma. *Nat Rev Cancer,* 12(5), 349-61.

[59] Smith, A. G., Beaumont, K. A. et. al. (2009).PPARy agonists attenuate proliferation and modulate Wnt/ β-catenin signaling in melanoma cells. *Int J Biochem Cell Biol,* (41), 844-52.

[60] Rubinfeld, B., Robbins, P. et. al. (1997). Stabilization of beta-catenin by genetic defects in melanoma cell lines. *Science,* 275, 1790-1792.

[61] Lucero, O. M., Dawson, D. W. et. al. (2010). A re-evaluation of the "oncogenic" nature of Wnt/beta-catenin signaling in melanoma and other cancers. *Curr. Oncol. Rep,* (12), 314-318.

[62] Damsky, W. E., Curley, D. P. et. al. (2011). β-Catenin Signaling Controls Metastasis in Braf-Activated Pten-Deficient Melanomas. *Cancer Cell,* 20(6), 741-754.

[63] Larue, L., Delmas, V. (2006). The WNT/Beta-catenin pathway in melanoma. *Front Biosci,* 11, 733-742.

[64] Lau, E. & Ronai, Z. A. (2011). *Chapter 7 Altered Signal Transduction Pathways in Melanoma.* In Bosserhoff, A., Melanoma Development (137-163). New York, New York: Springerwien.

[65] Sansal, I. & Sellers, W. R. (2004). The biology and clinical relevance of the PTEN tumour suppressor pathway. *J Clin Oncol,* 22, 2954–63.

[66] Guldberg, P., thor Straten, P. et al. (2007). Disruption of the MMAC1/PTEN gene by deletion or mutation is a frequent event in malignant melanoma. *Cancer Res,* 57, 3660–3.

[67] Tsao, H., Zhang, X. et al. (1998). Identification of PTEN/MMAC1 alterations in uncultured melanomas and melanoma cell lines. *Oncogene,* 16, 3397–402.

[68] Wu, H., Goel, V. et. al. (2003). PTEN signaling pathways in melanoma. *Oncogene,* 22, 3113–22.

[69] Trotman, L. C., Niki, M. et. al. (2003). PTEN dose dictates cancer progression in the prostate. *PLoS Biol,* 1(3), E59.

[70] Lopez-Bergami, P., Fitchman, Boris. et. al. (2008). Understanding Signaling Cascades in Melanoma. *Photochem Photobiol,* 84(2), 289-306.

[71] Chudnovsky, Y., Adams, A. E. et. al. (2005). Use of human tissue to assess the oncogenic activity of melanoma-associated mutations. *Nat Genet,* 37, 745–749.

[72] Dhawan, P., Singh, A. B. et. al. (2002). Constitutive activation of Akt/protein kinase B in melanoma leads to upregulation of nuclear factor-kappaB and tumour progression. *Cancer Res,* 62, 7335–42.

[73] Govindarajan, B., Sligh, J. E. et. al. (2007). Overexpression of Akt converts radial growth melanoma to vertical growth melanoma. *J Clin Invest,* 117, 719-29.

[74] Sauroja, I., Smeds, J., et. al. (2000). Analysis of G(1)/S checkpoint regulators in metastatic melanoma. *Genes Chromosom Cancer,* 28, 404–414.

[75] Smalley, K. S., Haass, N. K. et. al. (2006). Multiple signaling pathways must be targeted to overcome drug resistance in cell lines derived from melanoma metastases. *Br J Dermatol,* 156, 1204-13.

[76] Meister, M., Tomasovic, A., et al. (2013). Mitogen-Activated Protein (MAP) Kinase Scaffolding Proteins: A Recount. *Int. J. Mol.,* 14, 4854-4884.

[77] Krishna, M. & Narang, H. (2008). The complexity of mitogen-activated protein kinases (MAPKs) made simple. *Cell. Mol. Life Sci.,* 65, 3525 – 3544.

[78] Cargnello, M. & Philippe P. Roux. (2011). Activation and Function of the MAPKs and Their Substrates, the MAPK-Activated Protein Kinases. Microbiol. *Mol. Biol. Rev.*, 50–83.

[79] Duckworth, B. C. & Cantley, L. C. (1997). Conditional inhibition of the mitogen-activated protein kinase cascade by wortmannin.Dependence on signal strength. *J Biol Chem.* 272(44):27665-70.

[80] Aksamitiene, E., Kiyatkin, A. et al. (2012). Cross-talk between mitogenic Ras/MAPK and survival PI3K/Akt pathways: a fine balance. *Biochem Soc Trans.* 40(1):139-46.

[81] Castellano, E. & Downward, J. (2011). RAS Interaction with PI3K: More Than Just Another Effector Pathway. *Genes Cancer.* 2(3):261-74.

[82] Welch, H. C., Coadwell, W. J., et al. (2003). Phosphoinositide 3-kinase-dependent activation of Rac. *FEBS Lett.* 546(1):93-7.

[83] Ye, D. Z. & Field, J. (2012). PAK signaling in cancer. *Cell Logist.* 2(2):105-116.

[84] Chaudhary, A., King W. G., et al. (2000). Phosphatidylinositol 3-kinase regulates Raf1 through Pak phosphorylation of serine 338. *Curr Biol.* 10(9):551-4.

[85] Chiloeches, A., Mason, C. S., et al. (2001). S338 phosphorylation of Raf-1 is independent of phosphatidylinositol 3-kinase and Pak3. *Mol Cell Biol.* 21(7):2423-34.

[86] Zimmermann, S. & Moelling, K. (1999). Phosphorylation and regulation of Raf by Akt (protein kinase B). *Science.* 286(5445):1741-4.

[87] Moelling, K., Schad, K., et al. (2002). Regulation of Raf-Akt Cross-talk. *J Biol Chem.* 277(34):31099-106.

[88] Guan, K. L., Figueroa, C., et al. (2000). Negative regulation of the serine/threonine kinase B-Raf by Akt. *J Biol Chem.* 275(35):27354-9.

[89] Menges, C. W. & McCance, D. J. (2008). Constitutive activation of the Raf-MAPK pathway causes negative feedback inhibition of Ras-PI3K-AKT and cellular arrest through the EphA2 receptor. *Oncogene.* 27(20):2934-40.

[90] Sato, S., Fujita, N., et al. (2004). Involvement of 3-phosphoinositide-dependent Protein kinase-1 in the MEK/MAPK signal transduction pathway. *J Biol Chem.* 279(32):33759-67.

[91] Nasrazadani, A. & van den Berg C. L. (2011). c-Jun N-terminal Kinase 2 Regulates Multiple Receptor Tyrosine Kinase Pathways in Mouse Mammary Tumour Growth and Metastasis. *Genes Cancer.* 2(1):31-45.

[92] Logan, S. K., Falasca, M., et al. (1997). Phosphatidylinositol 3-kinase mediates epidermal growth factor-induced activation of the c-Jun N-terminal kinase signaling pathway. *Mol Cell Biol.* 17(10):5784-90.

[93] Zhou, H. Y., Wan, K. F., et al. (2008). Hepatocyte growth factor enhances proteolysis and invasiveness of human nasopharyngeal cancer cells through activation of PI3K and JNK. *FEBS Lett.* 582(23-24):3415-22.

[94] Merighi, S., Benini, A., et al. (2006). Modulation of the Akt/Ras/Raf/MEK/ERK pathway by A_3 adenosine receptor. *Purinergic Signal.* 2(4):627-32.

[95] Cheung, M., Sharma, A., et al. (2008). Akt3 and mutant V600E B-Raf cooperate to promote early melanoma development. *Cancer Res.* 68(9):3429-39.

[96] Chen, B., Tardell, C., et al. (2012). BRAFV600E negatively regulates the AKT pathway in melanoma cell lines. *PLoS One.* 7(8):e42598.

[97] Dankort, D., Curley, D. P., et al. (2009). Braf(V600E) cooperates with Pten loss to induce metastatic melanoma. *Nat Genet.* 41(5):544-52.

[98] Gilmore T. D. (2006). Introduction to NF-kappaB: players, pathways, perspectives. *Oncogene.* 25(51):6680-4.

[99] Ozes, O. N., Mayo L. D., et al. (1999). NF-kappaB activation by tumour necrosis factor requires the Akt serine-threonine kinase. *Nature.* 401(6748):82-5.

[100] Romashkova, J. A. & Makarov S. S. (1999). NF-kappaB is a target of AKT in anti-apoptotic PDGF signaling. *Nature.* 401(6748):86-90.

[101] Sizemore, N., Leung, S., et al. (1999). Activation of phosphatidylinositol 3-kinase in response to interleukin-1 leads to phosphorylation and activation of the NF-kappaB p65/RelA subunit. *Mol Cell Biol.* 19(7):4798-805.

[102] Madrid, L. V., Mayo, M. W., et al. (2001). Akt stimulates the transactivation potential of the RelA/p65 Subunit of NF-kappa B through utilization of the Ikappa B kinase and activation of the mitogen-activated protein kinase p38. *J Biol Chem.* 276(22):18934-40.

[103] Madrid, L. V., Wang, C. Y., et al. (2000). Akt suppresses apoptosis by stimulating the transactivation potential of the RelA/p65 subunit of NF-kappaB. *Mol Cell Biol.* 20(5): 1626-38.

[104] Burow, M. E., Weldon, C. B., et al. (2000). PI3-K/AKT regulation of NF-kappaB signaling events in suppression of TNF-induced apoptosis. *Biochem Biophys Res Commun.* 271(2):342-5.

[105] Hussain, A. R., Ahmed, S. O., et al. (2012). Cross-talk between NFkB and the PI3-kinase/AKT pathway can be targeted in primary effusion lymphoma (PEL) cell lines for efficient apoptosis. *PLoS One.* 7(6):e39945.

[106] Cuní, S., Pérez-Aciego, P., et al. (2004). A sustained activation of PI3K/NF-kappaB pathway is critical for the survival of chronic lymphocytic leukemia B cells. *Leukemia.* 18(8):1391-400.

[107] Li Y., Chinni, S. R., et al. (2005). Selective growth regulatory and pro-apoptotic effects of DIM is mediated by AKT and NF-kappaB pathways in prostate cancer cells. *Front Biosci.* 10:236-43.

[108] Julien, S., Puig, I., et al. (2007). Activation of NF-kappaB by Akt upregulates Snail expression and induces epithelium mesenchyme transition. *Oncogene.* (53):7445-56.

[109] Graham, T. R., Odero-Marah, V. A., et al. (2009). PI3K/Akt-dependent transcriptional regulation and activation of BMP-2-Smad signaling by NF-kappaB in metastatic prostate cancer cells. *Prostate.* 69(2):168-80.

[110] McNulty, S. E., del Rosario, R., et al. (2004). Comparative expression of NFkappaB proteins in melanocytes of normal skin vs. benign intradermal naevus and human metastatic melanoma biopsies. *Pigment Cell Res.* 17(2):173-80.

[111] Ueda, Y. & Richmond, A. (2006). NF-kappaB activation in melanoma. *Pigment Cell Res.* 19(2):112-24.

[112] Yang, J. & Richmond, A. (2001). Constitutive IkappaB kinase activity correlates with nuclear factor-kappaB activation in human melanoma cells. *Cancer Res.* 61(12):4901-9.

[113] McNulty, S. E., Tohidian, N. B et al. (2001). RelA, p50 and inhibitor of kappa B alpha are elevated in human metastatic melanoma cells and respond aberrantly to ultraviolet light B. *Pigment Cell* 14(6):456-65.

[114] Shattuck-Brandt, R. L., Richmond, A et al. (1997). Enhanced degradation of I-kappaB alpha contributes to endogenous activation of NF-kappaB in Hs294T melanoma cells. *Cancer Res.* 57(14):3032-9.

[115] Huang, S., de Guzman, A. et al. (2000). Nuclear factor-kappaB activity correlates with growth, angiogenesis, and metastasis of human melanoma cells in nude mice. *Clin Cancer Res.* 6(6):2573-81.

[116] Attisano, L & Wrana, J. L. (2002). Signal transduction by the TGF-beta superfamily. *Science.* 296(5573):1646-7.

[117] van Belle, P, Rodeck, U., et al. (1996). Melanoma-associated expression of transforming growth factor-beta isoforms. *Am J Pathol.* 148(6):1887-94.

[118] Krasagakis, K, Thölke, D., et al. (1998). Elevated plasma levels of transforming growth factor (TGF)-beta1 and TGF-beta2 in patients with disseminated malignant melanoma. *Br J Cancer.* 77(9):1492-4.

[119] Mohammad, K. S, Javelaud, D., et al. (2011). TGF-beta-RI kinase inhibitor SD-208 reduces the development and progression of melanoma bone metastases. *Cancer Res.* 71(1):175-84.

[120] Reed, J. A., McNutt, N. S., et al. (1994). Expression of transforming growth factor-beta 2 in malignant melanoma correlates with the depth of tumour invasion. Implications for tumour progression. *Am J Pathol.* 145(1):97-104.

[121] Javelaud, D., Delmas, V. et al. (2005). Stable overexpression of Smad7 in human melanoma cells inhibits their tumourigenicity *in vitro* and *in vivo*. *Oncogene.* 24(51): 7624-9.

[122] Javelaud, D., Mohammad, K. S., et al. (2007). Stable overexpression of Smad7 in human melanoma cells impairs bone metastasis. *Cancer Res.* 67(5):2317-24.

[123] di Vito, K. A., Trabosh, V. A., et al. (2010). Smad7 restricts melanoma invasion by restoring N-cadherin expression and establishing heterotypic cell-cell interactions *in vivo*. *Pigment Cell Melanoma Res.* 23(6):795-808.

[124] Fang, R, Zhang, G., et al. (2013). Nodal promotes aggressive phenotype via Snail-mediated epithelial-mesenchymal transition in murine melanoma. *Cancer Lett.* 333(1): 66-75.

[125] Fortini, M. E. (2009). Notch signaling: the core pathway and its posttranslational regulation. *Dev Cell.* 16(5):633-47.

[126] Hoek, K., Rimm, D. L., et al. (2004). Expression profiling reveals novel pathways in the transformation of melanocytes to melanomas. *Cancer Res.* 64(15):5270-82.

[127] Mauerer, A., Roesch, A., et al. (2011). Identification of new genes associated with melanoma. *Exp Dermatol.* 20(6):502-7.

[128] Massi, D., Tarantini, F., et al. (2006). Evidence for differential expression of Notch receptors and their ligands in melanocytic nevi and cutaneous malignant melanoma. *Mod Pathol.* 19(2):246-54.

[129] Pinnix, C. C., Lee, J. T., et al. (2009). Active Notch1 confers a transformed phenotype to primary human melanocytes. *Cancer Res.* 69(13):5312-20.

[130] Bedogni, B., Warneke, J. A., et al. (2008). Notch1 is an effector of Akt and hypoxia in melanoma development. *J Clin Invest.* 118(11):3660-70.

[131] Liu, Z. J., Xiao, M., et al. (2006). Notch1 signaling promotes primary melanoma progression by activating mitogen-activated protein kinase/phosphatidylinositol 3-kinase-Akt pathways and up-regulating N-cadherin expression. *M. Cancer Res.* 66(8): 4182-90.

[132] Heim, M. H. (1999). The Jak-STAT pathway: cytokine signaling from the receptor to the nucleus. *J Recept Signal Transduct Res.* 19(1-4):75-120.

[133] Aaronson, D. S. & Horvath, C. M. (2002). A road map for those who don't know JAK-STAT. *Science.* 296(5573):1653-5.

[134] Pansky, A., Hildebrand, P., et al. (2000). Defective Jak-STAT signal transduction pathway in melanoma cells resistant to growth inhibition by interferon-alpha. *Int J Cancer.* 85(5):720-5.

[135] Jackson, D. P, & Watling, D., et al. (2003). The JAK/STAT pathway is not sufficient to sustain the antiproliferative response in an interferon-resistant human melanoma cell line. *Melanoma Res.* 13(3):219-29.

[136] Guenterberg, K. D., Grignol, V. P., et al. (2010). Interleukin-29 binds to melanoma cells inducing Jak-STAT signal transduction and apoptosis. *Mol Cancer Ther.* 9(2):510-20.

[137] Krasilnikov, M., Ivanov V. N., et al. (2003). ERK and PI3K negatively regulate STAT-transcriptional activities in human melanoma cells: implications towards sensitization to apoptosis. *Oncogene.* 22(26):4092-101.

[138] Pópulo, H., Lopes, J. M., et al. (2012). The mTOR Signaling Pathway in Human Cancer. *Int J Mol Sci.* 13(2):1886-918.

[139] Laplante, M. & Sabatini, D. M. (2009). mTOR signaling at a glance. *J Cell Sci.* 122 (20):3589-94.

[140] Memmott, R. M. & Dennis, P. A. (2009). Akt-dependent and -independent mechanisms of mTOR regulation in cancer. *Cell Signal.* 21(5):656-64.

[141] Gulhati, P., Bowen, K. A. et al. (2011). mTORC1 and mTORC2 regulate EMT, motility, and metastasis of colorectal cancer via RhoA and Rac1 signaling pathways. *Cancer Res.* 71(9):3246-56.

[142] Guba, M., von Breitenbuch P., et al. (2002). Rapamycin inhibits primary and metastatic tumour growth by antiangiogenesis: involvement of vascular endothelial growth factor. *Nat Med.* 8(2):128-35.

[143] Guertin, D. A., Stevens, D. M., et al. (2009). mTOR complex 2 is required for the development of prostate cancer induced by Pten loss in mice. *Cancer Cell.* 15(2):148-59.

[144] Altomare, D. A., Wang, H. Q., et al. (2004). AKT and mTOR phosphorylation is frequently detected in ovarian cancer and can be targeted to disrupt ovarian tumour cell growth. *Oncogene.* 23(34):5853-7.

[145] Gao, N., Flynn, D.C., et al. (2004). G1 cell cycle progression and the expression of G1 cyclins are regulated by PI3K/AKT/mTOR/p70S6K1 signaling in human ovarian cancer cells. *Am J Physiol Cell Physiol.* 287(2):C281-91.

[146] Nishioka, C., Ikezoe, T., et al. (2008). Blockade of mTOR signaling potentiates the ability of histone deacetylase inhibitor to induce growth arrest and differentiation of acute myelogenous leukemia cells. *Leukemia.* 22(12):2159-68.

[147] Boulay, A., Rudloff, J., et al. (2005). Dual inhibition of mTOR and estrogen receptor signaling *in vitro* induces cell death in models of breast cancer. *Clin Cancer Res.* 11 (14): 5319-28.

[148] Zhang, Y. J., Dai, Q., et al. (2009). mTOR signaling pathway is a target for the treatment of colorectal cancer. *Ann Surg Oncol.* 16(9):2617-28.

[149] Panwalkar, A., Verstovsek, S. et al. (2004). Mammalian target of rapamycin inhibition as therapy for hematologic malignancies. *Cancer.* 100(4):657-66.

[150] Marinov, M., Fischer, B., et al. (2007). Targeting mTOR signaling in lung cancer. *Crit Rev Oncol Hematol.* 63(2):172-82.
[151] Chakraborty, S., Mohiyuddin, S. M., et al. (2008). Involvement of TSC genes and differential expression of other members of the mTOR signaling pathway in oral squamous cell carcinoma. *BMC Cancer.* 8:163.
[152] Karbowniczek, M., Spittle, C. S., et al. (2008). mTOR is activated in the majority of malignant melanomas. *J Invest Dermatol.* 128(4):980-7.
[153] Pópulo, H., Soares, P., et al. (2011). mTOR pathway activation in cutaneous melanoma is associated with poorer prognosis characteristics. *Pigment Cell Melanoma Res.* 24(1): 254-7.
[154] Aziz, S. A., Jilaveanu, L. B., et al. (2010). Vertical targeting of the phosphatidylinositol-3 kinase pathway as a strategy for treating melanoma. *Clin Cancer Res.* 16(24): 6029-39.
[155] Sinnberg, T., Lasithiotakis, K., et al. (2009). Inhibition of PI3K-AKT-mTOR signaling sensitizes melanoma cells to cisplatin and temozolomide. *J Invest Dermatol.* 129(6): 1500-15.
[156] Shapiro, L. & Weis, W. I. (2009). Structure and Biochemistry of Cadherins and Catenins. *Cold Spring Harb Perspectives in Biology.* 1(3), 1-21.
[157] Huber, A. H. & Nelson, W. J., et al. (1997). Three-Dimensional Structure of the Armadillo Repeat Region of β-Catenin. *Cell,* 90(5), 871-872.
[158] Xing, Y. & Takemaru, K., et al. (2008). Crystal Structure of a Full-Length β-Catenin, *Structure,* 16(3), 478-487.
[159] Huber, A. H., & Weis, W. I. (2001). The Structure of the B-Catenin/E-Cadherin Complex and the Molecular Basis of Diverse Ligand Recognition by B-Catenin. *Cell,* 105(3), 391-402.
[160] Maher, M. T. & Mo, R., et. al. (2010). β-Catenin Phosphorylated at Serine 45 is Spatially Uncoupled from β-Catenin Phosphorylated in the GSK3 Domain: Implications for Signaling. *PLoS One,* 5(4), 1-12.
[161] Hecht, A. & Litterst, C. M., et al. (1999). Functional characterization of multiple transactivating elements in beta-catenin, some of which interact with the TATA-binding protein *in vitro*. *J Biol Chem,* 274, 18017-25.
[162] Piedra, J. & Martinez, D., et. al. (2001). Regulation of B-Catenin Structure and Activity by Tyrosine Phosphorylation. *The Journ of Biol Chem,* 276(23), 20436-20443.
[163] Hecht, A. K. & Vleminckx, M. P., et al. (2000). The p300/CBP acetyltransferases function as transcriptional coactivators of β-catenin in vertebrates. *J EMBO,* 19, 1839-1850.
[164] Hülsken, J. & Birchmeier, W., et al. (1994). E-cadherin and APC complete for the interaction with beta-catenin and the cytoskeleton. *The Journ of Biol Chem,* 174, 2061-9.
[165] Roura, S. & Miravet, S., et al. (1999). Regulation of E-cadherin/Catenin association by tyrosine phosphorylation. *The Journ of Biol Chem,* 274,36734-40.
[166] Gumbiner, B. M. (2000). Regulation of cadherin adhesive activity. *J. Cell Biol,* 148, 399–404.
[167] Gottardi, C. J. & Wong, E., et al. (2001). E-Cadherin Suppresses Cellular Transformation by Inhibiting B-Catenin Signaling in an Adhesion-independent Manner. *The Journ of Cell Biol,* 153(5), 1049-1059.

[168] MacDonald, B. T. & Tamai, K., et al. (2009). Wnt/β-catenin signaling: components, mechanisms, and diseases. *Dev Cell,* 17(1), 9-26.

[169] Dajani, R. & Fraser, E., et al. (2003). Structural basis for recruitment of glycogen synthase kinase 3beta to the axin-APC scaffold complex. *EMBO J,* 22(3), 494-501.

[170] Amit, S. & Hatzubai, A., et al. (2002). Axin-mediated CKI phosphorylation of B-catenin at Ser 45: a molecular switch for the Wnt pathway. *Genes Dev,* 16, 1066–1076.

[171] Liu, J. & Xing, Y., et al. (2006). The third 20 amino acid repeat is the tightest binding site of APC for B-catenin. *J Mol Biol,* 360, 133–144.

[172] Kimelman, D., & Xu, W. (2006). beta-catenin destruction complex: insights and questions from a structural perspective. *Oncogene,* 25, 7482-91.

[173] http://www.stanford.edu/group/nusselab/cgi-bin/wnt/.

[174] Zeng, Y. A. & Rahnama, M. et al. (2008). Inhibition of Drosophila Wg Signaling Involves Competition between Mad and Armadillo/b-Catenin for dTcf Binding. *PLoS One,* 3(12), 1-9.

[175] Tamai K & Zeng X, et. al. (2004). A mechanism for Wnt coreceptor activation. *Molecular cell,* 13(1), 149-156.

[176] Davidson, G. & Wu, W., et. al. (2005). Casein kinase 1 gamma couples Wnt receptor activation to cytoplasmic signal transduction. *Nature,* 438(7069), 867-872.

[177] Mao, J. & Wang, J., et. al. (2001). Low-density lipoprotein receptor-related protein-5 binds to Axin and regulates the canonical Wnt signaling pathway. *Molecular cell,* 4, 801-809.

[178] Bilic, J. & Huang, Y.L., et. al. (2007). Wnt Induces LRP6 Signalosomes and Promotes Dishevelled-Dependent LRP6 Phosphorylation. *Science,* 316(5831), 1619-1622.

[179] Logan, C. Y., & Nusse, R. (2004). The Wnt Signaling Pathway in Development and Disease. Annu. Rev. *Cell Dev. Biol,* 20, 781-810.

[180] Xing, Y. & Clements, W. K. et al. (2003). Crystal structure of a beta-catenin/ axin complex suggest a mechanism for the beta-catenin destruction complex. *Genes Dev,* 17, 2753-64.

[181] Mo, R. & Chew, T., et al. (2000). The Terminal Region of B-Catenin Promotes Stability by Shiedling the Armadillo Repeats from the Axin-scaffold Destruction Complex. *The Journ of Biol Chem,* 284, 28222-28231.

[182] Staal, F. J. T. & Noort, Mv. M., et. al. (2002). Wnt signals are transmitted through N-terminally dephosphorylated B-catenin. *EMBO reports,* 3(1), 63-68.

[183] Kielhorn, E. & Provost, E., et. al. (2003). Tissue Microarray-Based Analysis Shows Phospho-Beta-Catenin Expression In Malignant Melanoma Is Associated With Poor Outcome. *Int J. Cancer,* 103, 652-656.

[184] Krieghoff, E. & Behrens, J., et al. (2006). Nucleo-cytoplasmic distribution of beta-catenin is regulated by retention. *J Cell Sci,* 119, 1453–1463.

[185] Behrens, J. & Jerchow, B. et. al. (1998). Functional interaction of an axin homolog, conductin, with beta-catenin, APC, and GSK3-beta. *Science,* 280(5263), 596-599.

[186] Simcha, I. & Shtutman, M. et. al. (1998). Differential Nuclear Translocation and Transactivation Potential of B-Catenin and Plakoglobin. *The Journ of Cell Biol,* 141(6), 1433-1448.

[187] Simcha, I. & Geiger, B., et. al. (1996). Suppression of Tumourigenicity by Plankoglobin: An Augmenting Effect of N-Cadherin. *The Journ of Cell Biol,* 133(1), 199-209.

[188] Zhurinsky, J. & Shtutman, M., et al. (2000). Differential Mechanisms of LEF/TCF Family-Dependent Transcriptional Activation of B-Catenin and Plankoglobin. *Mol and Cell Biol,* 20(12), 4238-4252.

[189] Fagotto, F. & Gluck, U., et al. (1998). Nuclear localization signal-independent and importin/karyopherin-independent nuclear import of B-catenin. *Current Biology,* 8, 181-190.

[190] Yokoya, F. & Imamoto, N., et. al. (1999). Beta-catenin can be transported into the nucleus in a Ran-unassisted manner. *Mol Biol Cell,* 10, 1119-1131.

[191] Polakis, P. (2000). Wnt Signaling and cancer. *Genes Dev,* 14, 1837-1851.

[192] Armengol, C. & Cairo, S., et. al. (2009). Wnt signaling and hepatocarcinogenesis: the hepatoblastoma model. *Int J Biochem Cell Biol,* 43, 265–270.

[193] El Wakil, A. & Lalli, E. (2011). The Wnt/beta-catenin pathway in adrenocortical development and cancer. *Mol Cell Endocrinol,* 332, 32–37.

[194] Zardawi, S. J. & O'Toole, S. A., et. al. (2009). Dysregulation of Hedgehog, Wnt and Notch signaling pathways in breast cancer. *Histol Histopathol,* 24, 385–398.

[195] Tycko, B. & Li, C. M., et al. (2007). The Wnt/beta-catenin pathway in Wilms tumours and prostate cancers. *Curr Mol Med,* 7, 479–489.

[196] Ge, X., & Wang, X. (2011). Role of Wnt canonical pathway in hematological malignancies. *J Hematol Oncol,* 3, 33.

[197] Laurent-Puig, P. & Zucman-Rossi, J. (2006). Genetics of hepatocellular tumours. *Oncogene,* 25, 3778–3786.

[198] Satoh, S. & Daigo, Y., et. al. (2000). AXIN1 mutations in hepatocellular carcinomas, and growth suppression in cancer cells by virus-mediated transfer of AXIN1. *Nat Genet,* 24(3), 245-250.

[199] Neufeld, K.L. & Zhang, F., et. al. (2000). APC-mediated downregulation of β-catenin activity involves nuclear sequestration and nuclear export. *EMBO Reports,* 1, 519-523.

[200] Morin, P. J. & Sparks, A.B., et al. (1997). Activation of β-catenin-Tcf signaling in colon cancer by mutations in β-catenin or APC. *Science,* 275, 1787-1790.

[201] Kageshita, T. & Hamby, C. V., et. al. (2001). Loss of b-catenin expression associated with disease progression in malignant melanoma. *British Journal of Dermatology,* 145, 210-216.

[202] Demunter A. L. & Libbrecht, H. et. al. (2002). Loss of membranous expression of beta-catenin is associated with tumour progression in cutaneous melanoma and rarely caused by exon 3 mutations. *Mod Pathol,* 15, 454-461.

[203] Persad, S. & Troussard, A. A., et. al. (2001). Tumour Suppressor PTEN Inhibits Nuclear Accumulation of Beta-Catenin and T Cell/Lymphoid Enhancer Factor 1–mediated Transcriptional Activation. *J Cell Biol,* 153(6), 1161-1174.

[204] Pap, M., & Cooper, G. M. (1998). Role of Glycogen Synthase Kinase-3 in the Phosphatidylinositol 3-Kinase/ Akt Cell Survival Pathway. *The Journ of Biol Chem,* 273(32), 19929-19932.

[205] Ng, S. S. & Mahmoudi, T., et. al.(2009). Phosphatidylinositol 3-Kinase Signaling Does Not Activated the Wnt Cascade. *The Journ of Biol Chem,* 284(51), 35308-35313.

[206] Sharma, M. & Chuang, W. W., et al. (2002). Phosphatidylinositol 3-kinase/Akt stimulates androgen pathway through GSK3beta and inhibition and nuclear beta-catenin accumulation. *Journ of Biol Chem,* 277, 30935-41.

[207] Blume-Jensen, P., & Hunter, T. (2001). Oncogenic kinase signaling. *Nature,* 411, 355-365.

[208] Mulholland, D. J. & Dedhar, S. et al. (2006). PTEN and GSK3β: key regulators of progression to androgen-independent prostate cancer. *Oncogene,* 25, 329-337.

[209] Cross, D. A. & Alessi, D. R. et al. (1995). Inhibition of glycogen synthase kinase-3 by insulin mediated by protein kinase B. *Nature,* 378(6559), 785-9.

[210] Ding, V. W. & Chen, R. H., et al. (2000). Differential regulation of glycogen synthase kinase 3beta by insulin and Wnt signaling. *J Biol Chem,* 275(42), 32475-81.

[211] Patel, S. & Doble, B. W., et al. (2008). Tissue-Specific Role of Glycogen Synthase Kinase 3 β in Glucose Homeostasis and Insulin Action. *Molecular and Cellular Biology,* 28(20), 6314-6328.

[212] Doble, B. W. & Patel, S., et al. (2007). Functional Redundancy of GSK-3α and GSK-3β in Wnt/β-Catenin Signaling Shown by Using an Allelic Series of Embryonic Stem Cell Lines. *Developmental Cell,* 12, 951-971.

[213] Fukumoto, S. & Hsieh, C., et al. (2001). Akt Participation in the Wnt Signaling Pathway through Dishevelled. *J Biol Chem,* 276(20), 17479-83.

[214] Fang, D. & Hawke, D., et al. (2007). Phosphorulation of β-Catenin by AKT Promotes β-Catenin Transcriptional Activity. *J Biol Chem,* 282(15), 11221-11229.

[215] He, X. C. & Yin, T., et al. (2007). PTEN-deficient intestinal stem cells initiate intestinal polyposis. *Nature Genetic,* 39(2), 189-198.

[216] Tian, Q. & Feetham, M. C., et al. (2004). Proteomic analysis identifies that 14-3-3ζ interacts with β-catenin and facilitates its activation by Akt. *PNAS,* 101(43), 15370-15375.

[217] Ann, S. & Kloor, M. (2005). Regulation of AKT1 expression by beta-catenin/TCF/Lef signaling in colorectal cancer cells. *Carcinogenesis,* 26(9), 1503-1512.

[218] Espada, J. & Peinado, H., et al. (2005). Direct metabolic regulation of β-catenin activity by the p85α regulatory subunit of phosphorinosite 3-OH kinase. *Experimental Cell Research,* 305, 409-417.

[219] Tanwar, P. S. & Zhang, L., et al. (2011). Mammalian target of rapamycin is a therapeutic target for muring ovarian endometriod adenocarcinomas with dysregulated Wnt/β-catenin and PTEN. *PLoS One,* 6(6), e20715.

[220] Shen, W. H. & Boyle, D. W., et al. (2005). Insulin and IGF-I stimulate the formation of the eukaryotic initiation factor complex and protein synthesis in C2C12 myotubes independent of availability of external amino acids. *J Endocrinol,* 185(2), 275-89.

[221] Harwood, F. C. & Shu, L., et al. (2008). mTORC1 signaling can regulate growth factor activation of p44/42 mitogen-activated protein kinases through protein phosphatase 2A. *J Biol Chem,* 283(5), 2575-85.

[222] Liu, H. & Remedi, M. S., et al. (2009). Glycogen synthase kinase-3 and mammalian target of rapamycin pathways contribute to DNA synthesis, cell cycle progression, and proliferation in human islets. *Diabetes,* 58(3), 663-72.

[223] Walsh, L. A., & Damjanovski, S. (2011). IFG-1 increases invasive potential of MCF 7 breast cancer cells and induces activation of latent TGF-β1 resulting in epithelial to mesenchymal transition. *Cell Commun Signal,* 9(1), 1-11.

[224] Vincent, T. & Neve, E. P., et al. (2009). A SNAIL1-SMAD ¾ transcriptional repressor complex promotes TGF-beta mediated epithelial-mesenchymal transition. *Nat Cell Biol,* 11(8), 943-50.

[225] Sayat, R. & Leber, B., et al. (2008). O-GlcNAc-glycosylation of beta-catenin regulates its nuclear localization and transcriptional activity. *Exp Cell Res,* 314(15), 2774-87.

[226] http://www.cancer.gov/cancertopics/pdq/treatment/melanoma/ HealthProfessional.

[227] http://www.cancer.gov/cancertopics/pdq/treatment/melanoma/HealthProfessional/Page 9#Reference9.6.

[228] Hideshima, T., Catley, L., et al. (2006). Perifosine, an oral bioactive novel alkylphospholipid, inhibits Akt and induces *in vitro* and *in vivo* cytotoxicity in human multiple myeloma cells. *Blood.* 107(10), 4053-62.

[229] Patel, V., Lahusen, T., et al. (2002). Perifosine, a novel alkylphospholipid, induces p21(WAF1) expression in squamous carcinoma cells through a p53-independent pathway, leading to loss in cyclin-dependent kinase activity and cell cycle arrest. *Cancer Res.* 62(5), 1401-9.

[230] Kondapaka, S. B, Singh, S. S. et al. (2003). Perifosine, a novel alkylphospholipid, inhibits protein kinase B activation. *Mol Cancer Ther.* 2(11):1093-103.

[231] Gaitonde, S., De, S. K. et al. (2009). BI-69A11-mediated inhibition of AKT leads to effective regression of xenograft melanoma. *Pigment Cell Melanoma Res.* 22(2):187-95.

[232] Sharma, A., Sharma, A. K. et al. (2009). Targeting Akt3 signaling in malignant melanoma using isoselenocyanates. *Clin Cancer Res.* 15(5):1674-85.

[233] Hainsworth, J. D., Infante, J. R. et al. (2010). Bevacizumab and everolimus in the treatment of patients with metastatic melanoma: a phase 2 trial of the Sarah Cannon Oncology Research Consortium. *Cancer.* 116(17), 4122-9.

[234] Niessner, H., Beck, D. et al. (2011). The farnesyl transferase inhibitor lonafarnib inhibits mTOR signaling and enforces sorafenib-induced apoptosis in melanoma cells. *J Invest Dermatol.* 131(2), 468-79.

In: Melanoma
Editor: Alexander C. Jones

ISBN: 978-1-62808-608-9

Chapter 2

CUTANEOUS MELANOMA: MOLECULAR BIOLOGY, RISK FACTORS AND TREATMENT OPTIONS

Mariana Aris[1], Ivana Jaqueline Tapia[1], José Mordoh[1,2,3] and María Marcela Barrio[1]

[1]Centro de Investigaciones Oncológicas, Fundación Cáncer FUCA, Buenos Aires, Argentina

[2]Instituto Médico Especializado Alexander Fleming, Buenos Aires, Argentina

[3]Instituto de Investigaciones Bioquímicas de Buenos Aires, Fundación Instituto Leloir, Buenos Aires Argentina

ABSTRACT

Cutaneous Melanoma is the neoplasia with the fastest growing incidence worldwide. Early diagnosed tumors are mostly curable by surgery. However, when it metastasizes, only a minority of patients can be cured; treatment options are still limited, in part due to its refractory nature to conventional therapies. In this section we will revisit the main risk factors associated to this disease and will perform an integral analysis of its biology, taking into consideration key signatures and signaling pathways. In light of the increasing knowledge about Cutaneous Melanoma biology and its immunogenic nature, we will go through new therapies that focus on targeted therapies and immunotherapy, including vaccines.

1. THE BIOLOGY OF CUTANEOUS MELANOMA

Cutaneous melanoma (CM) is a form of skin cancer that originates in melanocytes of the skin (National Cancer Institute, 2010). Most common types of melanoma are superficial spreading melanoma (SSM), nodular melanoma (NM) and lentigo maligna melanoma (LMM). The latter type is most prevalent in older-age groups and chronically photodamaged skin, whereas SSM and NM are more common among younger and white skin patients (van der Spek-Keijser, van der Rhee et al. 1997). SSM presents a phase with slow radial growth, followed by a fast vertical growth phase. In contrast, NM presents a fast vertical growth, without a previous phase of radial growth. Because of this feature, the latter type has worse prognosis than the superficial type. *Lentigo maligna* is refered to *in situ* benign stage of LMM. This type of melanoma usually begins like a brownish macula with a slow growth that in about 5% of cases progress to invasive melanomas. Acral lentiginous melanoma is the most common type of CM diagnosed in people with dark skin, but it has a low incidence in the total cases.

Fortunately, most CM types are pigmented; this feature is an advantage for clinical diagnosis of the disease. The cases of CM that do not present a pigmented appearence are called amelanotics. All the previously mentioned subtypes can have their amelanotic correlate.

The Clark Model of clinical and histological progression for melanoma proposes a gradual transition from normal melanocytes to nevi (moles); and transformation into malignant melanoma, including proliferation through the epidermis (radial growth phase or surface), invasion of the dermis (vertical growth phase) and from there to other organs (metastasis) (Clark, Elder et al. 1989). Melanoma staging is based on primary tumor size; whether cancer cells have spread to nearby lymph nodes or to other part of the body. Stages of CM (National Cancer Institute, 2010) are:

- Stage 0 (Melanoma *in situ*): melanoma involves only the top layer of skin.
- Stage I: the tumor is not more than 1 mm thick and the surface may be ulcerated; or the tumor is beetwen 1 and 2 mm thick, and the surface is not ulcerated.
- Stage II: the tumor is between 1 and 2 mm thick, and the surface appears ulcerated. Or, the thickness of the tumor is more than 2 mm, and the surface may be ulcerated.
- Stage III: The melanoma cells have spread to at least one nearby lymph node, or they have spread from the primary site to tissues nearby.
- Stage IV: Cancer cells have spread to the lung or other organs, skin, or lymph nodes far away from the original tumor growth site.

The international TNM staging system established by the American Joint Committee on Cancer (AJCC) (Balch, Gershenwald et al. 2009; Mordoh 2009) is commonly used for CM patients. While each cancer has its own classification depending on the organ of origin, the TNM system gathers the following basic aspects: the size of the primary tumor (T); lymph node involvement or positive regional lymph nodes (N); and the presence of spread to distance from the primary tumor or metastasis (M). Note that for prognosis, it is necessary to take into account the clinical and histologic evaluation of the patient in conjunction with age, sex and anatomic site of the tumor.

Nowadays, histopathology still remains the methodology of choice for the diagnosis of CM, although there are different complementary molecular diagnostic techniques, such as immunohistochemistry and DNA sequencing. The characteristic feature of CM is heterogeneity. Typically, an asymmetrical melanoma is poorly circumscribed, characterized by nests variable in shape and size. Lymphocytic infiltrate may be observed. Melanoma cells show morphological spectrum including round shapes, polygonal, tapered, fibroblastoid, multinucleated or dendritic.

The annual incidence of CM among whites has increased steadily more than 60% over the past 30 years. Increases have been most rapid among white women aged 15 to 39 years, in whom incidence has increased by 3% annually since 1992; and among white men older than 65, in whom incidence has increased by 5.1% annually since 1975 (National Cancer Institute, 2012). Jones Wo *et al.* predicted that this disease will continue increasing during this century due to the local depletion of ozone and the time between exposure and emergence of the disease (Jones, Harman et al. 1999).

The incidence of CM varies with ethnicity: it is rare among African Americans, being the lifetime risk of developing melanoma 23 times higher among whites. CM is expected to be diagnosed in about 76,690 persons in 2013 and 9,480 individuals are estimated to die from CM in the USA (Cancer Facts & Figures, American Cancer Society, 2013). Incidence rates for melanoma in Australia are the highest in the world and their levels are only matched by New Zealand. In Australia, CM is the second most prevalent cancer as a result of its high incidence and good survival (Australian Institute of Health and Welfare & Australasian Association of Cancer Registries, 2012). In contrast, the lowest incidence rates occur in asian populations: China, India, Japan and Singapore (Elwood 1989; Lee, Chay et al. 2012).

In Europe, approximately 26,100 males and 33,300 females are diagnosed each year with CM, and around 8,300 males and 7,600 females die of it (Parkin, Bray et al. 2001). Incidence rates vary substantially among regions, with highest rates in Northern and Western Europe, whereas mortality rates are more similar between regions. This pattern is probably related to lighter skin types and a higher intermittent sun exposure in many Northern European countries. Many Northern Europeans spend their summer holidays in the Mediterranean area, increasing their amount of sun exposure without being used to the amount of sun received during this period (de Vries, Bray et al. 2003).

1.1. Risk Factors

Risk factors for melanoma include both endogenous and exogenous factors. The more important factors are:

- Skin phototype: people with a sun-sensitive skin have the highest CM risks. Gandini *et al* studied the eye color and the risk of developing melanoma. A meta-analysis was performed and they found that blue, green and hazel eyes have a relative risk (RR) higher than dark eyes (1.47, 1.61 and 1.52 respectively). A similar analysis was performed in order to study the influence of hair color. Differents hair colors were compared to dark color, and red hair was found to have the highest RR of developing CM (3.64) (Gandini, Sera et al. 2005).
- Clinical atypical nevi: the presence of nevi with more than 0.5 cm diameter, dark or irregularly pigmented and undefined borders is a risk factor for developing melanoma (Gandini, Sera et al. 2005).
- Number of nevi: a recent meta-analysis performed in 2010 found that having more than 25 nevi may be a risk factor for CM (Olsen, Carroll et al. 2010). In this study, 42% of CM cases were associated with having over 25 nevi. Taking into account also the presence of clinical atypical nevi, they identified patients with 25 or more common nevi and/or 1 or more atypical nevi, as the high-risk group.
- Personal History: People who have already had melanoma have an increased risk of developing other melanomas (Tsao, Atkins et al. 2004).

- Family history of skin cancer and genetic factors: a meta-analysis was performed in order to evaluate the association between CM and family history. People with a positive family history had a RR of 1.74 for developing CM (Gandini, Sera et al. 2005). Susceptibility to CM is related to specific genotypes, which are reflected in the family history; between 6-12% of CM present a familiar pattern (Acosta, Fierro et al. 2009). In families with CM, two genes, CDKN2A and CDK4 have been discovered, of which CDKN2A (p16) is the most prevalent. Germline mutations in this gene have been found in up to 25% of melanoma families worldwide. Both CDKN2A and CDK4 are important in controlling cell division. Other genes, such as MC1R, are likely to play a role in susceptibility to melanoma. This gene is involved in skin and hair pigmentation and in senescence and immunity (Bishop, Demenais et al. 2002; Bataille 2003; Tucker and Goldstein 2003).
- Exposure to UV radiation: it is the most important exogenous risk factor (Armstrong and Kricker 1993; Gilchrest, Eller et al. 1999), although its association with melanoma depends on skin characteristics, with highest risk in people with a sun-sensitive skin. The RR of developing CM with high UV exposure is around 2, but when skin characteristics are taken into account, the RR increases markedly for those with a sun-sensitive skin (Brenner, Lubin et al. 2002; Tucker and Goldstein 2003). As it is known, sunbeds are a UV light source and are thought to be a potential contributor to the increasing incidence of CM among young people (Reed, Brewer et al. 2012). Several studies were performed in order to determine the RR of developing CM in people who have ever used tanning booths (Han, Colditz et al. 2006; Lazovich, Vogel et al. 2010; Cust, Armstrong et al. 2011; Gandini, Autier et al. 2011; Boniol, Autier et al. 2012). All these studies found differents values for RR, but in all cases, this parameter indicated that the risk of developing melanoma was higher in people who have ever been exposed to sunbeds. Furthermore, Boniol *et al* stratified the population of study and found that the risk for those people younger than 35 years is higher (Boniol, Autier et al. 2012).

1.2. Development of Cutaneous Melanoma

A key question is whether nevi are necessary for CM development (Aris, Barrio et al. 2010). A retrospective medical study of patient records diagnosed with melanoma found that CM arose from nevi at least in half of the cases (n = 377). Indeed, a dose–response pattern was established with an increase in risk for developing CM as a patient's number of common nevi increased (Gandini, Autier et al. 2011). Thus, a melanoma may develop *de novo*, without requiring a precursor nevus (Weatherhead, Haniffa et al. 2007). A nevus can be described as a benign proliferation of cells of clonal origin expressing the melanocytic phenotype. Nevi may develop as congenital or acquired during life. It is accepted that nevi might originate in a precursor stem cell, and cells tend to proliferate, migrate and differentiate from the dermis to the epidermis. However, experiments with cultures of transformed melanocytes show that these cells can penetrate the dermal component in a transplant, suggesting that migration from the epidermis to the dermis is possible (Chudnovsky, Adams et al. 2005).

There are different patterns of nevi and corresponding growth and survival is considered a consequence of the underlying mutation and its microenvironment. NRAS mutations are often found in congenital nevi, while BRAF mutations in acquired nevi (Ichii-Nakato, Takata et al. 2006; Bauer, Curtin et al. 2007). NRAS activation leads to the activation of several signaling pathways including the MAPK and PI3K pathway. In fact, culture of nevus cells requires less growth factors than normal melanocytes, thus these cells have an increased independence of homeostatic mechanisms (Alanko, Rosenberg et al. 1999).

It is unclear why some melanomas develop from a nevus and why others do not. One possibility is that melanoma can develop from the transformation of a melanocyte stem cell. Initially, mutations may accumulate in melanocytic quiescent stem cell. Eventually, appropriate environmental signals could trigger aberrant cell proliferation, because of previous mutations. Depending on the nature of the original mutation, there could be a benign nevi phase, requiring additional transforming mutations, or a melanoma *ab initio* could develop. In this scenario, nevi stage may be possible but not necessary for the development of melanoma. Transformed cells would try to follow normal differentiation pathways, including migration to the epidermis. Epidermal growth factors could lead to greater proliferation and differentiation, whereas accumulated mutations may result in different subclones that are more independent from substrate and growth factors, with aberrant migration patterns to the dermis, including nerves and vessels. Eventually, non-adherent clonogenic cells could enter and be removed outside the lymphatic system and the systemic circulation, where under appropriate conditions could restart the process in other organs. If melanoma develops migrating to or from the dermis is still under discussion. However, in either scenario, the deeper is the dermal tissue tumor, the smaller the epidermal factor requirements, and it has an increased risk to proliferate beyond the skin and metastasize.

1.2.1. Models for heterogeneity in Cutaneous Melanoma

There are several models to explain tumor growth and heterogeneity in CM. The cancer stem cell (CSC) model suggests a hierarchy within the tumor wherein, analogous to renewable tissues, only the minor fraction of CSC have unlimited proliferative potential, capable of self-renewal and generating a differentiated progeny, with limited proliferative potential, constituting the tumor mass (Reya, Morrison et al. 2001). CSC could arise from melanocyte stem cells or transformed cells that subsequently acquired this phenotype. Still, in this model the CSC would be the only population able to form new tumors after grafting. Therefore, it would be crucial to target the CSC population or tumor-initiating cells to eradicate tumors efficiently. In contrast, the stochastic model proposes that most cells within a tumor have the potential to proliferate extensively and result in new tumors. In relation to this point, a more dynamic model of Phenotypic Plasticity (PP), where the proliferative potential of the cells varies with time is lately gaining momentum (Quintana, Shackleton et al. 2010).

Several works have reported evidence supporting the different models. Several putative CSC markers were described in melanoma. It was shown that $ABCB5^+$ cells were capable of proliferation, self-renewal and differentiation in a competitive model of tumor development in immunodeficient NOD/SCID mice (Schatton, Murphy et al. 2008). It was also reported the isolation of CSC in melanoma tumors at different sites and stages enriched in the CD271/NGFR marker. Only $CD271^+$ cells initiated tumors in 90% in immunosuppressed $Rag2^{-/-}$ $c^{-/-}$ mice, with ability to form metastases (Boiko, Razorenova et al. 2010).

On the other hand, it was reported that depending on experimental conditions employed for CM xenografting, tumorigenic potential can be increased by several orders of magnitude

(Quintana, Shackleton et al. 2008). It was showed in immunosuppressed NOD/SCID IL2RG$^{-/-}$ mice and using matrigel as substrate, that one out of four melanoma cells form tumors without any prior selection. Thus, tumorigenic cells would be common in all primary and metastatic melanoma tumors. Other study also described the tumorigenic potential of melanoma cells at different stages without previous selection in NOD/SCID IL2RG$^{-/-}$ mice, and that phenotypic plasticity, even in markers as CD271 and ABCB5, would be a source of heterogeneity in CM (Quintana, Shackleton et al. 2010). In our experience, we observed in experimental models and in CM biopsies that cells present considerable antigenic plasticity in representative CM-Ag such as MART-1 and gp100, and in CSC marker CD271 (Aris, Zubieta et al. 2012). This means that expression of these Ag varies over time without affecting neither proliferative nor clonogenic potential of tumor cells, contributing to antigenic heterogeneity observed in the CM, and constituting a mechanism of tumor escape.

1.2.2. Pathways Involved in Cutaneous Melanoma Development and Progression

CM transformation and progression involves multiple tumor-promoting events, including activation of oncogenes and inactivation of tumor-suppressor genes. CM is the tumor pathology with most frequency of mutations (Bis and Tsao 2013). Most of them are consequence of skin exposure to UV rays (C>T/G>A), but there are also non-related mutations. Whole-genome sequence studies reveal that levels of point mutation depends on exposure to UV, with highest rates on patients with a documented history of chronic sun exposure (Berger, Hodis et al. 2012). Most frequent mutations in all types of melanoma include loss of PTEN (25-50%) and CDKN2A (10-30%); amplification of MITF (10-15%), CDK2/4 (20%), Cyclin D (30%) and Bcl-2 (90%). In particular, CM are enriched in mutations for GRIN2 (33%), NRAS (15%) and BRAF (50-65%). However, it is believed that pathogenesis of CM is sustained by the combination of genetic changes (Wangari-Talbot and Chen 2012; Bis and Tsao 2013).

Cell Proliferation and Angiogenesis Pathways

Growth factor Receptors: CM cells express several growth factor receptors from the Tyrosine Kinase family, including EGFR, PDGFR and c-KIT. c-KIT is altered by amplification and mutation, and it is involved in the development and maintenance of melanocytes. It is ubiquitously expressed in mature melanocytes, activating MAPK, PI3K-AKT and JAK-STAT proliferation and survival pathways (Jiang, Zhou et al. 2008). More recently, Ephrin type-A receptor 2 was described with a dual rol, even decreasing viability of less-adapted populations or promoting tumor aggressiveness (Udayakumar, Zhang et al. 2011). On the other hand, a large mutational analysis of receptor tyrosine kinases (RTKs) was performed in metastatic melanoma, where growth factor receptor ERBB4 was found in 19% of the samples. This receptor would be involved in AKT signaling, as either knockdown of ERBB4 or inhibition by Lapatinib downregulates this pathway (Prickett, Agrawal et al. 2009).

With the development of next generation sequence technologies, several studies analyzing whole-genome and exome sequences where performed. From these studies, mutations in the ionotropic glutamate receptor GRIN2A (25%) (Wei, Walia et al. 2011); and a mutational hotspot in E870K in GRM3, a G-coupled glutamate receptor (16.3%) were found. Functional assays revealed GRM3 roll in MEK activation; and use of Selumetinib

MEK1/2 inhibitor resulted in preferential inhibition of mutant GRM3 melanoma cells (Prickett, Wei et al. 2011).

MAPK pathway: *Mitogen-activated protein kinase* signaling pathways promote survival, growth, migration and resistance to apoptosis. MAPK pathway initiates in the cell membrane, either by ligand interaction with a Receptor Tyrosine Kinase receptor, or by adhesion of integrins to extracellular matrix, leading to RAS activation. The canonical pathway is RTK-RAS-RAF-MEK-ERK. BRAF mutations are exclusive with NRAS mutations; however, MEK mutations might occur simultaneously.

Protein BRAF is a member of the serine-threonine protein kinase families RAF, also with ARAF and CRAF isoforms. It is mainly expressed in neuronal tissue and in melanocytes. The most frequent mutation in CM is the mutation T1799A, wherein the transversion T A converts glutamic acid for valine at position 600 of the primary sequence (GTG GAG), $BRAF^{V600E}$, whereby the protein adopts a constitutively active configuration (40-60% clinical cases) (Davies, Bignell et al. 2002). There are other less frequent variants, as $BRAF^{V600K}$ and $BRAF^{V600R}$. Activating mutation in BRAF is a driver mutation that leads to the constitutive activation of the MAPK pathway and therefore proliferation (Davies, Bignell et al. 2002). However, mutations in BRAF would not be associated with sun exposure as prevailing in skin areas with intermittent sun exposure (Curtin, Fridlyand et al. 2005). Neither correlation was found sufficient to consider an inherited gene predisposition to melanoma (Jackson, Harland et al. 2005). BRAF mutations were associated with benign transformations of melanocytes to dysplastic nevi (Kumar, Angelini et al. 2004), although BRAF mutations were also detected in advanced stages (Dong, Phelps et al. 2003). Studies in inducible-expressing $BRAF^{V600E}$ mice confirm that its expression is associated with development of nevi. In general, these mutant mice are stable over time, although they can develop melanoma with long latencies. However, the introduction of additional mutations, such as inactivation of the tumor-suppressor genes CDKN2A, PTEN or p53, leads to progression to invasive melanomas (Chudnovsky, Adams et al. 2005; Patton, Widlund et al. 2005). Recently, it has been described that $BRAF^{V600E}$ would promote an invasive phenotype involved in tumor progression by induction of the T-Box3 Transcriptional Represor, which downregulates E-Cadherin (Boyd, Mijatov et al. 2013).

RAS family proteins are G protein-exchangers, including HRAS, KRAS, and NRAS isoforms. They exchange GTP for GDP, with GTPase activity. These proteins alternate between an active (GTP) and an idle state (by hydrolysis of GTP to GDP). Oncogenic disruption of RAS involves loss of hydrolytic activity, therefore it can no longer hydrolyze GTP, adopting a stable active configuration (Mitin, Rossman et al. 2005). In melanoma, activating mutations in NRAS are usually mutually exclusive with BRAF mutation, which speaks of redundancy in signaling pathways (Davies, Bignell et al. 2002).

Sequencing studies reveals presence of MEK1 and MEK2 mutations (8%), frequently coexpressed with BRAF (60%) or NRAS (10%) mutations. Functional studies of most frequent mutants MEK^{1P124S} and MEK^{1E203K} revealed constitutive phosphorylation of Erk. Although the oncogenic activity of MEK1 mutants was lower than that of $BRAF^{V600E}$, the potential of combinatorial BRAF and MEK inhibitor treatment warrants further investigation (Nikolaev, Rimoldi et al. 2012).

PI3K-AKT pathway: This pathway is involved in mechanisms of survival and suppression of apoptosis (Downward 2004). The canonical pathway is PIP3-PI3K-AKT-mTOR, although PI3K (phosphatidylinositol 3-kinase) may also be activated by RAS-GTP. AKT is usually found amplified in CM, and presents multiple effector functions. It blocks anti-apoptotic protein BAX, promotes protein synthesis and induces degradation of FOXO-mediated ubiquitination. AKT activation also stimulates NFB, a pleiotropic transcription factor that inhibits apoptosis and promotes cell proliferation.

Protein mTOR (mammalian target of rapamycin) functions downstream in the pathway and regulates the activity of AKT through formation of complexes (Ko and Fisher 2011). mTOR1 complex suppresses AKT signaling (negative feedback), whereas mTOR2 complex stimulates AKT through its phosphorylation, providing a therapeutic window.

Protein PTEN (Phosphatase and tensin homolog) is a negative regulator of PI3K-AKT pathway. It has phosphatase activity in lipids and proteins, interrupting PI3K and AKT signaling. Mutations resulting in loss of PTEN contribute significantly to the development of invasive melanomas (Wu, Goel et al. 2003), especially in cooperation with BRAF mutations (Tsao, Goel et al. 2004).

Recently, whole-genome sequencing studies performed on metastatic samples reveal that PREX2 (phosphatidylinositol-3,4,5-trisphosphate-dependent Rac exchange factor 2), a negative regulator of PTEN, is frequently mutated in several positions in melanoma (Berger, Hodis et al. 2012).

Angiogenic factors: Angiogenic factors released by melanoma cells and their microenvironment include VEGF, IL-8, bFGF and PDGF (Rofstad and Halsor 2000). Mutations in BRAF promote angiogenesis by stimulating the release of autocrine VEGF, developing highly vascularized metastases (Velazquez and Herlyn 2003).

Genomic Stability and Immortality Pathways

During cellular senescence, arrest in cell cycle is induced, mainly caused by shortening of telomeres and stress signals as a consequence of excessive proliferation signals derived from oncogenic activation. To overpass senescence, telomerase is frequently re-expressed (Ramirez, D'Atri et al. 1999).

CDKN2A (Cyclin-Dependent Kinase Inhibitor 2A) is the primary melanoma predisposition gene and the main target of UV radiation. It encodes two proteins, $p16^{CDKN2A}$ and $p14^{CDKN2A}$. CDKN2A inactivation may occur by mutation, deletion or promoter silencing (de Snoo and Hayward 2005; Goldstein, Chan et al. 2007). $P16^{CDKN2A}$ gene induces cell G1-phase arrest by inhibition of cyclinD/CDK4, whose function is to direct enter into the cell cycle by phosphorylation of Rb. RB protein binds to the transcription factor E2F, and releases it when phosphorylated, thereby allowing transcription of genes necessary to enter a cell cycle. Tumor-suppressor gene $p14^{CDKN2A}$ blocks HDM2 function, promoting p53 degradation mediated by ubiquitin. This interferes with p53's role as "the guardian of the genome", arresting cell division at G1 phase to allow DNA repair or to induce apoptosis if damage is irreparable. HDM2 expression was found to be increased by *in situ*, invasive and metastatic melanomas (Polsky, Bastian et al. 2001). Although low levels of mutated p53 are found in melanoma (13%), half of these mutations are related to ultraviolet radiation mutagenic stress in the pathogenesis of melanoma. By suppressing p53 response, survival is promoted by increasing levels of anti-apoptotic proteins, such as Bcl-2, and prevents cells from sensing damage related to the transformation process, even increasing their resistance to genotoxic therapies (Hocker and Tsao 2007).

Pigment Synthesis Pathways

The MC1R receptor, which binds to α-MSH hormone (α-Melanocyte-stimulating hormone), stimulates BRAF activity by increasing intracellular cAMP levels. MC1R gene is a major genetic determinant of skin pigmentation, and is highly polymorphic in Caucasian populations. These allelic variants can result in partial or complete loss of MC1R signaling. Lack of MC1R functionality is associated with loss of generation of eumelanin pigment, only pheomelanin pigment is synthesized, typical of redheads. Associations between MC1R polymorphisms and BRAF mutations have been established in CM development, independently from sun exposure (Landi, Bauer et al. 2006).

WNT signaling in melanoma is complex (Webster and Weeraratna 2013). The canonical Wnt signalling pathway induces β-catenin/lymphoid enhancer transcription factors, promoting metastatic spread by increasing migration and invasion. β-catenin plays a dual function, it fortifies cadherin-based adhesion at the plasma membrane and promotes cell proliferation as a transcription factor. However, the role of β-catenin in melanoma metastasis remains unclear. Recent papers describe the roles of Wnt5A and ARF6 in driving β-catenin expression and melanoma metastasis. Binding of WNT5A to the Frizzled 4-LRP6 receptor complex activates ARF6, a small GTPase. ARF6 would liberate β-catenin from N-cadherin, increasing free protein and enhancing β-catenin-mediated transcription, promoting invasion (Grossmann, Yoo et al. 2013).

MITF expression is essential for proliferation and survival of melanoma cells. It is used as a CM marker due to its ubiquitous expression at different stages. Amplification of MITF copy number occurs in 10% of primary cutaneous and in 21-40% of metastatic melanoma tumors, but is not observed in benign melanocytic nevi (Garraway, Widlund et al. 2005). MITF has no transforming properties *per se*, but it cooperates with $BRAF^{V600E}$ transformation process (Garraway, Widlund et al. 2005). MITF expression levels are tightly regulated in melanoma, and different expression levels regulate different functions (Gray-Schopfer, Wellbrock et al. 2007). High levels of MITF induce cell cycle arrest and differentiation, reduce cell proliferation even in the presence of $BRAF^{V600E}$, and reduce tumorigenicity. Very low levels of MITF lead to cell cycle arrest and apoptosis. However, intermediate expression levels of MITF promote cell proliferation. ERK activation promotes MITF phosphorylation and degradation, thereby contributing to maintenance of MITF levels. Recently, the MITF E318K allele was found associated with a family history of melanoma, multiple primary melanomas, increased nevi count, and non-blue eye color, therefore reported as a risk gene in the predisposition to familial and sporadic melanoma. Functional studies of the E318K MITF mutant revealed impaired sumoylation and differential transcriptional activity of MITF target genes, including genes related to pigmentation (Yokoyama, Woods et al. 2011).

1.3. Cutaneous Melanoma and the Immune System

The theory of Cancer Immunoediting

Tumor evolution is the result of a continuous feedback between tumor cells and their environment. In this process, interactions between cancer cells and the immune system are complex, with both controlling and enabling functions. This stands for the theory of cancer immunoediting, where the immune system has a dual role, both suppressing and enabling cancer (Schreiber, Old et al. 2011). It can repress tumor growth by killing cancer cells or arresting proliferation, but it can also enable tumor growth, either by the selection of less immunogenic cells better adapted to survive in an immunocompetent host, or by the establishment of a tumor-permissive microenvironment that enables tumor growth. This is described by three phases: elimination, equilibrium and escape.

Elimination: the immune system prevents cancer development by different ways. For instance, it protects the host from viral infections; it prevents a chronic inflammatory environment that enables tumorigenesis by abruptly removing pathogens; and it eliminates tumor cells by effector cells from the innate and adaptive immune system. In the beginning of tumor development, dying tumor cells and damaged-surrounding tissues release factors like IFN-γ, IFN-α/β, and DAMPs (Street, Cretney et al. 2001; Dunn, Bruce et al. 2005; Sims, Rowe et al. 2010). These signals recruit cells from innate (NK, NKT, γδ T cells, macrophages, and dendritic cells) and adaptive immune system (CD4 and CD8 T cells). Tumor infiltrating NK cells and macrophages activate each other by production of IFN-γ and IL-12, and kill tumor cells by apoptosis via TRAIL, perforins and reactive oxygen and nitrogen species. Also, the activation and maturation of dendritic cells (DC) promotes the induction of an adaptive immune response, through tumor antigen (Ag) presentation to CD8 cytotoxic T cells (CTL) with help from CD4 cells, ideally generating a long-lasting immune response.

Equilibrium: this phase takes place when a group of tumor cells survive the initial attack from the immune system and move into an equilibrium phase, in which tumor cells are under control of the immune system but cannot be completely eliminated. In this way, tumors can be controlled by the immune system for long periods of time, encompassing the host's entire life. T cells, IL-12, and IFN-γ are known to sustain the dormancy state (Koebel, Vermi et al. 2007).

Escape: continuous pressure by the immune system on genetically unstable cells can lead to the generation of tumor variants that (i) are no longer recognized by the IS, (ii) become insensitive to effector mechanisms, and (iii) induce an immunosuppressor, tolerant microenvironment. Also, changes in the immune system are induced that might contribute to generate a tumor-permissive environment. All these events contribute to tumor progression.

Evidences of immunoediting in Cutaneous Melanoma

Tumor Ag: the presence of tumor Ag in humans was shown by modern methodologies, involving the use of antibodies and CTL derived from patients as probes, tested on autologous tumor cell libraries. Most outstanding CM Ag include melanocyte differentiation Ag (MD-

Ag) such as MART-1 (Coulie, Brichard et al. 1994; Kawakami, Eliyahu et al. 1994 a), gp100 (Kawakami, Eliyahu et al. 1994 b), tyrosinase (Brichard, Van Pel et al. 1993), tyrosinase related protein-1 (TRP1) (Cohen, Muller et al. 1990), TRP2 (Wang, Appella et al. 1996), and MELOE-1 (Godet, Moreau-Aubry et al. 2008); cancer-testis Ag from the MAGE superfamily (van der Bruggen, Traversari et al. 1991) and NY-ESO-1 (Chen, Scanlan et al. 1997); and tumor-mutated Ag such as BRAF (Davies, Bignell et al. 2002).

Spontaneous regressions: First studies just analyzed the presence and distribution of lymphocytes; more recent studies also focus on the immunophenotype of immune system cells, as it is known that the IS may move from an antitumor environment to a tumor-permissive one.

Immunosuppression: Although CM is highly immunogenic, tumors develop and progress in immunocompetent patients. One of the contributing factors is the induction of a local state of immune suppression and tolerance to tumors as a result of tumor interaction with its environment. Cancer cells develop different mechanisms for tumor escape, including evasion of Ag recognition by the IS and secretion of immunosuppressive and proapoptotic factors. Tumor cells would secrete immunosuppressor factors that would render IS effector cells into a tolerant phenotype, which in turn would secrete more immunosuppressor factors, preparing the niche for metastasis before tumor dissemination. An analysis of primary CM biopsies revealed that primary CM cells would secret TGF-2, that renders dendritic cells tolerogenic; and tolerogenic dendritic cells (tDC) and Treg were found at all stages, with increasing IDO and IL-10 secretion with CM progression (Polak, Borthwick et al. 2007). This immunomodulation induces regulatory T cells ($CD4^{+}CD25^{+}Foxp3+$), tDC, myeloid-derived suppressor cells (MDSC), plasmacytoid dendritic cells, and tolerance of effector cells (NK and T cells). Accordingly, development of tumors is favored in immunodeficient patients, eg HIV^{+}, with immunosuppressive permissive environments (Frisch, Biggar et al. 2001).

Inflammation: Chronic inflammation is a key factor involved in tumor development and progression (Grivennikov, Greten et al. 2010). Sun exposure promotes an inflammatory environment in the skin, increasing the risk of developing skin cancer, including CM (Kanavy and Gerstenblith 2011). Inflammation contributes to tumor initiation by increasing the DNA mutation rate, and through production of reactive oxygen and nitrogen species that induce DNA damage and instability. Upon transformation, inflammation stimulates angiogenesis and causes local immunosuppression, helping tumor cells to survive and accumulate additional mutations as well as epigenetic changes, enabling tumor progression. Immune cells involved include macrophages, myeloid-derived suppressor cells (MDSC), tumor-associated neutrophils (TAN) and mast cells. For example, tumor-associated neutrophils (TAN) were shown to promote CM cells migration via MAC-1/ICAM-1 interaction (Bins, Mallo et al. 2007), and to be associated with poor prognosis at all stages (Maeurer, Gollin et al. 1996; Fujimura, Ring et al. 2012).

As a consequence of the dynamic interaction of tumor cells with the IS, different therapeutic approaches have been proposed with the main purposes of overcoming chronic inflammation, immunosuppression, and tolerance induced by the own tumor and its environment; and to stimulate tumor Ag immunogenicity and effector function of immune cells in order to eradicate tumors.

2. CUTANEOUS MELANOMA TREATMENT AND MANAGEMENT

Tumor removal by surgery remains the ultimate treatment for CM. Early diagnosed tumors (stage I-II) are mostly cured by surgery. However, once CM has invaded the deep dermis, if ulcerated lesions or lymph node metastases occurs, the prognosis becomes somber. The 5-year survival for patients with distant metastases is less than 20% (Balch, Gershenwald et al. 2009). CM does not usually respond to conventional therapies such as radiation or chemotherapy. The use of radiotherapy in CM is mainly restricted as adjuvant treatment after surgery; and as a palliative in unresectable disseminations (Mordoh 2009). As regards to CM poor response to chemotherapy, it may be due either to a lack of primary response to the drug, or to the development of acquired resistance mechanisms to the drug, commonly called multi-drug resistance (MDR). The identification of specific genes involved in this process indicates that there are three main mechanisms of drug resistance: a) decreased uptake of drugs such as Cisplatin, nucleoside analogs and antagonists of folate metabolism due to alterations in transporters; b) alterations in tumor cells resulting in the inability of a drug to kill the cell, such as defects in apoptotic pathways; and c) an increase in active efflux of hydrophobic drugs that enter the cell by passive diffusion (La Porta 2007). Standard chemotherapy employs Dacarbazine (DTIC), a DNA crosslinker that disrupts DNA function, leading to cell cycle arrest and apoptosis. Phase III clinical trials indicate that treatment with DTIC induces a response rate of 7-12%, with a median survival of 5.6 to 7.8 months for patients with metastatic melanoma (Chapman, Hauschild et al. 2011). DTIC combination with other chemotherapeutic agents did not improve overall survival. Other family agents, such as Carmustine and Temozolomide, and other agents, such as taxanes and platinum analogs, have similar effects (Chapman, Einhorn et al. 1999; Lens and Eisen 2003; Lawson 2004).

2.1. Targeted Therapies

Targeted therapies include the new generation of drugs for cancer treatment, in which the idea is the use of drugs aimed at a specific molecular target, either to tumor cells or to the immune system (immunotherapy).

Given the prevalence of BRAF mutation in CM, specific inhibitors for the most representative mutant allele $BRAF^{V600E}$ were developed. Vemurafenib (PLX4032) was selected because it inhibits $BRAF^{V600E}$ 30 times more selectively than the wild-type protein (Ribas and Flaherty 2011). In the registrational Phase III clinical trial, therapeutic effect of Vemurafenib (960 mg twice daily) was compared to chemotherapeutic drug Dacarbazine (1000 mg/m^2 body surface area every 3 weeks) in non-treated metastatic melanoma patients stages IIIC-IV, carrying BRAFV600E mutation (Chapman, Hauschild et al. 2011). After six months, Vemurafenib produced increases in overall survival (84% vs. 64%) and disease-free survival (5.3 months versus 1.6 months), and a higher response rate compared to Dacarbazine therapy (48% vs. 5%), with manageable side effects. Additionally, patients with $BRAF^{V600K}$ mutation would also respond to PLX4032 therapy. However, although Vemurafenib can achieve significant remissions in patients with advanced stages (generally non-operable), these are of limited duration, as resistance appears (Bollag, Hirth et al. 2010). Currently, great efforts are being directed towards revealing mechanisms of resistance to BRAF inhibition to overcome them (Trunzer, Pavlick et al. 2013).

It was shown that administration of Vemurafenib does not interfere neither with the viability nor functionality of T cells, allowing the implementation of a combinatorial approach with immunotherapy (Comin-Anduix, Chodon et al. 2010). The increase in the flow of CD4 and CD8 cells to the tumor site after beginning of Vemurafenib administration further supports combinatorial strategies (Wilmott, Long et al. 2011).

Also, metastatic melanoma patients receiving combined therapy with BRAF and MEK inhibitors (Dabrafenib plus Tremetinib), showed an increase in immune response (Frederick, Piris et al. 2013). Treated patients presented increased MD-Ag expression, $CD8^{+}$ T-cell infiltrate and markers of T-cell cytotoxicity, and decreased expression of immunosuppressive cytokines, favoring an anti-tumor response. Reactivation of the MAPK pathway might be responsible for MD-Ag suppression and re-establishment of an immunosuppressive tumor microenvironment, as seen within relapses. Another observation was that the immune response induced by these inhibitors may be limited due to an increase in TIM-3 and PD-1 exhaustion markers on T cells, and an increase in immunosuppressive ligand PD-L1. These findings imply that successful combination therapy may require immune checkpoint blockade to enhance antitumor immunity.

To suppress the PI3K-AKT pathway, Rapamycin derivatives were tested in clinical trials, which showed inhibitory effect on the growth of melanoma cell lines (Molhoek, Brautigan et al. 2005). However, it did not show any significant activity in the context of a phase II clinical trial (Margolin, Longmate et al. 2005).

2.2. Immunotherapy

As previously described, CM is an immunogenic tumor *per excellence*, with evidence of of tumor Ag and immunoedition in patients (Aris, Barrio et al. 2012). Therefore, immunotherapy has emerged as an option of interest for the treatment of CM. Immunotherapy seeks to stimulate, restore, manage, and even complement the immune system of the own patient to control any tumor foci. The first immunotherapeutic drug approved for treatment of metastatic melanoma was Interleukin 2 (IL-2), which promotes activation of T, B and NK cells. Studies indicate that high doses of IL-2 allowed to obtain long-term responses in 16% of patients and a complete response in 6% of cases (Tarhini, Kirkwood et al. 2007). IL-2 was the first "proof of principle" that a drug directed towards the immune system can control CM at long-term. Later on, Interferon alpha 2b (IFN- 2b) was approved by the FDA (Food and Drug Administration) for post-surgical adjuvant treatment. Previous studies have shown that adjuvant treatment with IFN-α2b at intermediate doses for two years increases disease-free survival (DFS) of patients with high risk of recurrence (stages IIb, IIC and III) in 10%, with no significant effect on overall survival (OS) (Kirkwood, Manola et al. 2004), and it is associated to severe side effects. The proposed mechanism of action for IFN-α2b is the inhibition of angiogenesis in tumors and non-specific stimulation of immune effector cells.

The main routes employed to promote tumor-specific immunity include active immunomodulation through the use of therapeutic vaccines (*in vivo*), or passive immunomodulation by targeted therapy. Other strategies like Adoptive Cell Therapy (ACT) with autologous T cells are beyond the scope of this chapter (Hershkovitz, Schachter et al.

2010). One of the key points of immunotherapy is the possibility of generating immunological memory, providing a framework for the development of therapeutic vaccines.

2.2.1. Therapeutic Vaccines

Therapeutic vaccines are administered after surgery with the purpose of eliciting a long-lasting immunity and controlling micrometastatic foci. The rational base of vaccines is that tumor Ag must be captured by DC, which migrate to lymph nodes to activate CD4 and CD8 cells, triggering an adaptive immune response, ideally generating immunological memory. Therapeutic vaccines include *tumor-Ag vaccines*, with different sources of Ag, like peptides, proteins, nucleic acid, tumor lysates, recombinant virus, or whole irradiated cells; and *DC vaccines*, consisting of autologous DC stimulated *in vitro* with a proper Ag source, maturated *ex vivo*, and then perfused back into the patient.

The main objectives of active immunotherapy against cancer are to overcome immunosuppression produced by the tumor itself and its microenvironment; to stimulate specific immunity effectors to kill tumor cells; and to increase immunogenicity to tumor Ag. Preexisting antitumor T cells may be ineffective at rejecting the tumor either because their frequency is too low; because tumor cells were selected to escape recognition, or because such lymphocytes are functionally deficient. Vaccination induces cytokine cascades both locally and systemically, resulting in activation and proliferation of anti-melanoma Ag precursors, and infiltration of these effectors into tumors. Generally, low occurrence of anti-vaccine T cells that have the required functional properties to migrate to the tumor, resist the inhibitory tumor environment, and initiate focal activation. In general, vaccines require two critical components, the source of Ag and an adjuvant (Mordoh 2009). Below, we will refer to some phase III clinical studies in CM representative peptide and tumor cell vaccines.

Peptide vaccines are directed to one or several representative CM Ag. To induce T-cell responses, one needs to immunize with adjuvants or Toll-like receptor (TLR) ligands. Numerous clinical trials were conducted with this strategy, some with encouraging results. However, the risk of using peptide vaccines is promoting the selection of tumor Ag-negative resistant populations. In one trial, stages III -IV patients were treated with a peptide vaccine gp100, in combination with the adjuvant Montanide ISA-51 and IL-2 at high doses as compared to treatment with IL-2 alone. Peptide vaccine group showed a significant increase in DFS (2.2 months vs. 1.6 months) and clinical response rate, with a trend of increase in overall survival (OS) (Schwartzentruber, Lawson et al. 2011). In other study, stage II-IV patients were treated with a multi-peptide vaccine alone, in combination with GM-CSF (250 μg/day subcutaneously for 14/28 days of the month); or combined with IFN-2b (10 million U/m^2 3 times a week), or in combination with GM-CSF and IFN-2b. A correlation was found between immune response and an increase in OS (21,3 months vs. 13.4 months), although in this case no association was found with the use of GM-CSF or IFN-2b adjuvants (Kirkwood, Lee et al. 2009). Although peptide vaccination is a very specific approach, therapies that combine peptide immunization with monoclonal antibodies and cytokine therapy are expected to be more effective.

The use of vaccines with whole cells or cell lysates gives the immune system the chance to interact with a broad antigenic repertoire. This is a key point as tumors are heterogeneous, being CM not an exception. A meta-analysis combining results from 173 immunotherapy clinical trials on several cancers found that patients immunized with whole-tumor Ag, including irradiated tumor cells, modified tumor cells, tumor extracts, tumor mRNAs, and

DCs pulsed with tumor extracts, showed an 8.1% clinical response compared with 3.6% in patients immunized with synthetic or recombinant peptides and proteins (Neller, Lopez et al. 2008). Nowadays, whole-cell vaccines are still in the clinical trial setting. For example, GVAX vaccines, consisting of irradiated genetically-modified cell lines secreting GM-CSF, is currently being assayed in stage IIB-IV melanoma patients on a phase I study (clinicaltrials.gov NCT01435499).

DC vaccines consists of autologous systems, where Dc precursors are purified from patient and are stimulated *in vitro* with tumor Ag (irradiated cells), matured *ex vivo*, and are then re-infused into the patient (Steinman and Banchereau 2007; Mordoh 2009). The principle of this methodology is to improve the efficiency of Ag presentation, by directly stimulating DC with tumor Ag and mature before returning them to incorporate the patient, to fulfill their effector Antigen-Presenting Cell function, Ag processing pathways classical and alternative Ag presenting and expressing co-stimulatory molecules to activate naïve T lymphocytes. A big step was done in this field when in 2010 the FDA approved Sipuleucel-T vaccine for treatment of metastatic castrate-resistant hormone-refractory prostate cancer (Beer, Bernstein et al. 2011). Sipuleucel-T or Provenge is made of an autologous DC cell vaccine loaded with a Prostatic acid phosphatase and GM-CSF recombinant Ag. In case of melanoma, a phase I-II was conducted on stage IV patients with autologous dendritic cells, where a cocktail of 5 melanoma-associated synthetic peptides (gp100, tyrosinase, MAGE-A2, MAGE-A3 and MART-1 or MAGE-A1) restricted to HLA-A2 or A24 and KLH were used for DC pulsing. Clinical responses were observed, with an increase in OS of 13.6 vs 7.3 months (vaccinated vs non-vaccinated); and 21.9 vs 8.1 months (high vs low ELISPOT). Also, MAGE-A1 auto-antibody before vaccination was determined as a positive prognostic factor (Oshita, Takikawa et al. 2012).

2.2.2. Our Experience with Therapeutic Vaccines

Therapeutic Vaccines of Irradiated Allogeneic Cutaneous Melanoma Cells

Between 2002 and 2004, a Phase I study with a vaccine of irradiated allogeneic CM cells, using BCG as adjuvant and combined with Molgramostim (GM-CSF) or placebo was conducted (Barrio, de Motta et al. 2006). BCG stimulates immune response, mainly T lymphocytes and NK cells, while the major therapeutic use of BCG is described in bladder carcinoma. The Granulocyte and Macrophage Colony-Stimulating Factor (GM-CSF) stimulates myelopoiesis. In this study, recombinant GM-CSF was used for its effects on the local attraction of monocytes and their differentiation into dendritic cells *in vitro*. In this Phase I study, 20 patients with CM stage IIB (n = 2), III (n = 10) and IV (n = 8) were vaccinated post-surgery, which were disease-free (n = 16), or had minimal disease (n = 4). Five groups were established, receiving vaccine plus different doses of BCG and GM-CSF (placebo, 150μg, 300μg, 400μg and 600μg). With respect to clinical response, it was observed a significant increase in OS and DFS in stage IIB-III patients. However, stage IV patients progressed (Barrio, de Motta et al. 2006). Data updated to July 2012 indicate an OS and DFS of 67% in the 12 stage II-III patients, with a mean of 8 years *(José Mordoh, personal communication, 2013)*. Furthermore, combination of vaccine with BCG and GM-CSF was found safe, no serious adverse events were detected. Regarding the immune response, it was observed a significant increase in cellular immunity to a maximum dose of 400μg GM-CSF. This was evaluated according to different criteria, including an increase in the delayed hypersensitivity (DTH), and observing tumor responses mediated by the immune system after immunization.

Currently, a randomized clinical phase II-III trial in 108 patients is ongoing in Argentina, comparing CSF-470 Vaccine to IFN-α2b treatment. The main objective of this trial is to compare the safety and efficacy of allogeneic irradiated CSF-470 vaccine adjuvanted with BCG and Molgramostim (GM-CSF), with respect to IFN-α2b in CM stages IIB, IIC or III post-surgery patients. Secondary objectives include comparing quality of life between the two treatments, and immune responses correlate with clinical outcome. This study is currently still open and enrolling patients (www.anmat.gov.ar/ Clinical Study number 107/2010, title CASVAC 0401; Clinical Trials NCT01729663).

As regards to DC based vaccines, we demonstrated that autologous DC can capture apoptotic-necrotic gamma-irradiated allogeneic melanoma cells, allowing maturation of DC and migration in response to the lymph node homing CCL19 chemokine, both in a murine model (Goldszmid, Idoyaga et al. 2003) and with DC isolated from peripheral blood monocytes from healthy donors (von Euw, Barrio et al. 2007). Furthermore, DC loaded with irradiated melanoma cells (DC/Apo-Nec vaccine) are able to cross-present MART-1 and gp100 melanoma Ag to specific, HLA-A0201 restricted CD8 T lymphocyte clones (von Euw, Barrio et al. 2007). We conducted a Phase I clinical trial on 16 CM patients, finding that with a mean follow-up of 49.5 months post-surgery, one stage IIC patient and 7/8 stage III patients remain NED (no evidence of disease), but 7/7 stage IV patients have progressed (von Euw, Barrio et al. 2008). In that study, the presence of CD8+T lymphocytes specific to gp100 and Melan A/MART-1 Ags was determined by ELISpot and tetramer analysis in five HLA-A*0201 patients before and after vaccination; one patient had stable elevated levels before and after vaccination; two increased their CD8 + levels, one had stable moderate and one had negligible levels. Although it is very difficult to assess specific immune responses elicited in patients against their own tumors, in one patient we could verify a post-vaccination DTH response to her own irradiated tumor cells since we were able to establish an autologous melanoma cell from her tumor biopsy. Furthermore, we tested in vitro if lymphocytes were primed by DC/Apo-Nec vaccination and recognized autologous Ags by measuring pre- and post-vaccination PBMC proliferation after a five-day coculture of mononuclear cells with irradiated patient's tumor cells (patient´s Apo-Nec). Post-vaccination PBMC proliferated approximately 10-fold more than pre-vaccination lymphocytes in response to DC loaded with patient´s Apo-Nec, demonstrating that after vaccination with DC/ApoNec vaccine, lymphocyte clones recognizing Ags shared by the Apo-Nec mixture and the patient's tumor cells had expanded (von Euw, Barrio et al. 2008). In an updated analysis with a mean follow-up of 65 months, still 88.9 % stage II-III patients have no evidence of melanoma recurrence (*José Mordoh, personal communication, 2012*).

2.2.2. Targeting immunomodulatory molecules

Given the role of CTLA-4 and PD-1 in modulation of the immune response, antagonist mAb were developed to counteract immunosuppressive environment, favoring the action of the immune system over the tumor. CTLA-4 is a critical negative checkpoint molecule that controls the activation and proliferation of T cells, leading to development of antagonist mAb Ipilimumab. In MDX010-20 phase III trial, unresectable stage III-IV patients with metastatic melanoma were randomly assigned in a 3:1:1 ratio to receive Ipilimumab plus gp100 peptide vaccine, Ipilimumab alone (3 mg/kg/3 weeks/4 treatments) or gp100 alone. Patients receiving

Ipilimumab showed improved survival (10.1 months versus 6.4 months). In addition, no differences were observed when using Ipilimumab alone or in combination with gp100 peptide vaccine (10.1 months versus 10.0 months). Furthermore, complete regressions continued after 2 years of follow-up. Adverse-related events were detected in 10-15% of patients treated, with 7 related deaths (Hodi, O'Day et al. 2010). In CA184-024 trial, previously untreated patients with unresectable metastatic melanoma were randomly assigned in a 1:1 ratio to receive ipilimumab 10 mg/kg plus DTIC 850 mg/m^2 or placebo plus DTIC 850 mg/m^2 every three weeks for up to four treatments, followed by DTIC alone every three weeks (Robert, Thomas et al. 2011). OS was greater in patients treated with Ipilimumab plus DTIC (11.2 months vs 9.1 months). Also, it was observed a higher survival by one (47.6% vs 36.3%), two (28.5% versus 17.9%) and three years (20.8% vs. 12.2%). Adverse reactions of grade 3 and 4 in 56.3% of patients treated with Ipilimumab plus DTIC, compared to 27.5% of patients treated with DTIC plus placebo. In 2011, the FDA approved the use of Ipilimumab (Yervoy) for the treatment of unresectable metastatic melanoma.

In the case of PD-1, it was tested in a phase I clinical trial the therapeutic effect of mAb anti-PD-1 MDX-1106 antagonist function in patients with advanced metastatic melanoma, colorectal cancer, or renal cell carcinoma, refractory to pretreatments (Brahmer, Drake et al. 2010). As a result, MDX-1106 mAb was generally well tolerated, with partial and complete remissions of tumors. Pharmacodynamic studies indicated a greater than 70% occupation of the mAb in the PD-1 molecules in circulating T cells after 2 weeks of infusion. It was recently described results regarding dose, safety and response with BMS-936558 anti-PD-1 blocking antibody patients with advanced melanoma, non-small-cell lung cancer, castration-resistant prostate cancer, or renal-cell or colorectal cancer. The adverse-event profile observed would not appear to preclude its use. Cumulative responses were observed in 28% with melanoma. Only patients with PD-L1-positive tumors had an objective response (9 of 25), suggesting a relationship between PD-L1 expression on tumor cells and objective response. Safety, activity, and immune correlates of anti-PD-1 antibody in cancer (Topalian, Hodi et al. 2012). Also, blockade of anti-PD-L1 in an initial trial induced tumor regression (objective response rate of 6 to 17%) and stabilization of disease (rates of 12 to 41% at 24 weeks) in patients with advanced cancers, including non-small-cell lung cancer, melanoma, and renal-cell cancer (Brahmer, Tykodi et al. 2012).

2.2.3. Clinical Assessment of Immunotherapy Responses

Conventional guidelines for chemotherapy responses, like RECIST (Response Evaluation Criteria In Solid Tumors) are based on the direct cytotoxic mode of action of chemotherapeutic agents that produces rapid responses (Eisenhauer, Therasse et al. 2009). Responses to therapy are simply described by improvement (Partial or Complete Response), stabilization (Stable Disease) or progression (Progressive Disease). It considers that achieving a response after the initial cycles of therapy is predictive of complete remission and improved survival; and that an early increase in tumor growth and/or the appearance of new lesions signals progression, meaning drug failure and discontinuation of current treatment. However, responses to immunotherapeutic agents can differ from those observed with conventional chemotherapy. For example, some patients can experience disease progression before they respond to therapy, and others can develop new lesions at the same time that their index lesions are shrinking. A case report described a CM patient treated with Ipilimumab anti-CTLA-4 therapy that was undergoing simultaneously the three phases of cancer immunoediting, with regressing, stable, and progressing lesions (Yuan, Page et al. 2010). Also, problem with vaccines is that the time for clinical evaluation might be too short to expect prolongation of OS because the optimal immune response would have several weeks to operate and pass the cancer progression. A conventional clinical evaluation based on RECIST criteria is incompatible with OS benefit obtained only by continual administration of vaccine despite of clinical progression. As a result, modified response criteria were proposed for use when assessing immunotherapeutic approaches: the immune-related Response Criteria (irRC) (Wolchok, Hoos et al. 2009; Hoos 2012).

Four distinct patterns of response were observed for immunotherapeutic approaches:

i) Objective/complete response, with an immediate reduction in tumor burden. The tumor is invaded by immune cells and tumor lesions decrease in size.
ii) Stable disease, with a slow and steady decline in tumor burden.
iii) An initial increase in tumor volume over time, followed by a response. This might be patients with tumor lesions that become heavily infiltrated by immune cells, therefore there may be an initial increase in tumor burden.
iv) The development of new lesions during treatment, resulting in an initial increase in tumor burden that was followed by a reduction. Also, new lesions may be due to T-cell infiltration into established tumor deposits.

These two later patterns of response are specific to immunotherapy approaches. The immune-response Related Criteria proposes antitumor response based on total measurable tumor burden; time-point response assessment using irRC (irCR; irPR (>=50% total tumor burden), irSD, irPD (>=25% total tumor burden); and that tumor burden should be assessed at numerous time points to perform a suitable follow up.

Conclusion

CM continues to be a challenge for medicine, given the rapid progression of this disease and its refractory nature to conventional treatments. However, great steps have been made in the development of therapeutic strategies in recent years, thanks to increasing knowledge in CM epidemiology and molecular biology.

Melanoma incidence has increased considerably in the last years, mainly because of its early detection, and possibly the high UV exposure related to depletion of the stratospheric ozone layer is likely to have had an impact on CM risk. The relationship between CM development and solar UV exposure is, however, still unclear and needs to be clarified to optimise preventive measures and minimise mortality from skin cancers (Norval, Lucas et al. 2011).

As regards to CM biology, we are gaining knowledge about key signaling pathways involved in tumor development and progression, but we are still looking forward to a suitable model for tumor growth in CM. It is crucial to discern whether Ag heterogeneity is due to the presence of differentiated cells with limited proliferative potential (CSC model), or to Ag plasticity independent from proliferation (phenotypic plasticity model), accounting for resistance and escape from immune effectors. In our experience, we found Ag plasticity both in MD-Ag and CSC markers. Thus, if Ag expression varies in time, immunotherapeutic approaches should point towards plasticity or multitargeting of Ag, so at least some responder T-cell clones with proper migration capability and resistance to inhibitory factors would be obtained. With respect to CM and the immune system, there is a continuous feedback between the tumor and its microenvironment that determines tumor fate. Tumor evolution is dynamic, thus its study provides the possibility to interfere with tumor progression with different therapeutic approaches according to the tumor stage. Among contributing factors, it is key the specific blockade of the tumor immunosuppressor environment, preserving the immune repertoire from the patient. Also, it is relevant to overcome chronic inflammation, which fosters genomic instability, immunosuppression, growth, and angiogenesis in tumors.

In clinical practice, surgery still remains first-line therapy for CM treatment, achieving durable responses in early-stage patients. Conventional chemotherapy and radiotherapy have achieved limited responses. As tumors metasizes to lymph nodes and other organs, there is an increasing risk of recurrence after surgery, therefore an adjunvant treatment is recommended. This seems to be initially the most favorable setting for vaccines. Certainly, CM has paved the way for the development of immunotherapeutic approaches. Vaccines constitute an active mechanism of immunization, with independence from molecular mechanisms and low toxicity, which can lead to a long-term immune response. While displaying slower kinetics compared to other therapies, serial inoculations in time can cause antigenic waterfalls that generate an immune response that is sustainable over time. In the adjuvant setting, the main objective for vaccination is to achieve immunization in disease-free host inducing effective humoral and cellular response in magnitude sufficient to neutralize the growth and subsequent dissemination of CM cells that may had metastasized. Today it is still necessary to establish a suitable adjuvant treatment to reduce the risk of recurrence in high-risk post-surgery patients. In our experience, CSF-470 allogeneic irradiated whole-cell vaccine and autologous DC vaccines loaded with CSF-470 vaccines have proved in initial trials their potential for melanoma adjuvancy, increasing DFS and OS in high-risk recurrent CM stage II-III patients.

In advanced patients, the equilibrium phase has largely been displaced, with a highly tumor immunosuppressive environment, many times with unresectable tumors. However, with advent to targeted therapies to specific molecular targets, with humanized mAb and chemical compounds, a whole new spectrum has opened. Assessement of specific inhibitors of proliferation pathways, like BRAF mutated inhibitor Vemurafenib; or immunomodulating molecules, like anti-CTLA-4 antagonist mAb Ipilimumab, have significantly improve OS when used as first-line therapy in advanced-stage patients. However, there are key differences between Ipilimumab and Vemurafenib. Vemurafenib produces responses rapidly in the majority of patients who have the $BRAF^{V600E}$ mutation, while Ipilimumab can be used regardless of tumor features, with slower but more durable responses.

It is becoming standard practice for CM patients to have their tumour biopsies assessed using molecular genotyping for most frequent mutations, like BRAF and NRAS mutation, along with clinical symptoms, to make decisions about the most appropriate treatment for patients with melanoma.

Vemurafenib might be best suited for BRAF-mutant patients, with rapidly progressing and/or symptomatic disease, with a high tumour load and elevated LDH levels. If this fails, patients have the option of switching to Ipilimumab. By contrast, patients with a low tumour load and LDH levels may be more suitable for treatment with Ipilimumab. Also, BRAF *wild type* patients might be eligible for a clinical trial.

One of the current challenges is the design of combinatorial therapeutic approaches according to tumor stage, with complementary strengths in terms of response to achieve a complete and long-term response. This is mainly determined by the nature of the tumor and the influence of the tumor microenvironment, including the presence of immunosuppressive factors. In this regard, exciting approaches have arisen since it was discovered that the immune system would play a role in tumor regression upon oncogene inactivation, a process that was considered cell-autonomous, adding scientific rationale for combination therapeutic approaches. Immune system might be modulated by stimulatory cytokines, such as IL-2, or by immune checkpoint inhibitors targeting CTLA-4, PD1, or PD-L1; will probably act synergistically with the immune infiltrate elicited by BRAF inhibition in patients with metastatic melanoma. To overcome resistance, targeted therapies with BRAF and MEK inhibitors are being combined. Also, vaccines might be administered after advance disease management to achieve a long-term immunization.

Therefore, it is essential to improve the design of clinical trials, considering selection of the better drug or combined therapy to assay, drug doses, patient population and clinical parameters analyzed. The combined roll of targeted therapies and immunotherapy can be described as a combination of tumor knock down with straightening and education of the immune system to control cancer. We believe that we are on the road of combinatorial therapeutic approaches that will lead to CM control and eradication.

REFERENCES

A snapshot of melanoma, National Cancer Institute, 2012.

Acosta, A. E. & Fierro, E. et al. (2009). "Melanoma: patogénesis, clínica e histopatología." *Rev Asoc Col Dermatol*, *17*(2), 87, 108.

Alanko, T. & Rosenberg, M. et al. (1999). "FGF expression allows nevus cells to survive in three-dimensional collagen gel under conditions that induce apoptosis in normal human melanocytes." *J Invest Dermatol*, *113*(1), 111-116.

Aris, M. & Barrio, M. M. et al. (2010). "Cutaneous Melanoma: A Test Field for Immunotherapy and a Medical Challenge." *Current Cancer Therapy Reviews*, *6*, 229-242.

Aris, M. & Barrio, M. M. et al. (2012). "Lessons from cancer immunoediting in cutaneous melanoma." *Clin Dev Immunol*, 2012, 192719.

Aris, M. & Zubieta, M. R. et al. (2012). "MART-1- and gp100-expressing and -non-expressing melanoma cells are equally proliferative in tumors and clonogenic in vitro." *J Invest Dermatol*, *132*(2), 365-374.

Armstrong, B. K. & Kricker, A. (1993). "How much melanoma is caused by sun exposure?" *Melanoma Res*, *3*(6), 395-401.

Balch, C. M. & Gershenwald, J. E. et al. (2009). "Final version of 2009 AJCC melanoma staging and classification." *J Clin Oncol*, *27*(36), 6199-6206.

Barrio, M. M. & de Motta, P. T. et al. (2006). "A phase I study of an allogeneic cell vaccine (VACCIMEL) with GM-CSF in melanoma patients." *J Immunother*, *29*(4), 444-454.

Bataille, V. (2003). "Genetic epidemiology of melanoma." *Eur J Cancer*, *39*(10), 1341-1347.

Bauer, J. & Curtin, J. A. et al. (2007). "Congenital melanocytic nevi frequently harbor NRAS mutations but no BRAF mutations." *J Invest Dermatol*, *127*(1), 179-182.

Beer, T. M. & Bernstein, G. T. et al. (2011). "Randomized trial of autologous cellular immunotherapy with sipuleucel-T in androgen-dependent prostate cancer." *Clin Cancer Res*, *17*(13), 4558-4567.

Berger, M. F. & Hodis, E. et al. (2012). "Melanoma genome sequencing reveals frequent PREX2 mutations." *Nature*, *485*(7399), 502-506.

Bins, A. & Mallo, H. et al. (2007). "Phase I clinical study with multiple peptide vaccines in combination with tetanus toxoid and GM-CSF in advanced-stage HLA-A*0201-positive melanoma patients." *J Immunother*, *30*(2), 234-239.

Bis, S. & Tsao, H. (2013). "Melanoma genetics: the other side." *Clin Dermatol*, *31*(2), 148-155.

Bishop, D. T. & Demenais, F. et al. (2002). "Geographical variation in the penetrance of CDKN2A mutations for melanoma." *J Natl Cancer Inst*, *94*(12), 894-903.

Boiko, A. D. & Razorenova, O. V. et al. (2010). "Human melanoma-initiating cells express neural crest nerve growth factor receptor CD271." *Nature*, *466*(7302), 133-137.

Bollag, G. & Hirth, P. et al. (2010). "Clinical efficacy of a RAF inhibitor needs broad target blockade in BRAF-mutant melanoma." *Nature*, *467*(7315), 596-599.

Boniol, M. & Autier, P. et al. (2012). "Cutaneous melanoma attributable to sunbed use: systematic review and meta-analysis." *BMJ*, *345*, e4757.

Boyd, S. C. & Mijatov, B. et al. (2013). "Oncogenic B-RAF(V600E) Signaling Induces the T-Box3 Transcriptional Repressor to Repress E-Cadherin and Enhance Melanoma Cell Invasion." *J Invest Dermatol*, *133*(5), 1269-1277.

Brahmer, J. R. & Drake, C. G. et al. (2010). "Phase I study of single-agent anti-programmed death-1 (MDX-1106) in refractory solid tumors: safety, clinical activity, pharmacodynamics, and immunologic correlates." *J Clin Oncol*, *28*(19), 3167-3175.

Brahmer, J. R. & Tykodi, S. S. et al. (2012). "Safety and Activity of Anti–PD-L1 Antibody in Patients with Advanced Cancer." *New England Journal of Medicine*, *366*(26), 2455-2465.

Brenner, A. V. & Lubin, J. H. et al. (2002). "Instrumental measurements of skin color and skin ultraviolet light sensitivity and risk of cutaneous malignant melanoma: a case-control study in an Italian population." *Am J Epidemiol*, *156*(4), 353-362.

Brichard, V. & Van Pel, A. et al. (1993). "The tyrosinase gene codes for an antigen recognized by autologous cytolytic T lymphocytes on HLA-A2 melanomas." *J Exp Med*, *178*(2), 489-495.

Cancer in Australia: in brief 2012, Australian Institute of Health and Welfare & Australasian Association of Cancer Registries,Cancer series no. 72. Cat. no. CAN 69. Canberra: AIHW, 2012.

Chapman, P. B. & Einhorn, L. H. et al. (1999). "Phase III multicenter randomized trial of the Dartmouth regimen versus dacarbazine in patients with metastatic melanoma." *J Clin Oncol*, 17(9): 2745-2751.

Chapman, P. B. & Hauschild, A. et al. (2011). "Improved survival with vemurafenib in melanoma with BRAF V600E mutation." *N Engl J Med*, *364*(26), 2507-2516.

Chen, Y. T. & Scanlan, M. J. et al. (1997). "A testicular antigen aberrantly expressed in human cancers detected by autologous antibody screening." *Proc Natl Acad Sci U S A*, *94*(5), 1914-1918.

Chudnovsky, Y. & Adams, A. E. et al. (2005). "Use of human tissue to assess the oncogenic activity of melanoma-associated mutations." *Nat Genet*, *37*(7), 745-749.

Clark, W. H., Jr. & Elder, D. E. et al. (1989). "Model predicting survival in stage I melanoma based on tumor progression." *J Natl Cancer Inst*, *81*(24), 1893-1904.

Cohen, T. & Muller, R. M. et al. (1990). "Nucleotide sequence of the cDNA encoding human tyrosinase-related protein." *Nucleic Acids Res*, *18*(9), 2807-2808.

Comin-Anduix, B. & Chodon, T. et al. (2010). "The oncogenic BRAF kinase inhibitor PLX4032/RG7204 does not affect the viability or function of human lymphocytes across a wide range of concentrations." *Clin Cancer Res*, *16*(24), 6040-6048.

Coulie, P. G. & Brichard, V. et al. (1994). "A new gene coding for a differentiation antigen recognized by autologous cytolytic T lymphocytes on HLA-A2 melanomas." *J Exp Med*, *180*(1), 35-42.

Curtin, J. A. & Fridlyand, J. et al. (2005). "Distinct sets of genetic alterations in melanoma." *N Engl J Med*, *353*(20), 2135-2147.

Cust, A. E. & Armstrong, B. K. et al. (2011). "Sunbed use during adolescence and early adulthood is associated with increased risk of early-onset melanoma." *Int J Cancer*, *128*(10), 2425-2435.

Davies, H. & Bignell, G. R. et al. (2002). "Mutations of the BRAF gene in human cancer." *Nature*, *417*(6892), 949-954.

de Snoo, F. A. & Hayward, N. K. (2005). "Cutaneous melanoma susceptibility and progression genes." *Cancer Lett*, *230*(2), 153-186.

de Vries, E. & Bray, F. I. et al. (2003). "Changing epidemiology of malignant cutaneous melanoma in Europe 1953-1997: rising trends in incidence and mortality but recent stabilizations in western Europe and decreases in Scandinavia." *Int J Cancer*, *107*(1), 119-126.

Dong, J. & Phelps, R. G. et al. (2003). "BRAF oncogenic mutations correlate with progression rather than initiation of human melanoma." *Cancer Res*, *63*(14), 3883-3885.

Downward, J. (2004). "PI 3-kinase, Akt and cell survival." *Semin Cell Dev Biol*, *15*(2), 177-182.

Dunn, G. P. & Bruce, A. T. et al. (2005). "A critical function for type I interferons in cancer immunoediting." *Nat Immunol*, *6*(7), 722-729.

Eisenhauer, E. A. & Therasse, P. et al. (2009). "New response evaluation criteria in solid tumours: revised RECIST guideline (version 1.1)." *Eur J Cancer*, *45*(2), 228-247.

Elwood, J. M. (1989). "Epidemiology and control of melanoma in white populations and in Japan." *J Invest Dermatol*, *92*(5 Suppl), 214S-221S.

Frederick, D. T. & Piris, A. et al. (2013). "BRAF inhibition is associated with enhanced melanoma antigen expression and a more favorable tumor microenvironment in patients with metastatic melanoma." *Clin Cancer Res*, *19*(5), 1225-1231.

Frisch, M. & Biggar, R. J. et al. (2001). "Association of cancer with AIDS-related immunosuppression in adults." *JAMA*, *285*(13), 1736-1745.

Fujimura, T. & Ring, S. et al. (2012). "Regulatory T cells stimulate B7-H1 expression in myeloid-derived suppressor cells in ret melanomas." *J Invest Dermatol*, *132*(4), 1239-1246.

Gandini, S. & Autier, P. et al. (2011). "Reviews on sun exposure and artificial light and melanoma." *Prog Biophys Mol Biol*, *107*(3), 362-366.

Gandini, S. & Sera, F. et al. (2005). "Meta-analysis of risk factors for cutaneous melanoma: III. Family history, actinic damage and phenotypic factors." *Eur J Cancer*, *41*(14), 2040-2059.

Garraway, L. A. & Widlund, H. R. et al. (2005). "Integrative genomic analyses identify MITF as a lineage survival oncogene amplified in malignant melanoma." *Nature*, *436*(7047), 117-122.

Gilchrest, B. A. & Eller, M. S. et al. (1999). "The pathogenesis of melanoma induced by ultraviolet radiation." *N Engl J Med*, *340*(17), 1341-1348.

Godet, Y., Moreau-Aubry, A. et al. (2008). "MELOE-1 is a new antigen overexpressed in melanomas and involved in adoptive T cell transfer efficiency." *J Exp Med*, *205*(11), 2673-2682.

Goldstein, A. M. & Chan, M. et al. (2007). "Features associated with germline CDKN2A mutations: a GenoMEL study of melanoma-prone families from three continents." *J Med Genet*, *44*(2), 99-106.

Goldszmid, R. S. & Idoyaga, J. et al. (2003). "Dendritic cells charged with apoptotic tumor cells induce long-lived protective CD4+ and CD8+ T cell immunity against B16 melanoma." *J Immunol*, *171*(11), 5940-5947.

Gray-Schopfer, V. & Wellbrock, C. et al. (2007). "Melanoma biology and new targeted therapy." *Nature*, *445*(7130), 851-857.

Grivennikov, S. I. & Greten, F. R. et al. (2010). "Immunity, inflammation, and cancer." *Cell*, *140*(6), 883-899.

Grossmann, A. H. & Yoo, J. H. et al. (2013). "The small GTPase ARF6 stimulates beta-catenin transcriptional activity during WNT5A-mediated melanoma invasion and metastasis." *Sci Signal*, *6*(265), ra14.

Han, J. & Colditz, G. A. et al. (2006). "Risk factors for skin cancers: a nested case-control study within the Nurses' Health Study." *Int J Epidemiol*, *35*(6), 1514-1521.

Hershkovitz, L. & Schachter, J. et al. (2010). "Focus on adoptive T cell transfer trials in melanoma." *Clin Dev Immunol*, 2010, 260267.

Hocker, T. & Tsao, H. (2007). "Ultraviolet radiation and melanoma: a systematic review and analysis of reported sequence variants." *Hum Mutat*, *28*(6), 578-588.

Hodi, F. S. & O'Day, S. J. et al. (2010). "Improved survival with ipilimumab in patients with metastatic melanoma." *N Engl J Med*, *363*(8), 711-723.

Hoos, A. (2012). "Evolution of end points for cancer immunotherapy trials." *Ann Oncol*, *23* Suppl 8, viii47-52.

Ichii-Nakato, N. & Takata, M. et al. (2006). "High frequency of BRAFV600E mutation in acquired nevi and small congenital nevi, but low frequency of mutation in medium-sized congenital nevi." *J Invest Dermatol*, *126*(9), 2111-2118.

Jackson, S. & Harland, M. et al. (2005). "No Evidence for BRAF as a melanoma/nevus susceptibility gene." *Cancer Epidemiol Biomarkers Prev*, *14*(4), 913-918.

Jiang, X. & Zhou, J. et al. (2008). "Imatinib targeting of KIT-mutant oncoprotein in melanoma." *Clin Cancer Res*, *14*(23), 7726-7732.

Jones, W. O. & Harman, C. R. et al. (1999). "Incidence of malignant melanoma in Auckland, New Zealand: highest rates in the world." *World J Surg*, *23*(7), 732-735.

Kanavy, H. E. & Gerstenblith, M. R. (2011). "Ultraviolet radiation and melanoma." *Semin Cutan Med Surg, 30*(4), 222-228.

Kawakami, Y. & Eliyahu, S. et al. (1994) a. "Cloning of the gene coding for a shared human melanoma antigen recognized by autologous T cells infiltrating into tumor." *Proc Natl Acad Sci U S A, 91*(9), 3515-3519.

Kawakami, Y. & Eliyahu, S. et al. (1994) b. "Identification of a human melanoma antigen recognized by tumor-infiltrating lymphocytes associated with in vivo tumor rejection." *Proc Natl Acad Sci U S A, 91*(14), 6458-6462.

Kirkwood, J. M. & Lee, S. et al. (2009). "Immunogenicity and antitumor effects of vaccination with peptide vaccine+/-granulocyte-monocyte colony-stimulating factor and/or IFN-alpha2b in advanced metastatic melanoma: Eastern Cooperative Oncology Group Phase II Trial E1696." *Clin Cancer Res, 15*(4), 1443-1451.

Kirkwood, J. M. & Manola, J. et al. (2004). "A pooled analysis of eastern cooperative oncology group and intergroup trials of adjuvant high-dose interferon for melanoma." *Clin Cancer Res, 10*(5), 1670-1677.

Ko, J. M. & Fisher, D. E. (2011). "A new era: melanoma genetics and therapeutics." *J Pathol, 223*(2), 241-250.

Koebel, C. M. & Vermi, W. et al. (2007). "Adaptive immunity maintains occult cancer in an equilibrium state." *Nature, 450*(7171), 903-907.

Kumar, R. & Angelini, S. et al. (2004). "BRAF mutations are common somatic events in melanocytic nevi." *J Invest Dermatol, 122*(2), 342-348.

La Porta, C. A. (2007). "Drug resistance in melanoma: new perspectives." *Curr Med Chem, 14*(4), 387-391.

Landi, M. T. & Bauer, J. et al. (2006). "MC1R germline variants confer risk for BRAF-mutant melanoma." *Science, 313*(5786), 521-522.

Lawson, D. H. (2004). "Update on the systemic treatment of malignant melanoma." *Semin Oncol, 31*(2 Suppl 4), 33-37.

Lazovich, D. & Vogel, R. I. et al. (2010). "Indoor tanning and risk of melanoma: a case-control study in a highly exposed population." *Cancer Epidemiol Biomarkers Prev, 19*(6), 1557-1568.

Lee, H. Y. & Chay, W. Y. et al. (2012). "Melanoma: differences between Asian and Caucasian patients." *Ann Acad Med Singapore, 41*(1), 17-20.

Lens, M. B. & Eisen, T. G. (2003). "Systemic chemotherapy in the treatment of malignant melanoma." *Expert Opin Pharmacother, 4*(12), 2205-2211.

Maeurer, M. J. & Gollin, S. M. et al. (1996). "Tumor escape from immune recognition: lethal recurrent melanoma in a patient associated with downregulation of the peptide transporter protein TAP-1 and loss of expression of the immunodominant MART-1/Melan-A antigen." *J Clin Invest, 98*(7), 1633-1641.

Margolin, K. & Longmate, J. et al. (2005). "CCI-779 in metastatic melanoma: a phase II trial of the California Cancer Consortium." *Cancer, 104*(5), 1045-1048.

Mitin, N. & Rossman, K. L. et al. (2005). "Signaling interplay in Ras superfamily function." *Curr Biol, 15*(14), R563-574.

Molhoek, K. R. & Brautigan, D. L. et al. (2005). "Synergistic inhibition of human melanoma proliferation by combination treatment with B-Raf inhibitor BAY43-9006 and mTOR inhibitor Rapamycin." *J Transl Med, 3*, 39.

Mordoh, A. (2009). "Clínica del melanoma." *Acta Bioquímica Clínica Latinoamericana, 43*(3), 327-331.

Mordoh, J. (2009). "Melanoma cutáneo: un campo de ensayo para la inmunoterapia y un desafío médico." *Acta Bioquímica Clínica Latinoamericana*, *43*(3), 357-361.

Neller, M. A. & Lopez, J. A. et al. (2008). "Antigens for cancer immunotherapy." *Semin Immunol, 20*(5), 286-295.

Nikolaev, S. I. & Rimoldi, D. et al. (2012). "Exome sequencing identifies recurrent somatic MAP2K1 and MAP2K2 mutations in melanoma." *Nat Genet*, *44*(2), 133-139.

Norval, M. & Lucas, R. M. et al. (2011). "The human health effects of ozone depletion and interactions with climate change." *Photochem Photobiol Sci*, *10*(2), 199-225.

Olsen, C. M. & Carroll, H. J. et al. (2010). "Estimating the attributable fraction for cancer: A meta-analysis of nevi and melanoma." *Cancer Prev Res* (Phila), *3*(2), 233-245.

Oshita, C. & Takikawa, M. et al. (2012). "Dendritic cell-based vaccination in metastatic melanoma patients: phase II clinical trial." *Oncol Rep*, *28*(4), 1131-1138.

Parkin, D. M. & Bray, F. et al. (2001). "Estimating the world cancer burden: Globocan 2000." *International Journal of Cancer*, *94*(2), 153-156.

Patton, E. E. & Widlund, H. R. et al. (2005). "BRAF mutations are sufficient to promote nevi formation and cooperate with p53 in the genesis of melanoma." *Curr Biol*, *15*(3), 249-254.

Polak, M. E. & Borthwick, N. J. et al. (2007). "Mechanisms of local immunosuppression in cutaneous melanoma." *Br J Cancer*, *96*(12), 1879-1887.

Polsky, D. & Bastian, B. C. et al. (2001). "HDM2 protein overexpression, but not gene amplification, is related to tumorigenesis of cutaneous melanoma." *Cancer Res*, *61*(20), 7642-7646.

Prickett, T. D. & Agrawal, N. S. et al. (2009). "Analysis of the tyrosine kinome in melanoma reveals recurrent mutations in ERBB4." *Nat Genet*, *41*(10), 1127-1132.

Prickett, T. D. & Wei, X. et al. (2011). "Exon capture analysis of G protein-coupled receptors identifies activating mutations in GRM3 in melanoma." *Nat Genet*, *43*(11), 1119-1126.

Quintana, E. & Shackleton, M. et al. (2010). "Phenotypic heterogeneity among tumorigenic melanoma cells from patients that is reversible and not hierarchically organized." *Cancer Cell, 18*(5), 510-523.

Quintana, E. & Shackleton, M. et al. (2008). "Efficient tumour formation by single human melanoma cells." *Nature, 456*(7222), 593-598.

Ramirez, R. D. & D'Atri, S. et al. (1999). "Progressive increase in telomerase activity from benign melanocytic conditions to malignant melanoma." *Neoplasia, 1*(1), 42-49.

Reed, K. B. & Brewer, J. D. et al. (2012). "Increasing Incidence of Melanoma Among Young Adults: An Epidemiological Study in Olmsted County, Minnesota." *Mayo Clinic Proceedings*, *87*(4), 328-334.

Reya, T. & Morrison, S. J. et al. (2001). "Stem cells, cancer, and cancer stem cells." *Nature, 414*(6859), 105-111.

Ribas, A. & Flaherty, K. T. (2011). "BRAF targeted therapy changes the treatment paradigm in melanoma." *Nat Rev Clin Oncol*, *8*(7), 426-433.

Robert, C. & Thomas, L. et al. (2011). "Ipilimumab plus dacarbazine for previously untreated metastatic melanoma." *N Engl J Med*, *364*(26), 2517-2526.

Rofstad, E. K. & Halsor, E. F. (2000). "Vascular endothelial growth factor, interleukin 8, platelet-derived endothelial cell growth factor, and basic fibroblast growth factor promote angiogenesis and metastasis in human melanoma xenografts." *Cancer Res, 60*(17), 4932-4938.

Schatton, T. & Murphy, G. F. et al. (2008). "Identification of cells initiating human melanomas." *Nature, 451*(7176), 345-349.

Schreiber, R. D. & Old, L. J. et al. (2011). "Cancer immunoediting: integrating immunity's roles in cancer suppression and promotion." *Science, 331*(6024), 1565-1570.

Schwartzentruber, D. J. & Lawson, D. H. et al. (2011). "gp100 peptide vaccine and interleukin-2 in patients with advanced melanoma." *N Engl J Med, 364*(22), 2119-2127.

Sims, G. P. & Rowe, D. C. et al. (2010). "HMGB1 and RAGE in inflammation and cancer." *Annu Rev Immunol, 28*, 367-388.

Steinman, R. M. & Banchereau, J. (2007). "Taking dendritic cells into medicine." *Nature, 449*(7161), 419-426.

Street, S. E. & Cretney, E. et al. (2001). "Perforin and interferon-gamma activities independently control tumor initiation, growth, and metastasis." *Blood, 97*(1), 192-197.

Tarhini, A. A. & Kirkwood, J. M. et al. (2007). "Durable complete responses with high-dose bolus interleukin-2 in patients with metastatic melanoma who have experienced progression after biochemotherapy." *J Clin Oncol, 25*(25), 3802-3807.

Topalian, S. L. & Hodi, F. S. et al. (2012). "Safety, activity, and immune correlates of anti-PD-1 antibody in cancer." *N Engl J Med, 366*(26), 2443-2454.

Trunzer, K. & Pavlick, A. C. et al. (2013). "Pharmacodynamic Effects and Mechanisms of Resistance to Vemurafenib in Patients With Metastatic Melanoma." *J Clin Oncol.*

Tsao, H. & Atkins, M. B. et al. (2004). "Management of cutaneous melanoma." *N Engl J Med, 351*(10), 998-1012.

Tsao, H. & Goel, V. et al. (2004). "Genetic interaction between NRAS and BRAF mutations and PTEN/MMAC1 inactivation in melanoma." *J Invest Dermatol, 122*(2), 337-341.

Tucker, M. A. & Goldstein, A. M. (2003). "Melanoma etiology: where are we?" *Oncogene, 22*(20), 3042-3052.

Udayakumar, D. & Zhang, G. et al. (2011). "EphA2 is a critical oncogene in melanoma." *Oncogene, 30*(50), 4921-4929.

van der Bruggen, P. & Traversari, C. et al. (1991). "A gene encoding an antigen recognized by cytolytic T lymphocytes on a human melanoma." *Science, 254*(5038), 1643-1647.

van der Spek-Keijser, L. M. & van der Rhee, H. J. et al. (1997). "Site, histological type, and thickness of primary cutaneous malignant melanoma in western Netherlands since 1980." *Br J Dermatol, 136*(4), 565-571.

Velazquez, O. C. & Herlyn, M. (2003). "The vascular phenotype of melanoma metastasis." *Clin Exp Metastasis, 20*(3), 229-235.

von Euw, E. M. & Barrio, M. M. et al. (2007). "Monocyte-derived dendritic cells loaded with a mixture of apoptotic/necrotic melanoma cells efficiently cross-present gp100 and MART-1 antigens to specific CD8+ T lymphocytes." *J Transl Med, 5*, 19.

von Euw, E. M. & Barrio, M. M. et al. (2008). "A phase I clinical study of vaccination of melanoma patients with dendritic cells loaded with allogeneic apoptotic/necrotic melanoma cells. Analysis of toxicity and immune response to the vaccine and of IL-10 -1082 promoter genotype as predictor of disease progression." *J Transl Med, 6*, 6.

Wang, R. F. & Appella, E. et al. (1996). "Identification of TRP-2 as a human tumor antigen recognized by cytotoxic T lymphocytes." *J Exp Med, 184*(6), 2207-2216.

Wangari-Talbot, J. & Chen, S. (2012). "Genetics of melanoma." *Front Genet, 3*, 330.

Weatherhead, S. C. & Haniffa, M. et al. (2007). "Melanomas arising from naevi and de novo melanomas--does origin matter?" *Br J Dermatol*, *156*(1), 72-76.

Webster, M. R. & Weeraratna, A. T. (2013). "A Wnt-er Migration: The Confusing Role of beta-Catenin in Melanoma Metastasis." *Sci Signal*, *6*(268), pe11.

Wei, X. & Walia, V. et al. (2011). "Exome sequencing identifies GRIN2A as frequently mutated in melanoma." *Nat Genet*, *43*(5), 442-446.

What You Need To Know About Melanoma and Other Skin Cancers, National Cancer Institute Publication No.10-7625, 2010.

Wilmott, J. S. & Long, G. V. et al. (2011). "Selective BRAF inhibitors induce marked T cell infiltration into human metastatic melanoma." *Clin Cancer Res*.

Wolchok, J. D. & Hoos, A. et al. (2009). "Guidelines for the evaluation of immune therapy activity in solid tumors: immune-related response criteria." *Clin Cancer Res*, *15*(23), 7412-7420.

Wu, H. & Goel, V. et al. (2003). "PTEN signaling pathways in melanoma." *Oncogene*, *22*(20), 3113-3122.

Yokoyama, S. & Woods, S. L. et al. (2011). "A novel recurrent mutation in MITF predisposes to familial and sporadic melanoma." *Nature, 480*(7375), 99-103.

Yuan, J. & Page, D. B. et al. (2010). "Correlation of clinical and immunological data in a metastatic melanoma patient with heterogeneous tumor responses to ipilimumab therapy." *Cancer Immun*, *10*, 1.

In: Melanoma
Editor: Alexander C. Jones

ISBN: 978-1-62808-608-9

Chapter 3

MOLECULAR DETERMINANTS OF MELANOMA VASCULOGENIC MIMICRY

Amalia Vartanian and Anatoly Baryshnikov
N.N. Blokhin Russian Cancer Research Center, Russian Academy of Sciences, Moscow, Russian Federation

ABSTRACT

The rising incidence of melanoma makes this tumor an important public health problem. Standard systemic therapies have not been adequately effective in the management of melanoma. Moreover, melanoma is resistant to antiangiogenesis therapy suggesting the existence of alternative blood circulation system. For years sprouting angiogenesis has been considered as exclusive mechanism of tumor vascularization. However, in recent years another mechanism of tumor vascularization has been identified that does not involve endothelial cells, a process called vasculogenic mimicry (VM).VM describes the unique ability of highly aggressive tumor cells to express a multipotent, stem cell-like phenotype, and form capillary-like structures (CLS) and matrix-rich patterned network in three-dimentional culture that mimic embryonic vasculogenic network. VM occurrence is tumors strongly associated with poor prognosis.

This review will focus on molecular determinants and signaling pathways involved in melanoma VM. We will discuss the mechanisms that operate at the initial phase of CLS formation by melanoma cells. We will provide the experimental evidence that CLS formation requires apoptotic cell death through activation of caspase-dependent mechanism. In addition, we will describe the status of VM under the condition of angiogenesis blockage.

ABBREVIATIONS

vWF	Wllebrand factor
c-Kit	tyrosine protein kinase kit;
TF	tissue factor
TFPI1	tissue factor pathway inhibitor 1

VE-	cadhein, vascular endothelial cadherin
EphA2	epithelial kinase A2
MMP	matrix metalloproteinase
gal-3	galectin-3
ROS	reactive oxygen species
TNF	tumor necrosis factor
HIF-1α,	hypoxia-inducible factor-1α
FAK,	focal adhesion kinase
VEGFR	vascular endothelial growth factor receptor
VM	vasculogenic mimicry
PAS	periodic Acids-Schiff reagent
PKC	protein kinase C
EC	endothelial cells
PlGF	placental growth factor
TPA	Phorbol-12-myristate-13-acetate
ECM	extracellular matrix
GAPDH	glyceraldehyde-3-phosphate dehydrogenase
CLS	capillary-like structures
PTKI II	protein tyrosine kinase inhibitor II

1. Introduction

Melanoma accounts for only 4% of all skin cancer cases but most of skin cancer-related death [1]. The rising incidence of melanoma makes this tumor an important public health problem. Standard systemic therapies have not been adequately effective in the management of melanoma [2].

Malignant melanoma has been well documented as an angiogenic tumor type, clearly demonstrating new vessels formation as an important step in disease [3]. Neovascularization in melanoma has a poor prognostic significance: elevated serum levels of VEGF, VEGFR2 and VEGFR1 in patients with melanoma are associated with worse survival [4]. As such, inhibitors of angiogenesis may restrict primary tumor growth and metastasis, and potentially improve clinical outcomes. Recent reports of definitive clinical success with the use of angiogenesis inhibitors alone or in combination with cytotoxic chemotherapy have led to their approval for the treatment of metastatic colorectal cancer and renal cell carcinoma. Although this combination was well tolerated, few patients with disseminated melanoma responded to therapy [5]. Several other studies have equally identified either no correlation or a direct correlation, with increasing angiogenesis predicting paradoxical, and somewhat counter-intuitive, improved outcome [6]. Although there are several plausible explanations for this incongruity, a key factor may be the heterogeneity of the vascular supply in tumor [7-9]. In melanomas, traditional angiogenesis is observed in addition to vascular channels, cords and sinuses that lack endothelial cell (EC) lining. These vascular channels are formed by highly aggressive tumor cells, and have a basement membrane that stains positive with periodic-acid-Schiff (PAS) reagent. In contrast, less aggressive melanoma cell lines did not generate these patterns [10].

Channels, formed *in vitro,* were morphologically identical to PAS-positive channels in histological preparations from highly aggressive uveal and cutaneous melanomas found in patients. The generation of microvascular channels by aggressive tumor cells was termed “vasculogenic mimicry” (VM) to emphasize their *de novo* generation without participation by EC and independent of angiogenesis. Morphological characterization reveals that VM networks are rich in laminin and lined by tumor cells. The distinctive pattern of VM appears to recapitulate embryonic vasculogenesis networks. The resemblance of VM networks with embryonic vasculogenic structures suggest that aggressive tumor cells convert to an undifferentiated, embryonic-like phenotype. The microarray analyses studies of differential gene expression of highly aggressive melanoma cell lines revealed the co-expression of multiple phenotype-specific genes (VE-cadherin, EphA2, CD31, VEGF and different receptors for VEGF, vWF, TIE-1, MHC class II, KIT, desmin) [10]. In addition, aggressive VM positive tumors have a higher expression of the basement membrane extracellular matrix (ECM) component laminin5γ2, and metalloproteinase-1, 2, 9. The increased expression of these ECM components suggests that highly aggressive melanoma cells are able to modify their ECM in such way to initiate or promote VM [11]. The occurrence of VM is relatively rare within tumors but the presence of VM networks in patients’ tumor correlates with the increased risk of metastasis and, therefore, poor outcome suggestive of functional contribution of these networks [12-14].

This review will focus on key signaling molecules and cascades described to be implicated in the molecular mechanisms of melanoma VM. We will also discuss the status of VM under the conditions of angiogenesis blockage.

2. Functional Relevance of VM

Recent studies have shown that the presence of VM characteristic structures in patients’ tumor tissue correlates with rapid progression of tumor, elevation of metastasizing, and, as a consequence, short survival of patients.

A recent study contributing to the importance of VM was that among EC-associated markers upregulated by aggressive VM positive tumors are tissue factor (TF), tissue factor pathway inhibitor (TFPI)-1 and -2. All are crucial components for regulation of the coagulation pathway. Recently, Seftor et al. demonstrated high expression of blood clotting proteins in aggressive uveal melanoma [15]. It is known that blood coagulation is initiated by tissue factor (TF) [16]. Deposition of fibrin in tumor vessels and thrombosis are prevented by TFPI-1 and TFPI-2.

Both inhibitors are highly expressed in aggressive uveal melanoma and are negligible in low aggressive melanoma. Moreover, both TFPI-1 and TFPI-2 are localized along the VM channels [17]. The fact the VM-positive tumor, like ECs, supplies itself with an anticoagulation mechanism implies that VM channels are functionally active and can provide blood circulation within the tumor, particularly in zones of deep hypoxia.

By these means, VM channels could provide tumor with an additional vascularization mechanism, either dependent or independent of conventional vascularization ways. Involvement of tumor VM in blood microcirculation was demonstrated on a model of ischemic limbs [18].

Five days after injection of fluorescently labeled metastatic melanoma cells into the mouse ischemic limb, a formation of “mosaic” vessels composed of ECs and tumor cells, as well as vascular channels lined by melanoma cells was observed. This study has significantly altered our understanding of the role of VM.

Using dynamic resonance angiography and histological or immunohistochemical analysis a physiological connection between EC-lined vasculature and tumor cell-lined networks was revealed [19-20]. Microinjection of a fluorescent dye into arteria of experimental tumor established that the vasculogenic component is predominantly localized in the central area, whereas neoangiogenesis occurs on the periphery. Moreover, blood flow exists between neoangiogenesis and VM loci: a contrasting fluorescence dye stained both peripheral and central tumor area. The dye did not accumulate in the central area of tumor lacking VM. These data suggest that tumor cells might actually contribute to conducting blood in vasculogenic-like structures.

As VM networks are linked to the EC-lined vessels, the structures of VM channels in aggressive tumors might facilitate metastasis of tumor cells. The tumor cells lining the inner surface are directly exposed to the blood flow. Therefore, detachment of these tumor cells enables them to reach the blood stream and metastasize to other organs. It seems reasonable that there are at least two metastatic pathways: one directed by angiogenesis and one which is not, although it does co-opt with the existing vasculature.

3. Key VM Signaling Molecules

Historically, VE-cadherin was the first signaling molecule identified as an important key signaling molecule in VM. VE-cadherin is a transmembrane protein which is expressed in ECs and contributes to homotypic cell-cell interaction [21]. Its role in integration of ECs was confirmed in experiments with VE-cadherin knockout mouse; the animals died during midgestation due to vascular malformations [22]. High level of this protein was observed in aggressive melanoma cells. Melanoma cells lacking VE-cadherin were incapable of VM tube formation. In 2006, Hendrix et al. showed that knock-down of VE-cadherin in aggressive cutaneous or uveal melanoma reduced dramatically the cooperation of melanoma cells into CLS [23]. Additionally, loss of VE-cadherin by cultivation with monoclonal antibodies resulted in complete disability of highly aggressive melanoma cells to form CLS. Thus, vascular channel formation by melanoma cells follows the same regularity as formation of blood vessels by ECs: recognition of tumor cells that can enter VM occurs with involvement of VE-cadherin. In connection with this, VE-cadherin is now regarded as vasculogenic switch of melanoma VM. Another key molecule in melanoma VM is EphA2. EphA2 is a tyrosine kinase receptor that was shown to be overexpressed and constitutively active in aggressive melanoma cells [24]. Decrease EphA2 expression in melanoma cells was shown to inhibit VM tube formation *in vitro*. EphA2 co-localizes with VE-cadherin at area of cell—cell contact and these two molecules are able to directly interact during the process of VM [25].

As mentioned above, melanoma cells that are capable of forming vascular channels have a higher expression of the ECM component laminin 5γ2. Laminins are main components of basal membrane and play an active role in tumor invasiveness: they activate cell migration and are implicated in neoangiogenesis signal transduction [26].

Proteolytic cleavage of the laminin5γ2 chain by MMP-2 to γ2 and γ2x fragments regulates the integrin-mediated migration of tumor cells [10].

The data of numerous recent studies suggest that exactly these three molecules (VE-cadherin, laminin 5γ2 and MMP-2) as well as their ligands and receptors are necessary for formation and maintenance of blood vessel stability, because the absence of any of these leads to fetal death caused by defects in vascularization [13, 27].

High levels of these proteins are also observed in aggressive melanoma; poorly aggressive melanoma cells are characterized by low, if any, production of them [28]. Antibodies against MMP-2 blocked the cleavage of laminin 5γ2 and interrupted the process of vascular channel formation by melanoma cells. This fact confirms an idea that highly aggressive tumor cells "recognize" each other by means of VE-cadherin and like ECs, can modify the ECM and initiate vascular channel formation.

The putative role of cyclooxygenase (COX) in VM has been shown recently. COX is the enzyme catalizing the rate-limiting step in prostaglandin synthesis. There are two COX isoforms in humans: COX-1 and COX-2. COX-1 is constitutively expressed in normal cells and is involved in tissue homeostasis [29]. COX-2 is not found under the normal conditions but is associated with pathological hyperplastic and neoplastic processes [30]. COX-2 is now regarded as one of the key molecular targets in targeted anticancer therapy.

Recent studies have revealed that highly invasive breast cancer cells expressing COX-2 can develop vascular channels on Matrigel, while cells with low COX-2 expression lack this ability [31]. COX-2 inhibition by celecoxib or specific siRNA may inhibit vascular channels formation in vitro [32]. Vascular channel formation was abrogated by addition of exogenous prostaglandin E_2 (PGE_2).Therefore, the effect of celecoxib in inhibiting vascular channels is probably related to the dependence of prostaglandin E2.

Galectin-3 (Gal-3) was recently identified as a protein required for VM channel formation. Gal-3 is one of the 15 mammalian members of the galectin family of conserved carbohydrate-binding proteins that contributes to cell adhesion, cell cycle regulation, tumor growth and angiogenesis [33]. Gal-3 is not expressed in normal cells and most benign tumors, whereas it is almost always found in highly aggressive tumors.

During neoplastic progression Gal-3 accumulates in the tumor cells cytoplasm, induces transition of the tumor to more aggressive phenotype, and stimulates angiogenesis and metastasis formation [12]. Gal-3 can function both extracellularly, by interacting with ECM and cell-surface glycoproteins, and intracellularly, via interaction with various proteins thereby modulating signaling pathways [34].

In the aggressive cutaneous melanoma cell line C8161 the shRNA-induced decrease in Gal-3 expression abolished the capacity of these cells to form the CLS in 3D type 1 Collagen [35]. Activation of RAF kinase and PI3K was observed in cells with a low level of Gal-3. Microarray analysis showed that Gal-3 silencing had a negative influence on VE-cadherin and fibronectin.

Additionally, the production of the angiogenic Il-8 decreased following diminished Gal-3 expression. Il-8 is known to regulate the expression of MMP-2, which was described previously to be important for VM tube formation. Consistent with in vitro data, VE-cadherin, Il-8 and MMP-2 expression were downregulated in C8161 tumors xenografts. Summarizing the above, a novel key molecule is identified that is implicated in melanoma VM.

To determine the molecular mechanisms underlying the phenomenon of VM in disseminated melanoma, six cell lines from surgical species of patients with disseminated melanoma were derived in our lab: Mel P, Mel Cher, Mel Kor, Mel Il, Mel Si and Mel Ibr [36]. Melanoma status was confirmed by immunocytochemistry for four melanoma-associated markers (Melan-A, S-100, Tyrosinase and HMW). All melanoma cell lines expressed different levels of angiogenesis-associated markers including VEGF, VEGFR1, VEGFR2, FGF-2, FGFR, integrin $\alpha v\beta 3$. We also calculated the invasive potential of melanoma cells. Using the standardized short-term Matrigel in vitro assay, we showed that five cell lines expressing traditional endothelial markers and having high invasive potential were engaged in CLS formation [37]. Thus, disseminated melanoma as well as uveal and cutaneous melanomas adopts a vascular-related phenotype and engages in VM.

The time-dependent analysis indicated that CLS formation proceeds along three main stages. In the first stage (0-4 h) after being randomly seeded on Matrigel, melanoma cells start moving in different directions, interact and adhere with neighbors, spread and eventually form a multicellular network whose geometry is not substantially modified in the following stages. In the second stage (4-8 h) highly directorial movement toward zones of higher cell concentration was observed. In the third stage (8-16 h) individual cells fold up to form CLS along the previously formed network [37]. We propose that the main geometrical features of CLS are determined during the first stage of vascular network assembly and depend on individual molecular characteristic of tumor cells. The differences between CLS geometry formed by ovarian cancer cells (SKOV-3), breast cancer cells (MCF-7) or melanoma cells (Mel Cher) confirmed the hypothesis that VM like tumor angiogenesis is tissue-specific.

A reproducible feature of CLS formation was the gradual decrease in the cell number by the time when CLS formation was irreversible. This change is characteristic of transition of the cell population from proliferation to differentiation. Adhesion to Matrigel seems to activate differentiation signals, allowing the cells to imitate behavior of ECs, and decrease in cell number at the moment of melanoma cells organization into CLS can be explained by elimination of those cells that are unable to fulfill the EC-like functions. The Hoecht 33342 staining of cultures pointed to apoptotic cell death (Figure1, A). Time course analysis of apoptotic cell death during CLS formation showed an increase with time in PI-positive cells compared with control on plastic (Figure1, B). These findings suggest that apoptosis may be responsible for the decrease in cell number.

If apoptosis is indeed the driving force for VM establishment, inhibition of caspases should interrupt CLS formation. Supporting this, a broad range caspase inhibitor zVAD-fmk simultaneously inhibited CLS formation. In this case, 95% of cells remaining in the culture were alive, although no CLS was found (Figure1, C and D). To strengthen the role of apoptosis in CLS formation, we used another caspase inhibitor. DEVD, a specific caspase-3 inhibitor, induced malformation in CLS similar to that induced by zVAD-fmk (Figure 1, E and H).

In agreement with this conclusion, CLS formation was unaffected when zVAD-fmk was added delay 16 h after seeding the cells on Matrigel [37]. Our results with five melanoma cell lines extended this observation and indicated that apoptosis may be a general mechanism, probably, to eliminate the tumor cells, which failed to turn on the gene program that leads to the differentiation of melanoma cells to endothelial-like cells. Thus, we have identified a mechanism that participates at the early stages of melanoma cells assembly into CLS, before organization of cells for CLS.

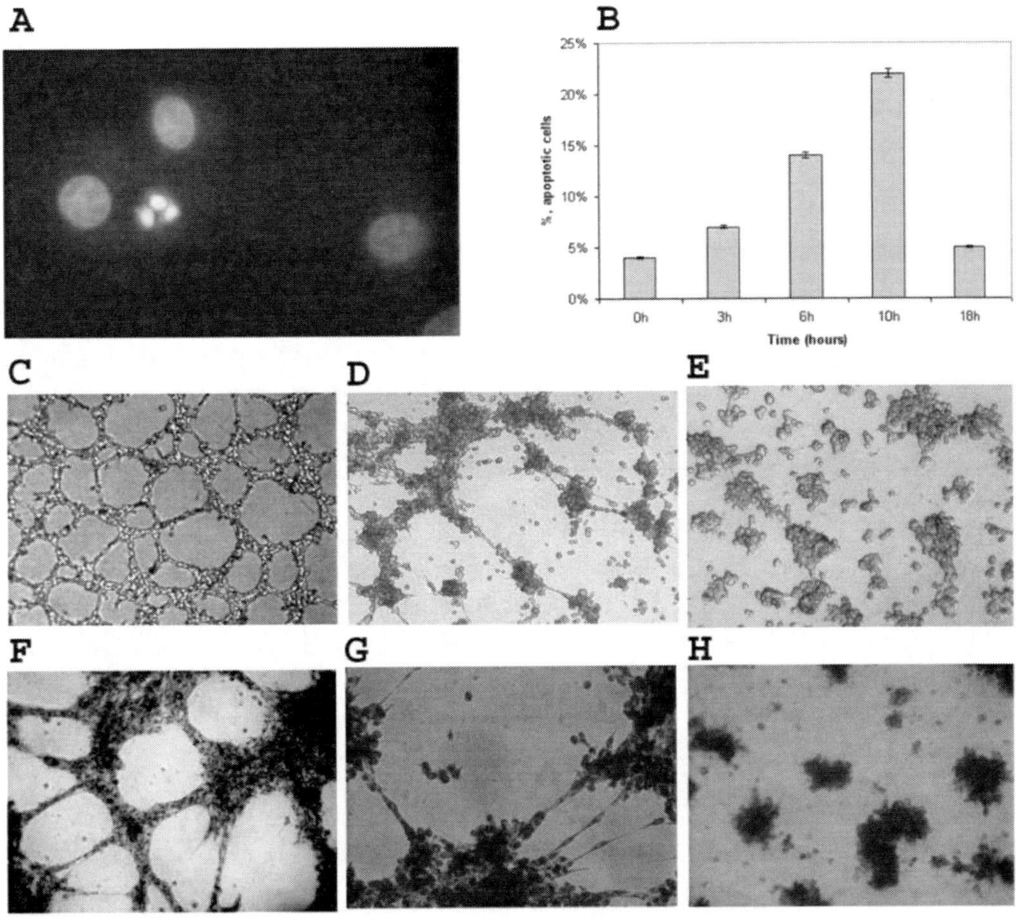

Figure 1. Apoptosis occurs during capillary-like structures (CLS) formation on Matregel. (A) Apoptotic Mel Il cells were visualized by Hoecht 33342. (B) Time curse analysis of apoptotic Mel Il cells by flow cytometry. (C) Control, non-treate dMel Il cells. (D) Mel Il cells were treated with 0.1 mmol/l zVAD-fmk. (E) Mel Il cells were treated with 0.2 mmol/l DEVD. MTT staining of mel Il cells during CLS formation. (F) Control. (G) zVAD-fmk, 0.1 mmol/l. (H) DEVD, 0.2 mmol/l. original magnification x100 (A), x40 (C-H).

Two closely related observations have prompted us to examine the effect of antioxidants (AO) on CLS formation. First, the development of melanoma is believed to be a result of excessive exposure to sunlight: a deleterious imbalance between the production and removal of reactive oxygen species (ROS) was observed in melanoma cells, possibly related to the disease status and progression [39]. Second, ROS is considered to be an important mediator of tumor vascularization [39]. We supposed that ROS also play an important role in vascular channel formation by melanoma cells. To be sure that the effect of antioxidants (AO) such as Resveratrol, Epigallocatechin gallate, N-acetyl cysteine, and Trolox, is not mediated by blocking melanoma cell proliferation, we excluded their effect on proliferative rate, or metabolic activity, or cell migration. Our data have shown that decrease in ROS levels by 50-70% caused non-toxic concentrations of AO completely blocked the ability of cells to form CLS. To confirm the hypothesis that AOs inhibit melanoma VM *in vivo*, we implanted the B16/F10 melanoma cells in C57/Bl/6 mice and anti-vasculogenic property of resveratrol was examined. Our results for the first time demonstrate that resveratrol act as an inhibitor of melanoma VM when administrated intraperitoneally [40]. The observed inhibition was dose-dependent (Figure 2, A-C). We believe that ROS level is a sensitive indicator of the ability of tumor cells to become involved in VM. Future work defining the nature of resveratrol inhibition of vasculiogenesis is necessary, however, we would propose that our study raises the exciting possibility of using this agent for both prevention and therapy of disseminated melanoma.

The importance of VEGF as tumor angiogenic factor in melanoma has been directly substantiated by experiments which show that VEGF expression is a prerequisite for melanoma tumor growth and metastasis [39]. As our findings suggested that ROS level might be a decisive step in CLS formation, initial experiments were designed to determine whether AO could influence the expression of "classical" EC markers. Our data based on immunocytochemical analysis and Western blot indicate that the level of VEGF, VEGFR1, VEGFR2 proteins in cells treated with AOs were significantly lower compared with control. Several reports showed that AOs inhibited VEGF expression in tumor cells [41-42]. It is of considerable value that AO also inhibited VEGFR1 and VEGFR2 expression. This clearly raises the possibility that AO might modulate the VEGF action in non-ECs. As discussed above the blockage of caspase activity resulted in destroyed CLS. To assess the mechanism involved in apoptosis activation, we asked a question as to which apoptotic pathway participates in CLS formation.

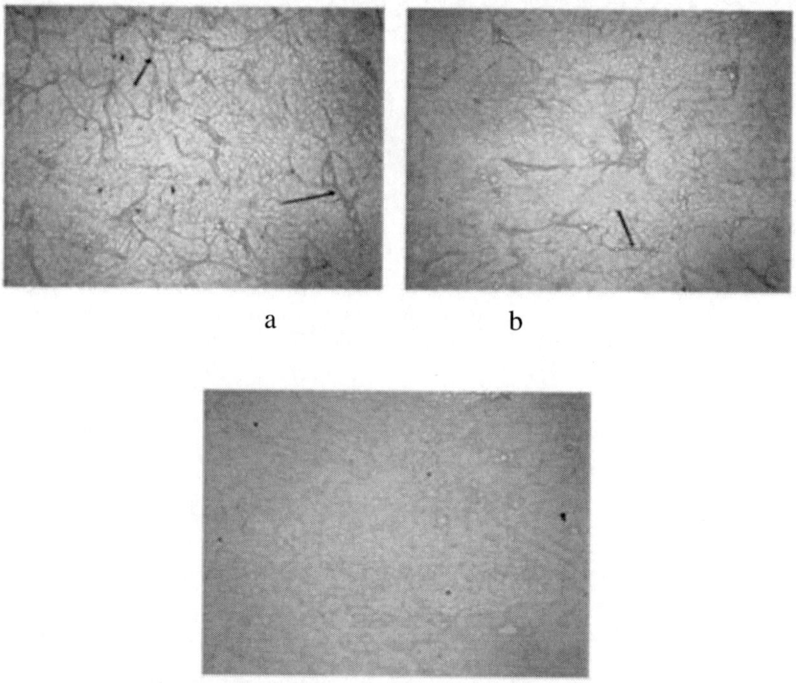

a b

c

Figure 2. The effect of resveratrol (RT) on VM channels formation in experimental tumor. (A) PAS-stained images of histological sextions of murine melanoma tumor obtained from control mice. (B and C) Mice were treated with 2.5 and 10 mg/kg body RT. The density of VM channels in tumor treated with RT was significantly lower compared with control. Original magnification x200.

Caspase-3 is an executioner, not an initiator caspase; thus it must be activated by another caspases, such caspase-2, caspase-8, caspase-10 (in case of TNF family death receptors) or caspase-9 (in case of intracellular stress and cytochrome release from mitochondria) [43-44]. Fas-FasL interaction was exclude, as an antagonistic anti-Fas antibody did not block the apoptotic process and CLS were observed. We found that initially undetectable caspase-3 appeared delay of several hours: activation was initiated followed by cytochrome *c* release from mitochondria [45]. We conclude from these data that in the first step of CLS formation the intrinsic apoptotic pathway is activated in melanoma cells. It is of interest that AO were very effective at decreasing active caspase-3 level. Caspases play a central role in most cell death pathway leading to apoptosis. Nevertheless, cytosolic cytochrome *c* has been associated also to vital functions (i.e. differentiation), suggesting that its release not always occurs in all-or-nothing fashion and that mitochondria outer membrane permeabilization might not invariably lead to cell death. It is unclear how apoptosis is induced under the conditions we used; we can only suggest that downregulation of pathways in which caspases exert non-apoptotic function (by AO in our experiments) is suspected to alter the tumor vascularization.

3. Signaling Cascades Involved in Melanoma V*M*

Hypoxia, HIF-1α, VEGFA/VEGFR1 Signaling Pathway, and VM

The tumor spheroid beyond a diameter of 2 mm (dormant tumor) is avascular. "Tumor dormancy" describes a prolonged quiescent state in which tumor cells are present, but tumor progression is not clinically apparent. Switching of the tumor to the angiogenic program depends on the general balance between pro- and anti-angiogenic signals which is more often shifted to tumor proliferation. VEGF secreted by tumor cells plays a crucial role in tumor angiogenesis and lymphangiogenesis [51]. Moreover, VEGF is the most potent endothelial-specific mitogen; it directly participates in angiogenesis by recruiting EC into avascular areas and stimulating their proliferation. Tumor angiogenesis is stimulated by hypoxia, the usual state of growing tumor cells having insufficient blood supply [52]. In response to hypoxia, tumor cells activate the synthesis of hypoxia-inducible factors HIF-1α and HIF-2α. HIF-1α is considered to be the main player in tumor vascularization.

Its binding to the enhancer sequence of the *VEGF* gene activates VEGF expression, thus stimulating new vessel formation. Once the tumor enters the vascular stage, new vessels continue to form during tumor growth. Recently, it was shown that HIF-1α is localized along the VM channels and is not stained in the CD31 zone of blood vessels [53-54]. These results were confirmed by staining with pimonidozole, a marker of hypoxia. Severe hypoxia was observed in the tumor zones where VM channels are localized, thus indicating association of VM with HIF-1α. In 2007, we first demonstrated that melanoma VM, as well as tumor angiogenesis, are under the control of VEGFA [37]. The next year our data were confirmed by two independent groups. Wang et al have shown that HIF-1α inhibitor, rapamican, blocked VEGF expression, decreased the level of VE-cadherin, EphA2, and MMP-2 and prevent VM channel formation by ovarian cancer cells [55]. Mei et al. have shown that inhibition of VEGF expression by siRNA can suppress VM channels formation in osteocarcoma cells [56].

VEGF binds and activates two tyrosine kinase receptors on EC – VEGFR1 and VEGFR2 [57]. Despite high homology between these two receptors, they transmit different signals. VEGFR1 possesses high affinity to VEGF and low kinase activity; the affinity of VEGF to VEGFR2 is lower, but the kinase activity of VEGFR2 is higher than that of VEGFR1. At present, the concept that VEGFA/VEGFR2 signaling pathway controls tumor angiogenesis is accepted by everybody [58]. Hiratsuka et al. showed that deletion of the VEGFR1 tyrosine kinase domain had no effect on embryonic and postnatal development of mice [59]. This indicated that the VEGFR1 intracellular domain is not essential for EC function. A complete surprise was that the specific VEGFR2 kinase inhibitor, PTKI, does not influence CLS formation. On the other hand, siRNA-mediated suppression of VEGFR1 expression made the melanoma cells unable to form CLS suggesting that the VEGFa/VEGFR1 signaling pathway exerts a control in VM and does not depend on VEGFR2 tyrosine kinase activity [60]. Placental growth factor (PlGF) also binds to VEGFR1 and induces EC tubulogenesis [61]. In our experiments, PlGF failed to induce CLS formation, but its effect on clustering and shape of Matrigel-plated melanoma cells was clearly observed. This added to the evidence that PlGF and VEGFA may transmit distinct signals through VEGFR1 [62]. In a series of *in vitro* experiments we have shown that PKCα and PKCδ are under the control of VEGFA/VEGFR1 signaling pathway in melanoma VM. Nock-down of PKCα and PKCδ isozymes using siRNA transfection strategy has shown that transfection of melanoma cells with PKCα siRNA abrogated CLS formation, but PKCδ siRNA had no effect suggesting that PKCα is the main player in melanoma VM (Figure 3, a-c). To test whether the activation of PKC may solely trigger CLS formation, melanoma cells were treated with VEGF-neutralizing antibody and then seeded on Matrigel in the presence of TPA, PKC activator. No early signs of CLS formations were observed. These results indicated that PKC activation is apparently not sufficient to substitute for VEGF. To confirm the hypothesis that VEGF/VEGFR1/PKCα signaling controls melanoma VM, *in vivo* animal testing was performed. Our data for the first time show that selective PKCα inhibitor, Ro32-0432 significantly inhibits the signs of melanoma VM when administrated intraperitonealy [60]. While activation of VEGFR2 is required to initiate tumor angiogenesis by promoting EC proliferation and survival, VEGFR1 signal transduction pathway may act through activation of PKCα to drive melanoma cells to form VM channels.

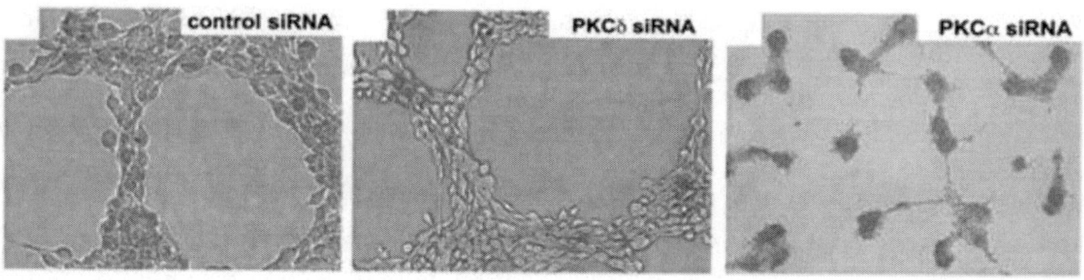

a b c

Figure 3. The effect of PKCα and PKCδ genes silencing on CLS formation. PKCα and PKCδ differently participate in CLS formation. (a) Mel Cher cells were transfected with control siRNA and grown on Matrigel for 14-16 h. (b) Transfection of Mel Cher cells with PKCδ siRNA had no effect on CLS formation. (c) Cells lose their ability to form CLS after transfection with PKCα siRNA. Representative images from three independent experiments are shown. Original magnification x40.

The presence of tumor cell-lined channels provides a potential additional route by which metastases may escape from a tumor or a lymph node into the blood stream. On the other hand, they may provide or supplement the exchange of nutrients, oxygen and growth factors at least in some areas of the tumor. Finally, it has been suggested that the blood vessels in the sites of metastatic growth are being formed from within of the tumor utilizing occasional EC incorporated into the tumor [63]. Therefore the first blood vessels in metastases would be composite ones formed by both tumor and EC. Arguably, the tumor capable of VM may more readily form such composite vessels as well. Current antiangiogenesis strategies, which are directed mainly against tumor endothelium, had no effect on VM [64]. Moreover, when the density of endothelium-dependent vessels is reduced by the antiangiogenesis therapy, the hypoxia of tumor cells caused by antiangiogenesis may induce a compensatory increase in VM to maintain the tumor blood supply. As a result, anticancer therapy targeted at EC might have the unintended effect of promoting tumor growth and metastasis by increasing VM.

EphA2, FAK, VE-Cadherin and Melanoma VM

In 2006, Hess et al. demonstrated that in sites of cell-cell contacts VE-cadherin is co-localized with epithelial kinase EphA2, and cooperation of these two molecules is necessary for VM channels formation [65]. They proposed a possible signal transduction pathway establishing VM. According to their model, the homotypic binding of VE-cadherin molecules on adjacent tumor cells leads to translocation of EphA2 to membrane and binding to its ligand ephrin-A1, suggesting that VE-cadherin and EphA2 activation occur sequentially. The binding of EphA1 to ephrinA-1 results in the phosphorylation of the receptor. The phosphorylated EphA2 induces conversion of inactive GDP-bound Rac1 small GTPase; (membrane GTPase) form and Cdc42 in their GTP-bound active forms. This is consistent with the fact that in highly aggressive melanoma cells, the levels of Rac1 and Cdc42 are considerably higher than in melanoma cells that do not form CLS on Matrigel, and inhibition of Rac or Cdc42 synthesis using siRNA technology completely blocked the melanoma cell assembly into CLS [66]. Activated Rac and Cdc42 are involved both in lamellipodia and filopodia formation required for cell migration and in translocation of focal adhesion kinase (FAK) to the newly formed focal adhesion sites. When localized on a membrane, FAK can phosphorylate EphA2 and, possibly, integrins, which in turn facilitate cell migration via paxillin. Although FAK expression shows little differences among highly and poorly aggressive melanoma cells, FAK activation is enhanced in aggressive melanoma cells due to increased phosphorylation [67]. Activated FAK mediates its signal via enhanced phosphorylation of ERK1/2, which subsequently enhances MMP-2 and MT1-MMP activity. Blockage of FAK phosphorylation at tyrosine 397 and 576 makes the enzyme inactive, and this completely eliminates the CLS forming ability of highly aggressive melanoma cells. FAK is now regarded as the VM trigger [68].

Signaling pathway triggered by VE-cadherin and EphA2 can also activate phophatidylinositol 3-kinase (PI3K), which parcipitates in branched reaction cascades implicated in cell survival and proliferation, differentiation and metabolism. In highly aggressive melanoma cells PI3K is important adjustor of VM directly affecting the cooperative interactions of MT1-MMP and MMP-2 activity [69]. Both enzymes may promote the cleavage of the laminin-5γ2 into pro-migratory γ2 and γ2x fragments.

The deposition of these fragments in extracellular milieu, results in increased invasion and VM. As mentioned above, γ2 and γ2x fragments are molecular messenger triggering VM. Specific PI3K inhibitors decreased both activity of metalloproteinases and accumulation of γ2 and γ2x, eventually resulting in blockage of vascular network formation. Expression of VE-cadherin and EphA2 by highly aggressive melanoma cells and triggering signaling pathways involving FAK and PI3K are consistent with the hypothesis of the ability of highly aggressive tumor cells to imitate the behavior of ECs.

cAMP Signaling Pathway and Melanoma VM

cAMP is a second messenger controlling cell growth, and differentiation. cAMP is produced from ATP following activation of adenyl cyclases, due to ligand binding to G-protein-coupled receptors (GPR) [70]. Perhaps, the very important role of cAMP is activation of cAMP-dependent protein kinases. The most studied is serine-threonine protein kinase A (PKA). Being activated, PKA uses ATP to phosphorylate one or another of many biologically active cell proteins, such as enzyme, receptors, and channel proteins, nuclear histones, transcirption factors, etc. As a rule, serine, threonine, or tyrosine residues undergo phosphorylation. It is worth noting that besides PKA-mediated cAMP signaling, a PKA-independent cAMP signaling pathway also exists. PKA-independent responses are mediated by exchange proteins directly activated by cAMP (Epac)-1 and Epac-2, although Epac responses can cooperate with PKA response [71]. *In vitro* study demonstrated that cAMP signaling is implicated in the ability of aggressive melanoma cells (MUM-28 and C8161) to form CLS [72]. The adenylate cyclase activator forskolin increased the cAMP level and reversibly inhibited CLS formation. This effect was mediated by activation of Epac/Rap1 and did not depend on PKA. Forskolin also inhibited the PI3K-dependent phosphorylation of Akt. In addition, accumulation of cAMP in melanoma cells led to inhibition of ERK1/2, the pharmacological inhibitors of which counteract VM channel formation. Although the role of cAMP in tumor angiogenesis is not clearly presented in literature, it was recently reported that cAMP is important for endothelial cell differentiation and this effect involves cooperation with the Notch signaling pathway [73]. Besides implication in EC differentiation, the cAMP signaling also controls localization of VE-cadherin in EC. It was shown on Human umbical vein endothelial cells (HUVEC) that forskolin and prostacyclin, agents that can elevate cAMP level, enhanced accumulation of VE-cadherin at the cell-cell contact region. Elevated expression of VE-cadherin elevates EC adhesion to the matrix. In relation to diminished VM tube, the role of cAMP on VE-cadherin remains unknown. One could speculate that, although a cAMP signaling is involved in vascular channels formation by melanoma cells, this process is likely under the control of several signaling pathways whose balance depends on cellular context and, possibly, on the nature of the signal.

Ca^{2+} Signaling Pathway, Integrins and Melanoma VM

CLS formation, which is considered to be *in vitro* reconstitution of VM, occurs on Matrigel, but not on plain plastic substrate, and is dependent on autocrine VEGFA production [37] and Ca^{2+}-dependent PKCα activity [60].

Thus, VM requires cooperation of signals from ECM usually transduced by integrins and VEGFA signaling. Tube formation in 3D gels occurs as a consequence of a number of biological activities, including cell migration, cell-cell junction formation, and cell elongation. The sprouting cells stop proliferation, recognize each other by forming a VE-cadherin contact along their apposing basolateral surfaces, then align, communicate with ECM and form tubes. The flexible changes between adhesive and non-adhesive states of a cell, as well as the cytoskeletal rearrangements are regulated by proteins that are present in the focal adhesions [74]. It is known that interaction between cells occurs via subapical junctional complex consisting of several structurally and functionally distinct sites. Several independent lines of evidences demonstrated that the junction complex is highly Ca^{2+}-dependent and that depletion of extracellular Ca^{2+} leads to a rapid destruction of the entire junction complex [75]. Putative Ca^{2+}-binding sites were identified on the extracellular domain of cadherins, F-actin, tubulin and integrins suggesting that the presence of Ca^{2+} is needed for homophilic binding as well as for tight junction formation [76-77]. These observations led us to investigate more closely the contribution of Ca^{2+} in melanoma VM. Our experiments confirm that the levels of both intracellular and extracellular Ca^{2+} are crucial for CLS formation [78]. It should be noted that chelation of extracellular Ca^{2+} does not necessarily mean that the effect of the low Ca^{2+} concentration on integrins and cadherins primarily affect CLS formation: a reduction in extracellular Ca^{2+} probably reduced the availability of intracellular Ca^{2+}. Therefore, it is possible that the reduction of intracellular Ca^{2+} is responsible for the disruption of CLS. Our experiments also confirm an expected participation of actin cytoskeleton in CLS formation [79]. Of note was the previously unreported requirement for intact microtubule network, which can be explained by its involvement in integrin recycling [80]. Impairment of some integrin-dependent functions in response to microtubule-disrupting drugs has been reported [81]. Little is known about the potential roles for integrins in the process of melanoma VM. In our study we focused on αvβ3 and avβ5 integrins and used β1 integrins as a control. Both αvβ3 and β1 integrins are able to activate PKCα [82], which is required for CLS formation and maintenance. αvβ3 is shown to be correlated with metastatic potential in melanoma and seems to regulate the adhesion of melanoma cells to EC. β1 is in control of adhesion and motility in multiple myeloma [83]. Therefore, we tried to evaluate their respective roles. Our results indicate that integrins αvβ3 and avβ5 are primarily involved in initial CLS formation.

The β1 subunit does not play an important role in the process because the blocking antibody had no effect [78]. This evidence suggests that the contributions provided by different integrins are not necessarily of the same kind and perhaps have to be carefully regulated. The initial formation of CLS is associated with cell migration and the formation of proper cell-cell contacts. One may speculate that at this stage it is required that the attachment sites should be flexible; therefore the contribution of β1 integrin known to glue cells to ECM molecules is not crucial for CLS formation. The αvβ3 integrin can be detected in focal contact while αvβ5 can be found in spots other than focal contacts; however, both integrins are primarily responsible for CLS.

To confirm the hypothesis that Ca^{2+} signaling controls melanoma VM, *in vivo* animal testing was performed. Our data demonstrate for the first time that intracellular Ca^{2+}-chelator BAPTA-AM inhibits melanoma VM when administrated intraperitoneally [78].

In summary, we for the first time provided evidence that Ca^{2+}-sensitive cross-talk between integrins, actin, and functional cytoskeleton is central to VM channel formation.

The later phenomenon involves coordinated cytoskeleton rearrangements including cell shape changes as well as creation and dispersal of adhesion sites required for motility, cell-cell alignment and contacts. The exact roles of the each mechanism are to be further elucidated. Evidence that Ca^{2+}/integrin signaling pathway controls melanoma VM suggests that reduction of intracellular Ca^{2+} level might be therapeutically beneficial.

6. Notch Signalling Pathway and Melanoma VM

The Notch pathway is a highly conserved intercellular signalling mechanism that is activated by the interaction of trans-membrane ligands of the Jagged (Jagged1 and 2) and Delta (Delta-like 1, 3 and 4) families with Notch receptors (Notch1 to -4) expressed on adjacent cells [84]. Upon ligands' binding, Notch receptors are activated by proteolytic cleavage of the single trans-membrane domain releasing the Notch intracellular domain, which translocates to the nucleus, where it associates with DNA-binding transcription factors, CSL (CBF1, LAG-1 or Su(h) and MAML. The forming trimeric complex has been shown to activate the expression of basic Helix-loop-helix transcription factors Hes1 and Hes5, and Hey1 and Hey2 thus affecting the regulation of their downstream target genes. Accumulating data indicate that dis-regulated Notch activity is involved in a variety of human cancers, including gliomas, breast cancers, pancreatic cancers, colorectal and cervical carcinomas and hematopoietic malignancies and serves as a trigger for tumor progression to more aggressive phenotype, which is a prerequisite for vascular channels formation by tumor cells [85-89]. On the other hand, expression of Notch and its ligands is also observed in EC, and activation of this signaling pathway in EC terminates proliferation and allows differentiation of cells [90]. Blockage of Notch signaling pathway in endothelium was shown to promote non-productive angiogenesis thus inhibiting tumor growth [91].

The change of angiogenic phenotype in melanomas during the transition from primary tumor to metastatic stage is not sufficiently studied. The development of human metastatic melanoma is marked by the progression from radial to vertical growth phase, when cells acquire the ability to penetrate through the dermal layer and basal membrane into the underlying connective tissue and blood vessels [92].

This progression signals a change to the potentially metastatic phenotype of malignant melanomas and correlates with the appearance of VM channels in tumors.

The crucial role of Notch isoforms in vascular development, together with the knowledge that Notch signaling is implicated in several human cancers, suggests a function for the Notch signaling in the process of VM.

Thus far, only Notch4 was reported to be increasingly expressed in uveal melanoma in the context of VM [93]. Enhanced Notch4 expression was speculated to increase the expression of Nodal in these aggressive melanoma cells which is known to support VM. We observed the high expression of three Notch signaling molecules, Notch3, Notch4 and Jagged1 in melanoma cells derived from surgical species of patients with disseminated melanoma [94]. As mentioned above, activation of Notch pathway directly depends on the functional state of γ-secretase. Inhibition of this enzyme by DAPT or benzodiazepine (BZ) stabilizes CLS *in vitro*. These data were confirmed by blocking the ligand-receptor binding linkage.

Anti-Jagged1 neutralizing antibodies also stabilized CLS. It becomes obvious that attenuation of Notch signaling is necessary for maintenance of CLS integrity. It is worth noting that we did not specify the individual contributions of the respective Notch signaling molecules since chemical compounds that specifically inhibit the proteolytic activity of γ-secretase affect all Notch receptors.

The data obtained *in vitro* were confirmed in xenograft tumor model. We used Mel Cher melanoma cells for melanoma formation in nude mice. Experimental tumor expressed melanoma-associated antigens, CD63, HMB45, Melan A or Tyrosinase, and angiogenesis-associated markers, VEGF, VEGFR1, VEGFR2, VIII as.ag, laminin 5γ2. Thus, our mouse model recapitulates the pathophisiological aspects of human melanomas and allows detailed studies of tumor angiogenesis and VM.

During the early stage of melanoma growth, both mosaic blood vessel and VM channels formation were observed, with prevalence of VM. As the tumor expand the density of endothelium-lined vessels increased and that of VM decreased. At the later stages blood vessels become the predominant blood supply structures in the tumors. Of interest, a VM channels were present mostly in low vascularized areas of tumors. Analysis of xenografts has shown that DAPT increases the signs of VM in experimental melanoma model: VM channels became larger and more branched. Furthermore, we have shown that the increased formation of VM channels is associated with the up-regulation of VEGFR1 and MMP-2, proteins known to trigger VM. Finally, the necrosis areas were not observed in PAS-positive patterns zones suggesting that VM channels are functional and support tumor growth. Altogether, in accordance with our *in vitro* 3D CLS formation assay and *in vivo* data, we suggest that disruption of Notch signaling accounts for the development of neovasculature independent of EC. Our data are in line with the recent observations indicating that anti-angiogenesis treatment causes tumor adaptation and progression to stages of greater malignancy as indicated by increased invasion and metastasis [95]. This would imply that such treatment, although initially resulting in tumor reduction allows the tumor to select for cells capable of surviving when angiogenesis is hampered. These aggressive tumor cells adopt an endothelial-like morphology (VM) and VM may provide tumors with an escape mechanism. It seems reasonable that under the angiogenesis blocking conditions, tumor relapses to the alternative vascularisation mechanism by changing tumor cells characteristics. Taken together, our results give additional rationale to an attempt to use a combination of angiogenesis and VM drug therapies.

Prognostic Significance of PAS-Positive Patterns in Melanoma

A major problem in management of patients with melanomas is predicting tumor behaviour. Although stage, grade, and histologic subtype are well known prognostic factors, patients with histologically comparable tumors can have completely different outcomes. Futhermore, despite the increasing rate of incidental detection of melanomas, the rate of mortality in these patients has remained the same and increasing parallel to the incidence rate. This has led to an extensive search for new tumor characteristics that might influence patients' outcomes.

Recently, Maniotis et al. showed that aggressive primary and metastatic uveal melanoma cells reconstituted PAS-positive patterns *in vitro* in the absence of EC, fibroblasts, or soluble growth factors; less aggressive cells did not generate these patterns in vitro [96]. The generation of these patterns was, therefore, linked to aggressive tumor cell phenotype. Microinjection experiments demonstrated that portions of the *in vitro* tumor cell-generated patterns were capable of conducting dye. Highly aggressive primary and metastatic melanomas, unlike non-aggressive melanomas, have been shown to form a pattern of matrix-rich, tumor cell-lined circulation channels, similar to embryonic vasculogenic patterned networks, VM. In tissue sections, the basement membrane of VM channels stains positive with PAS and this can take the form of several morphological patterns: straight channels, parallel straight channels, cross-linked straight channels, arcs (incompletely closed loops), closed loops, and networks (that can be defined as at least three, back-to back, closed PAS-positive loops) [97]. In a study of 234 patients a strong statistical association was established between the presence of PAS-positive patterns and outcome in primary uveal melanoma [98]. Specifically, the presence of closed loops of PAS-positive material encircling small clusters of tumor cells, networks, and cross-linked parallel PAS-positive linear structures was strongly linked to death from metastatic uveal melanoma. The identification of these patterns was reproducible, and the prognostic significance of these patterns has been confirmed by others [11-13]. The fact that aggressive melanoma cells make not only loops and networks, but also cross-linked parallel patterns, suggests that each of these patterns in tissue sections reflects the presence of an aggressive tumor cell phenotype. It seems reasonable, that the appearance of these architectural characteristics seems to reflect a distinctive gene expression.

The results obtained in a study of 96 patients with primary cutaneous melanoma are consistent with previous observations. The presence of parallel with cross-linking or neyworks carried prognostic significance: patients whose tumors contained either of these patterns had a worse outcome than patients whose tumors lacked these patterns. The stepwise Cox model suggests that both thickness and the presence of parallel with cross-linking or networks exert an independent effect on DFS [99].

When studying a smaller data set of patients with disseminated melanoma, we have also discovered a relationship between the appearence of either the parallel with cross-linking pattern or networks in patients' sections and outcome [11].

To date, little functional data exist that show that tumor cell-lined channels contribute to the overall survival of the tumor. However, even among researches who have questioned the concept of VM as a crucial circulatory system, there is generally a consensus that the prognostic significance of PAS-positive patterns is valid.

The presence of looping patterns in histological sections of primary tumor has been repeatedly shown to have an exceptionally strong association with death from metastatic cancer. The findings of our recent study are entirely in agreement with the literature data suggesting that prominent VM patterns are a feature of more aggressive tumors [14]. We believe that this correlation could become much stronger if the tymidine phosphorylase (TP) expression, a marker of tumor angiogenesis, is also taken into account [14]. Perhaps, the simultaneous presence of these factors may be required to turn on a "malignant switch". If this is confirmed in larger studies, the prognostic significance of the networks/TP phenotype may suggest the possibility of real cooperation between a VM network and angiogenesis in the metastatic process, which in turn suggests that a combination of VM-inhibiting substances and angiogenesis-inhibiting drugs (such as TP inhibitors) might offer therapeutic benefit.

Clinical Significance of VM

The observation that tumor cells can form tubular networks, together with expression of genes associated with an endothelial phenotype, may suggest that VM could be inhibited by angiogenesis inhibitors similar to the way they inhibit EC-driven angiogenesis. However, treatment with angiogenesis inhibitors did not inhibit tube formation of aggressive uveal and cutaneous melanoma cells *in vitro*, thereby showing that plastic tumor cells do not acquire sensitivity [64]. In contrast to this, the anti-angiogenesis drug, thalidomide was reported to diminish the presence of VM vessels (visualized by CD34/PAS double staining) and reduce tumor growth in C57/Bl/6 mice subcutaneously injected with B16/F10 murine melanoma cells [100]. These experiments are crucial for studying the phenomenon of VM in clinics and open a new page in the evaluation of physiological significance of angiogenesis and consideration of vasculogenic component in the blood microcirculation in tumor.

Recent findings indicate that antiangiogenesis treatment may elicit malignant progression of tumors. VEGF receptor inhibition in mouse model of syngenic melanoma reveals an initial anticancer response indicated by vascular withdraw and tumor stasis. However, these conditions elicit an "evasive resistance" response causing tumor adaptation and progression to stages of greater malignancy as indicated by increased invasion and metastasis. Continuous treatment of mice with sunitinib, an approved tyrosine kinase inhibitor with potent antiangiogenic activity, induced a more aggressive tumor phenotype following 5 weeks of treatment [101].

Moreover, the *in vivo* experiments have demonstrated that prolonged treatment with angiostatin, natural inhibitor of angiogenesis, induced resistance to the treatment in mice [102]. Histological analysis of samples insensitive to the drug indicated the presence of VM, unlike samples that were sensitive to the treatment. Thus, the resistance of many tumors to antiangiogenic therapy can be explained, at least partially, by the appearance of a vascular networks formed by tumor cells.

These data indicate that antiangiogenesis treatment also initially resulting in tumor stasis, allows the tumor to select for those cells capable of surviving when angiogenesis is hampered. This escape mechanism is possibly mediated by plastic tumor cells gaining endothelial characteristics, i.e. VM. In our experiments, necrosis was absent in those tumor areas in which high density of VM channels was observed. This fact assuredly confirms the functional activity of VM channels and their ability to maintain tumor growth.

The relationships between VM channels, mosaic blood vessels, endothelium-lined vessels, and lymphatic tube need to be elucidated. Mosaic blood vessels contribute 4% of the total surface area of tumor microcirculation and at present mosaic blood vessels are considered to be a transient phenomenon. Zhang et al. [103] and later in our lab [94] have shown that during early stage of transplanted melanoma, both mosaic blood vessel and VM channels formation were observed, with prevalence of VM. As the tumor expand the density of endothelium-lined vessels increased and that of VM decreased. At the later stages blood vessels become the predominant blood supply structures in the tumors. Of interest, a VM channels were present mostly in low vascularized areas of tumors.

VM serves as a selective advantage for rapid growing tumors in need of perfusion. As a tumor is comprised of a highly heterogeneous cell population, the assumption that tumors are capable of adaptation and even progression by means of selection is not impossible.

The correlation of VM with tumor grade suggests a functional contribution of plastic tumor cells to increase malignancy. These considerations may contribute to develop more accurate antivascular and anticancer strategies.

It seems that tumor VM is regulated by the same pathways that are involved in motility and invasiveness. This may suggest that tumor VM may not be causative for an aggressive phenotype but both are manifestations of increased motility and invasiveness characteristic of de-differentiated cells. Hence, tumor VM may not in any part contribute to the aggressiveness but is just a marker of it. Then it should be possible to switch VM off but retain an aggressive phenotype. On the other hand, it is possible that VM is an indicator of metastatic potential and the one cannot be switched off without ruining the other, as they share common functional links. In either case VM can be easily tested *in vivo* and therefore would serve as a valuable prognostic factor. Our preliminary studies indicate that its prognostic significance may be greatly enhanced by combination with other independent prognostic factors [14], pointing at the possibility that VM-involved oncogenic events are insufficient to induce the aggressive phenotype and require the cooperation with other factors.

CONCLUSION

The term of VM was introduced in 1999 [97]. Over the years, research on VM has increased our knowledge of the molecular events causing aggressive tumor cells to gain plasticity resulting in their ability to mimic vasculature. On one hand, aggressive tumor cells demonstrate high expression of genes encoding VEGF receptor/ligand system proteins, Tie-1, Tie-2, EphA2, VE-cadherin and MMP-2, which are necessary for tumor cells acquiring the endothelium-like characteristics, and on the other hand, Notch and its target genes, *Nodal* expression is observed, enabling the aggressive tumor cells simulate the behavior of embryonic cells. As tumor progress to a more aggressive stage there is a constant selection for cells providing advantage to the tumor. The ability for transdifferentiation combined with a highly invasive, and, hence, metastatic potential in a number of cells allows them to form a channel network within the tumor, which can partially compensate insufficiently development of the microcirculation network and create conditions for survival and proliferation of tumor cells by preventing necrosis within the tumor.

As a result, a small fraction of cells appears and develops in the tumor that is capable of invasive growth and, due to this feature, possesses elevated ability of distant metastasis formation.

Interestingly, VM is not equally presented in different tumor types: in melanoma 60-62% of blood supply occurs via VM channels; in soft tissue sarcoma 35-37%; in renal cell carcinoms 30-32%, in ovarian, breast and prostate cancers 15-18%; and in colorectal cancer 10-12% (our unpublished data). It is worth noting that the vascular system of the tumor is strikingly different from that of healthy tissue: in tumor the vessels are either greatly widened or barely visible. These vessels are not always connected with each other and are poorly stabilized by pericytes, which elevates the risk of bleeding. Their chaotic structure also decelerates the bloodstream. Against the background of the extreme imperfection of the blood circulation in the tumor, 10-12 % of VM channels are unlikely to significantly alter the situation, but 60-62% clearly can be significant.

In our experiments, we selectively inhibited VM in experimental melanoma model in three ways: antioxidants, Ca^{2+} chelators, and PKC inhibitor. In all three cases neither the weight nor tumor volume was significantly changed, while the VM channels density significantly decreased. However, the number of metastases in lung dramatically reduced. Nobody doubts today that the cancer patients do not die from a large tumor, but rather of metastasis. It is the presence of metastases that makes extremely difficult a full recover from cancer. Identification of markers that are tightly associated with the metastasizing potential of each individual tumor is necessary not only for rational therapy of cancer patients, but also for the individualization of treatment ("the right drug for right therapy").

It appears that the process of VM does not rely on a sole signaling pathway, but rather the similar outcome of different signaling events resulting in the activation/expression of VM key signal transduction molecules. The exploration of drugs targeted at molecular signaling pathways in VM is a field of challenges and hopes. Therapy targeted VM has only been attempted in experimental research till date. Research on molecular mechanisms underlying VM and functional relevance will allow not only better understanding the interaction between the metastatic cell, its environment, and malignant switch, but also will offer a novel approach to diagnosis and treatment of malignant tumor. Perhaps, the combination of anti-VM with other therapy strategies, such as chemotherapy, anti-angiogenesis will prove to be promising option.

ACKNOWLEDGMENTS

This work was supported from Russian Ministry of Education and Science 02.512.11. 2195. The authors are grateful to I. Alexandrov for valuable comments, good advice and critical reading the MS.

REFERENCES

[1] Forguson, K. Melanoma. J *Cont. Educ. Nurs.* 2005, 36(6), 242-243.

[2] Mandara, M., Nortilli, R., Sava, T., and Cetto, G. L. Chemotherapy for metastatic melanoma. *Expert Rev. Anticancer Ther.* 2006, 6(1), 121-130.

[3] Marneros, A. C. Tumor angogenesis in melanoma. *Hematol. Oncol. Clin. North Am.*, 2009, 23(3), 431-446.

[4] Brychtova, S., Bezdekova, M., Brychta, T., Tichy, M. The role of vascular endothelial growth factors and their receptors in malignant melanoma. *Neoplasma*, 2008, 55(4), 273-279.

[5] Zaki, K. A., Basu, B., Corrie, P. The role of angiogenesis inhibitors in the management of melanoma. *Curr. Top. Med. Chem.* 2012, 12(1), 32-49.

[6] Wu, S., Singh, R. K. Resistance to chemotherapy and molecularly targeted therapies: rationale for combination therapy in malignant melanoma. *Curr. Mol. Med.*, 2011, 11 (7), 559-563.

[7] Helfrich, A. C., Schadendorf, D. Blood vessel maturation, vascular phenotype and angiogenic potential in malignant melanoma: one step forward for overcoming anti-angiogenic drug resistance. *Mol. Oncol.*, 2011, 5(2), 137-149.

[8] Hiratsuka, S. Vasculogenesis, angiogenesis and special features of tumour blood vessels. *Front Biosci.* 2011; 16:803-814.

[9] Chang, Y. S., DiTomaso, E., McDonald, D. M., Jones, R., Jain, R. K., Munn, L. L. Mosaic blood vessels in tumors: frequency of cancer cells in contact with flowing blood. *Proc. Natl. Acad. Sci. US*, 2000; 97,14608-14613.

[10] Hendrix, M. J., Seftor, E. A., Hess, A. R., and Seftor, R. E. Molecular plasticity of human melanoma cells. *Oncogene*, 2003, 22, 3070-3075.

[11] Vartanian, A. Signaling pathways in tumor vasculogenic mimicry. *Biochemistry*. 2012, 77(9), 1258-1272.

[12] Fan, Y. Z., Sun, W. Molecular regulation of vasculogenic mimicry in tumours and potential tumor-target therapy. *World J. Gastrointest. Surg*. 2010, 2(4), 117-124.

[13] Paulis, Y. W., Soetekouw, P. M., Verheul, H. M., Tjan-Heijnen, C. G., Griffioen, A. W. Signaling pathways in vasculogenic mimicry. *Biochem. Biophys. Acta*, 2010; 1806(1): 18-28.

[14] Vartanian, A., Stepanova, E., Baryshnikov, A., Gutorov, S., Lichinitser, M., Grigorieva, I., Sokolova, I., Solomko, E. Prognostic significance of Periodic Acid-Shiff-positive patterns in clear cell renal cell carcinoma. *The Canadian Journal of Urology*, 2009, 16(4), 4726–4731.

[15] Raf, W., Seftor, E. A., Petrovan, R. J., Gruman, L. M., Margaryan, N. V., Seftor, R. E., Myagi, Y., Hendrix, M. J. Differential role of tissue factor pathway inhibitors 1 and 2 in melanoma vasculogenic mimicry. *Cancer Res.*, 2003, 63, 5381-5389

[16] Mackman, N. Role of tissue factor in hemostasis, thrombosis, and vascular development. *Arterioscler. Throm. Vasc. Biol.*, 2004, 24, 1015-1022.

[17] Daisy, W. J, Hillen, F., Pauwels, P., Kirschman, D. A., Delatte, O., Sciot, R., Maxwell, P. H., Hendrix, M. J., Griffioen, A. W. Tumor cell plasticity in Ewing sarcoma, an alternative circulatory system stimulated by hypoxia. *Cancer res.*, 2005, 65(24), 11520-11528.

[18] Hendrix, M. J., Seftor, R. E., Seftor, A. E., Gruman, L. M., Lee, L. M., Sheriff, D. D., Schatterma, G. C. Transendothelial function of human metastatic melanoma cells: role of the microemvironment in cell-fate determination. *Cancer Res.*, 62(3), 665-668.

[19] Shirakawa, K., Kobayashi, H., Heike, Y., Kawamoto, S., Kasumi, F., Iwanaga, T., Konishi, F., Tarada, M., Wakasigi, H. Hemodynamic of an inflammatory breast cancer xenograft model. *Breast Cancer Res.*, 2003, 5, 136-138

[20] Clarijs, R., Otte-Holler, J., Ruiter, D. J., de Waal, R. M. Presence of fluid-conducting meshwork in xenografted cutaneous and primary human uveal melanoma. *Invest. Ophtalmol. Vis. Sci.*, 2002, 43, 912-918.

[21] Dejana, E., Gianpietro, C. Vascular cadherin and vascular stability. *Curr. Opin. Hematol.,* 2012, 19(3), 218-223.

[22] Gory-Fauer, S., Prandini, M. H., Pointu, H., Roullot, V., Pignot-Paintrand, I., Vernet, M., Huber, P. Role of vascular endothelial cadherin in vascular morphogenesis. *Development*, 1999, 126, 2093-2012.

[23] Hendrix, M. J., Seftor, E. A., Meltzer, P. S., Gardner, L. M., Hess, A. R., Kirshmann, D. A., Schatterman, G. C., Seftor, R. E. Expression and functional significance of VE-

cadherin in aggressive human melanoma cells: role in vasculogenic mimicry. *Proc. Natl. Acad. Sci. US,* 2001, 98, 8018-8023.

[24] Hess, A. R., Seftor, E. A., Gruman, L. M., Kinch, M. S., Seftor, R. E., Hendrix, M. J. VE-cadherin regulates EphA2 in aggressive melanoma cells through a novel signalling pathway: implications for vasculogenic mimicry. *Cancer Biol. Ther.*, 2006, 5 , 228-233.

[25] Margaryan, N. V., Strizzi, L., Abbot, D. E., Seftor, E. A., Rao, M. S., Hendrix, M. J., Hess, A. R. EphA2 as a promoter of melanoma tumorogenity. *Cancer Biol. Ther.*, 2009, 8, 279-288.

[26] Gianneli, G., Falk-Maeziller, J., Schialdi, O., stettler-Stevenson, W. G., Quaranta, V. Induction of cell migration by matrix metalloprotease-2 cleavage of Laminin-5. *Science*, 1997, 277, 225-228

[27] Koshikawa, N., Gianelli, G., Cirulli, V., Quaranta, V. Role of cell surface metalloprotease MT1-MMP in epithelial cell migration over Laminin-5. *J. Cell Biol.,* 2000,148, 615-624.

[28] Seftor, R. E., Seftor, E. A., Koshikawa, N., Meltzer, P. S., Gardner, L. M., Bilban, M., Stetler-Stevenson, W. G., Quaranta, V., Hendrix, M. J. Cooperative interactions of Laminin 5gamma 2 chain, matrix metalloproteinase-2 and membrane type-1-matrixmetalloproteinase are required for mimicry of embryonic vasculogenesis by aggressive melanoma. *Cancer Res.*, 2001, 61, 6322-6327.

[29] Gasparini, G., Longo, R., Sarmicento, R., Mibabito, A. Inhibitors of cyclooxygenase-2: a new class of anticancer agents? *Lancet Oncol.*, 2003, 4(10), 605-615.

[30] Liao, Z., Mason, K. A., Milas, L. Cyclo-oxygenase-2 and its inhibition in cancer. *Drugs*, 2007, 67(6), 821-845.

[31] Basu, G. D., Pathangey, L. B., Tinder, T. L., Gendler, S. J., Mukherijee, P. Mechanism underlying the growth inhibitory effects of the cyclo-oxygenase-2 inhibitor celecoxib in human breast cancer. *Breast Cancer Res.*, 2005, 7, R422-R435.

[32] Basu, G. D., Pathangey, L. B., Tinder, T. L., Gendler, S. J., Mukherijee, P. Mechanism underlying the growth inhibitory effects of the cyclo-oxygenase-2 inhibitor celecoxib in human breast cancer. *Breast Cancer Res.,* 2005, 7, R422-R435.

[33] Krizslak, A., Lipinska, A. Galectin-3 as a multifunctional protein. *Cell. Mol. Biol. Lett.*, 2004, 9, 305-328.

[34] Ochieng, J., Furtak, V., Lukyanov, P. Extracellular functions of galectin-3. *Glycoconj J.*, 2004, 19, 527-535.

[35] Mourad-Zeidan, A. A., Weinkova, V. O., Wang, H., Raz, A., Bar-Eli, M. Expression profiling of Galectin-3-depleted melanoma cells reveals its major role in melanoma cell plasticity and vasculogenic mimicry. *Am. J. Pathol.*, 2008, 173, 1839-1852.

[36] Mikhailova, I. N., Lukashina, M. I., Baryshnikov, A. Yu, Morozova, L. F., Burova, O. S., Kiselev, S., and Georgiev, G. P. Melanoma cell line as a basis for antitumor vaccine preparation. *Vest. Ross. Akad. Med. Nauk*, 2005, 7, 37-40.

[37] Vartanian, A., Burova, O., Stepanova, E., Baryshnikov, A. Yu, Lichinitser, M. R. The involvement of apoptosis in melanoma vasculogenic mimicry. *Mel. Res.*, 2007; 17(1), 1-8.

[38] Meykens, F. L., Farmer, P., Fruehanf, J. P. Redox regulation in human melanocytes and melanoma. *Pigm. Cell Res.*, 2001, 14, 148-152.

[39] Galanis, A., Pappa, A., Giannakakis, A., Lanitis, E., Sandaltzopoulos, R. Reactive oxygen species and HIF-1alpha signaling in cancer. *Cancer Lett.*, 2008, 266(1), 12-20.

[40] Vartanian, A., Burova, O., Stepanova, E., Baryshnikov, A. Yu, Lichinitser, M. R. Melanoma vasculogenic mimicry is strongly related to reactive oxigen species level. *Mel. Res.*, 2007, 17(6), 370-379.

[41] Brakenhielm, E., Cao, R., Cao, Y. Suppression of angiogenesis, tumor growth and wound healing by resveratrol, a natural compound in red wine and grapes. *FAZED J.*, 2002, 15, 1798-1800.

[42] Lamy, S., Gingras, D. and Beliveau, R. Green tea catechins inhibit vascular endothelial growth factor receptor phosphorylation. *Cancer Res.*, 2002, 62, 381-385.

[43] Meier, P., Finch, A., Evan, G. Apoptosis in development. *Nature*, 2002, 407, 796-801

[44] Schulze-Osthoff, K., Ferrari, D. and Loss, M. Apoptosis signaling by death receptors. *Eur. J. Biochem.*, 1998, 17, 1675-1687.

[45] Vartanian, A., Baryshnikiv, A. Yu. Crosstalk between apoptosis and antioxidants in melanoma vasculogenic mimicry. *Adv. Exp. Med. Biol.*, 2007, 601, 145-153.

[46] De Botton, S., Sabri, S., Daugas, E., Zermati, Y., Gudorti, J. E., Hermine, O., and Debili, N. Platelet formation is the consenquence of caspase activation within megakariocytes. *Blood*, 2002, 100, 310-317.

[47] Fernando, P., Kelly, J. F., Balazsi, K., Slack, R. S., and Megeney, L. A. Caspase-3 activity is required for skeletal muscle differentiation. *Proc. Natl. Acad. Sci US*, 2002, 99, 11025-11030.

[48] Garrido, C. and Kroemer, G. Life's smile, death grin: vital function of apoptosis-executing proteins. *Curr. Opin. Cell. Biol.* 2004, 16(6), 639-646.

[49] Mogi, M., and Togari, A. Activation of caspases is required for osteoblastic differentiation. *J. Biol. Chem.*, 2003, 278, 47477-47482.

[50] Sordet, O., Rebe, C., Plenchette, S., Hermine, O., Vanchenker, W., and Dubrez-Daloz, L. Specific involvement of caspases in the differentiation of monocytes into macrophages. *Blood*, 2002, 100, 4446-4453.

[51] Tallquist, M. D., Soriano, P. and Klinghoffer, R. Growth factor signalling pathways in vascular development. *Oncogene*, 1999, 18(55), 7917-7932.

[52] Semenza, G. L. Expression of hypoxia-inducible factor 1: mechanism and consequences. *Biochem. Pharmacol.*, 2000, 59, 47-53.

[53] Van der Schaft, D. W., Hillen, F., Pauwels, P., Kirshmann, D. A., Castermans, A., Tran, M. G., Sciot, R., Hauben, E., Hogendoorn, P. C., Maxwell, P. H., Hendrix, M. J., Griffioen, A. W. Tumor cell plasticity in Ewing sarcoma, an alternative circulatory system stimulated by hypoxia. *Cancer Res.*, 2005, 65, 11520-11528.

[54] Sun, B., Zhang, D., Zhang, S., Zhang, W., Guo, H., Zhao, X. Hypoxia influences vasculogenic mimicry channel formation and tumor invasion-related protein expression in melanoma. *Cancer Lett.*, 2007, 249(2), 188-197.

[55] Wang, J. X., Sun, T., Zhao, X. L., Zhang, S. W., Zhang, D. F., Wang, X. H., Qie, S., Sun, B. C. Functional significance of VEGF-A in human ovarian carcinoma: role in vasculogenic mimicry. *Cancer Biol. Ther.*, 2008, 7(5), 758-766.

[56] Mei, J., Gao, Y., Zhang, L., Cai, X., Qian, Z., Huang, H., Huang, W. VEGF-siRNA silencing induces apoptosis, inhibits proliferation and suppresses vasculogenic mimicry in vitro. *Exp. Oncol.*, 2008, 30(1), 29-34.

[57] Shibuya, M. Differential roles of Vascular Endothelial Growth Factor Receptor-1 and Receptor-2 in angiogenesis. *Biochem. Mol. Biol.*, 2006, 9(5), 469-478.

[58] Waltenberger, J., Claesson-Welsh, L., Siegbahn, A., Shibuya, M., Heldin, C. H. Different signal transduction properties of KDR and Flt1, two receptors for vascular endothelial growth factor. *J. Biol. Chem.*, 1994, 69(43), 26988-26995.

[59] Hiratsuka, S., Minova, O., Kuno, J., Noda, T., Shibuya, M. Flt-1 lacking the tyrosine kinase domain is sufficient for normal development and angiogenesis in mice. *Proc. Natl. Acad. Sci. US,* 1998, 95(16), 9349-9354.

[60] Vartanian, A., Stepanova, E., Grigorieva, I., Solomko, E., Baryshnikov, A., Lichinitser, M. VEGFR1 and PKCα signaling control melanoma vasculogenic mimicry in a VEGFR2 kinase-independent manner. *Melanoma Research*, 2011, 21(2), 91-98.

[61] Hauser, S., Weich, H. A. A heparin-binding form of placenta growth factor (PlGF) is expressed in human umbilical vein EC and in placenta. *Growth Factor*, 1993, 9(4), 259-268.

[62] Autiero, M., Waltenberger, J., Communi, D., Kranz, A., Moons, L., Lambrechts, D. Role of PlGF in the intermolecular cross-talk between the VEGF receptors Flt1 and Flk1. *Nat. Med.,* 2003, 9(7), 936-943.

[63] Elzarrad, K., Haroon, A., Reed, D., Al-Meidi, A. B. Early incorporated endothelial cells as origin of metastatic tumor vasculogenesis. *Clin. Exp. Metastasis*, 2009, 26(6), 589-598.

[64] Van der Schaft, W., Seftor, R. E., Seftor, E. A., Hess, A. R., Gruman, L. M., Kischmann, D. A. Effect of angiogenesis inhibitors on vascular network formation by human endothelial and melanoma cells. *J. Natl. Cancer Inst*., 2004, 96(19), 1473-477.

[65] Hess, A. R., Seftor, E. A., Gardner, L. M., Carles-Kinch, K., Schneider, G. B., Seftor, R. E., Kinch, M. S., Hendrix, M. J. Molecular regulation of tumor cell vasculogenic mimicry by tyrosine phosphorylation: role of ephitelial cell kinase (Eck/EphA2). *Cancer Res*., 2001, 61, 3250-3255.

[66] Hess, A. R., Margaryan, N. V., Seftor, E. A., Hendrix, M. J. Deciphering the signalling events that promote melanoma tumor cell vasculogenic mimicry and their link to embryonic vasculogenesis: role of the Eph receptors. *Dev. Dyn*., 2007, 236, 3283-3296.

[67] Hess, A. R., Hendrix, M. J. Focal adhesion kinase signalling and the aggressive melanoma phenotype. *Cell Cycle*, 2006, 5, 478-480.

[68] Hess, A. R., Postovit, L. M., Margaryan, N. V., Seftor, E. A., Schneider, G. B., Seftor, R. E., Nickoloff, M. J. Focal adhesion kinase promotes the aggressive melanoma phenotype. *Cancer Res*., 2005, 65, 9851-9860.

[69] Hess, A. R., Seftor, E. A., Seftor, R. W., Hendrix, M. J. Phosphoinositide 3-kinase regulates membrane Type 1-matrix metalloproteinase (MMP) and MMP-2 activity during melanoma cell vasculogenic mimicry. *Cancer Res*., 2003, 63, 4757-4762.

[70] Kamenetsky, M., Middelhaufe, S., Bank, E. M., Levin, L. R., Buck, J., Streggborn, C. Molecular details of cAMP generation in mammalian cells: a tale of two systems. *J. Mol. Biol.*, 2006, 623-639.

[71] Bos, J. L. Epac proteins: multi-purpose cAMP targets. *Trends Biochem. Sci*., 2006, 31, 680-686.

[72] Lissitzky, J. C., Parriaux, D., Ristorcelli, E., Verine, A., Lombardo, D., Verrando, P. Cyclic AMP signaling as a mediator of vasculogenic mimicry in aggressive human melanoma cells in vitro. *Cancer Res*., 2009, 69, 802-809.

[73] Yuguri-Kobayashi, T., Itoh, H., Schneider, T., Nakano, A., Narazaki, G., Kita, F., Hiraoka-Kanie, M., Ara, T., Nagasawa, T., Just, U., Nakao, K., Yamashita, J. K. Cyclic

AMP pathway induces Notch activation and differentiation of arterial endothelial cells from vascular progenitors. *Arterioscler. Thromb. Vas. Biol.*, 2006, 26, 1977-1984.
[74] Cheng, H., Lederer, W. J. Calcium sparks. *Physiol. Rev.*, 2008, 88, 1491-1545.
[75] Brown, R. C., Davis, T. P. Calcium modulation of adherens and tight junction function. *Stroke*, 2002, 33, 1706-1711.
[76] Munaron, L., Fiorio, P. A. Endothelial calcium machinery and angiogenesis: understanding physiology to interfere with pathology. *Curr. Med. Chem.*, 2009, 16(35), 4691-4703.
[77] Patton, A. M., Kassis, J., Dhong, H., Kohn, E. C. Calcium as molecular target in angiogenesis. *Curr. Pharm. Res.*, 2003, 9, 543-551.
[78] Vartanian, A., Stepanova, E., Grigorieva, I., Solomko, E., Belkin, V., Baryshnikov, A., Lichinitser, M. Melanoma vasculogenic mimicry capillary-like structure formation depends on integrin and calcium signaling. *Microcirculation*, 2011, 18(5), 390-399.
[79] Stricker, J., Falzone, T., Gardel, M. L. Mechanics of the F-actin cytoskeleton. *J. Biomech.,* 2010, 43, 9-14.
[80] Pasquior, E., Kavallaris, M. Microtubules: a dynamic target in cancer therapy. *IUBMB Life*, 2008, 60, 165-170.
[81] Sjaactad, M. D., Nelson, W. J. Integrin-mediated Ca^{2+} signaling and regulation of cell adhesion by intracellular Ca^{2+}. *Bioassay*, 1997, 19(1), 47-55.
[82] Podar, K., Tai, Y. T., Lin, B. K., Narsimhan, R. P., Satter, M., Salgia, R., Gupte, D., Anderson, K. C. Vascular endothelial growth factor-induced migration of multiple myeloma cells is associated with beta 1 integrin and phosphotidylinositol 3-kinase-dependent PKC alpha activation. *J. Biol. Chem.*, 2002, 277, 7875-7881.
[83] Pellinen, T., Ivaska, J. Integrin traffic. *J. Cell Sci.*, 2006, 19(Pt18), 723-731.
[84] Schwanbeck, R., Martini, S., Bernoth, K., Just, U. The Notch signalling pathway: Molecular basis of cell content dependency. *Eur. J. Cell. Biol.*, 2011, 90(6-7), 572-581.
[85] Koch, U., Radtke, F. Notch signaling in solid tumor. *Curr. Top Dev. Biol.,* 2010, 92, 367-409.
[86] Guo, S., Liu, M., Gouzalez-Perez, R. R. Role of Notch and its oncogenic signaling crosstalk in breast cancer. *Biochem. Biophys. Acta*, 2011, 1815(2), 197-213.
[87] Aster, J. C., Blacklow, S. C., Pear, W. S. Notch signalling in T-cell lymphoblastic leukaemia/lymphoma and other haematological malignancies. *J. Pathol.*, 2011, 223(2), 262-273.
[88] Sjolund, J., Johanson, M., Manna, S., Norin, C., Pietras, A., Beckman, S. Suppression of renal cell carcinoma growth by inhibition of Notch signalling in vitro and in vivo. *J. Clin. Invest.,* 2008, 118(1), 217-228.
[89] Massi, D., Tarantini, F., Franchi, A., Paglierani, M., Di Serio, A., Pellerito, S. Evidence for differential expression of Notch receptors and their ligands in melanocytic nevi and cutaneous malignant melanoma. *Modern Pathol.*, 2006, 19, 246-254.
[90] Jabobsson, L., Bentley, K., Gerhardt, U. VEGFRs and Notch: a dynamic collaboration in vascular patterning. *Biochem. Soc. Trans.*, 2009, 37(pt6), 216-233.
[91] Kame, T. Novel insights into the differential functions of Notch ligands in vascular formation. *J. Angiogeneisi Res.*, 2009, 16, 1-8.
[92] Ko, J. M., Verez, N. F., Tsao, H. Pathways to melanoma. *Semin. Cutan. Med. Surg.,* 2010, 29(4), 210-217.

[93] Hardy, K. M., Kirschmann, D. A., Seftor, E. A., Margaryan, N. V., Postovit, L. M., Hendrix, M. J. Regulation of the embryonic morphogen Nodal by Notch facilitates manifestation of the aggressive melanoma phenotype. *Cancer Res.*, 2010, 70(24), 10340-10350.

[94] Vartanian, A., Gatsina, G., Grigorieva, I., Solomko, E., Dombrovsky, V., Baryshnikov, A., Stepanova, E. The involvement of Notch signaling in melanoma vasculogenic mimicry. *Clin. Exp. Med.*, 2012, 12(3), 121-128.

[95] Paez-Ribes, M., Allen, E., Hudock, J., Takeda, T., Okuyama, H., Vinals, F. Antiangiogenic therapy elicits malignant progression of tumors to increased local invasion and distant metastasis. *Cancer Cell*, 2009, 15, 220-231.

[96] Maniotis, A. J., Chen, X., Garcia, C., de Christopher, P. J., Wu, D., and Folberg, R. Control of melanoma morphogenesis, endothelial survival and perfusion by extracellular matrix. *Lab. Invest.* 2002, 82, 1031-1043

[97] Maniotis, A., Folberg, R., Hess, A., Seftor, E. A., Gardner, L. M., Pe'er, J., and Hendrix, M. J. Vascular channel formation by human melanoma cells in vivo and in vitro: vasculogenic mimicry. *Am. J. Pathol.*, 1999, 55, 739-752.

[98] Clarijs, R., Otte-Holler, I., Ruiter, D. J., de Waal, R. M. Prognostic significance of periodic acid—Schiff-positive patterns in human uveal melanoma. *Invest Ophtalmol. Vis. Sci.,* 2002, 43, 912-918

[99] Warso, M. A., Maniotis, A. J., Chen, X., Majumdar, D., Patel, M. K., Shikaltis, A., Gupta, T. K., Folberg, R. Prognostic significance of periodic acid—Schiff-Positive patterns in cutaneous melanoma. *Clin. Cancer Res.*, 2001, 7, 473-477.

[100] Zhang, S., Li, M., Gu, Y., Liu, Z., Zu, S., Cui, Y., Sun, B. Thalidomide influences growth and vasculogenic mimicry channel formation in melanoma. *J. Exp. Clin. Cancer Res.*, 2008, 27, 60-65.

[101] Ebos, J. M., Lee, C. R., Cruz-Munoz, W., Bjarnason, G. A., Christensen, J. C., Kerbel, R. S. Accelerated metastasis after short-term treatment with a potent inhibitor of tumor angiogenesis. *Cancer Cell.*, 2009, 15, 232-238.

[102] Lloyd, R. V., Vidal, S., Horvath, E., Kovacs, K., Scheithauer, B. Angiogenesis in normal and neoplastic pituitary tissue. *Microsc. Res. Tech.*, 2003, 60(2), 244-250.

[103] Zhang, S., Guo, H., Zhang, W., Zhao, X., Ren, Z., Sun, B. Microcirculation patterns in different stages of melanoma growth. *Oncol. Rep.*, 2006, 15, 15-20.

In: Melanoma
Editor: Alexander C. Jones

ISBN: 978-1-62808-608-9

Chapter 4

NEW ASPECTS OF THE MOLECULAR BIOLOGY OF MELANOMA METASTASIS

***Frédérique Deshayes*[1] *and Stéphanie Ghislin*[2]**
[1]Equipe : « Morphogenèse, homéostasie et pathologies » Institut Jacques Monod CNRS-Université Paris Diderot Bât.Buffon, Paris Cedex 13, France
[2]Lorraine University. Faculty of Medicine. Stress Immunity Pathogens Laboratory, Vandœuvre-lès-Nancy, France

ABSTRACT

Metastatic melanoma is a highly aggressive tumor and compared to other types of skin cancer, it has recently shown the highest increase in incidence and studies in several countries indicate that this increase is expected to continue over the next two decades. If this type of cancer has of good prognosis when diagnosed during the early stages of development (5-year survival estimated at 88-98%), the metastatic 5-year survival is less than 20%, the currently used chemotherapy protocols having a poor efficiency. It is therefore necessary to better understand the process of metastatic spread of this type of cancer in order to identify new targets and to gain better insight into potentially efficient therapies. The metastatic dissemination of tumor cells can be divided in four main steps intravasation, adhesion, extravasation and secondary tissue colonization. Many attempts have been made to identify molecules involved in the three first steps and some mechanisms are now beginning to be better understood. The interactions with the endothelium have notably been described by different groups, and seem to involve several immune molecules.

To colonize secondary tissue, the last step but not the least, cells must adapt to their new microenvironment before proliferating. This is a critical step for the spread of metastases and melanoma particularly succeeds in it. Among the several models that have been suggested to explain these properties one is particularly of interest suggesting that melanoma progression may be driven by phenotype-switching. This would be triggered by cell adaptation to changes in tumor microenvironment, made possible by an important plasticity of melanoma cells. Therefore, melanoma would regularly shift between aggressive/proliferative phases and invasive phases. All this progress in the understanding of melanoma biology highlights different aspects of the development of metastatic melanoma (i.e. plasticity and immune mimetic mechanisms) and might hopefully help to develop new therapeutic strategies.

I. INTRODUCTION

Cutaneous melanoma, which has shown an increased incidence rate in the last few decades, is held to be the most aggressive skin cancer due to its propensity to metastasize and to its poor response to different treatments. Although it represents only 4% of skin cancer, this tumor is responsible for 80% of deaths from these cancers [1]. The survival rate at 5 years was 93% in 1999-2005 [2]. However, this figure depends critically on the stage at the time of diagnosis. Three stages can be identified as stage I: Localized tumor without lymph node or metastasis, stage II: reaching one regional lymph node and stage III: Lymph node metastasis beyond the first relay and / or visceral metastasis. If the 5-year survival is 98% when melanoma is diagnosed while still localized (stage I), it is only about 15% when the melanoma has metastasized (stage III) with a median survival of 6 months [2], [3].

In the case of melanoma, the progression model that has been established is based on clinical and histological observations and is commonly called "model of Clark". It describes the different stages of malignant transformation of a melanocyte to melanoma which are respectively a phase of proliferation and radial growth (RGP) followed by a phase of vertical growth (VGP).

The first step of this model is the appearance of a benign nevus. Melanocytes must then acquire new mutations allowing them to escape the control of proliferation and therefore present abnormal growth. Nevi then show cytological abnormalities, and are thus called dysplastic nevi. This type of nevus may be asymmetrical, with irregular borders, a heterogeneous pigmentation and an increase in diameter. The cells then expand in the epidermis: this is the radial growth phase (Figure 1).

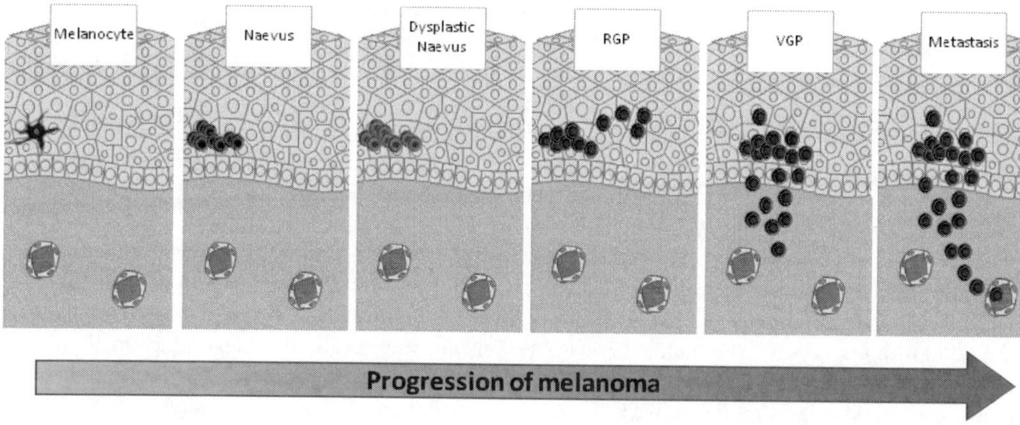

Figure 1. Melanoma progression according to the model of Clark. Schematic representation of the different stages of development of melanoma.

Vertical growth phase is observed when the cells acquire the capacity to invade. They can then pass through the basement membrane and invade the dermis. The invasion of the dermis can be done either by individual migration or by collective migration [4]. In the dermis, the cells will be able to reach the blood and lymph vessels and metastasize to colonize other organs (Figure 1).

This step of metastasis is considered as the final step in the development of cancers. In the case of melanoma, this metastatic step represents a barrier to treatment.

II. Metastasis

In order to colonize new organs metastatic cells must pass through many stages including a neo-vascularization due to hypoxia, intravasation and survival in the circulation, adhesion to the vessel, extravasation and neo-colonization (Figure 2). In this section, we will describe these steps and focus on adhesion and extravasation through blood vessels.

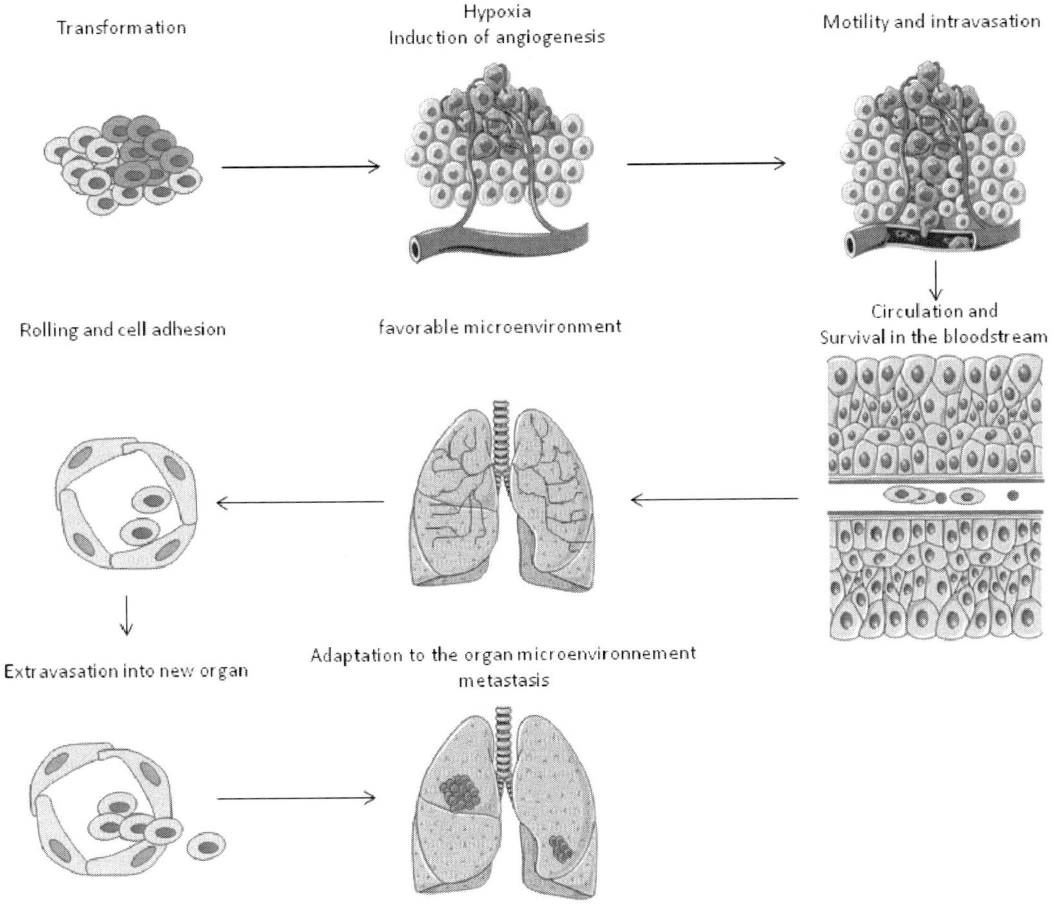

Figure 2. Development of metastasis. Schematic representation of the selective series of steps of the metastatic process.

1.) Hypoxia and Neo-Vascularization

During tumor growth, the increase in size of the tumor leads to a distance from the vessels and thus a deprivation of oxygen for the cells within the tumor. The existence of a hypoxic center induces a selection pressure on cells and promotes the survival and the development of resistant cells and the selection of the most aggressive cells [5]. In agreement with these observations, pronounced hypoxia detected in a tumor is usually associated with a poor prognosis for survival [6] and has been reported to be an essential cofactor for melanoma development [7]. Hence, melanoma is able to induce the formation of new blood vessels, mainly by the production of endothelial cells growth factors. Adaptation to hypoxia is mainly by means of the HIF (Hypoxia Inducile Factors) family of transcription factors. Briefly, when in low oxygen conditions, HIF1-α is stabilized and its fixation as a heterodimer with HIF1-β on HRE (Hypoxia Responsive Element) site triggers the expression of the target genes. More than a hundred of these genes have been identified as far as now, included apoptotic genes, VEGF (Vascular Endothelial Growth factor), PDGF (Platelet Derived Growth Factor) and importantly for melanoma, MITF (Microphtalmia-associated transcription factor), the master gene in melanocyte differentiation.

Thus hypoxia will stimulate neovascularization allowing nutrient and oxygen intake within the tumor. In vivo, the work of Gimbrone et al in 1972 has shown that beyond 1mm^3 tumor developed vasculature to continue its proliferation [8].

In 1999, Maniotis et al. [9] discovered a new phenomenon in the biology of tumor vascularization known as vasculogenic mimicry (VM). Under appropriate matrix microenvironment conditions, highly aggressive and metastatic cutaneous melanoma cells can form highly patterned vascular channels. The discovery of VM by Manitotis remains a debatable subject, and several researchers believe that the findings are neither persuasive nor novel. Tumor cells can obtain oxygen and nutriment through VM and mosaic vessels besides endothelium-dependent vessels [10]. McDonald et al [11] argued that the VM phenomenon discovered by Maniotis exists in uveal and metastatic cutaneous melanomas only and is not associated with all tumor types. Immunohistochemical staining, histochemical staining and electron microscopy have confirmed that tumor cells constitute only 3% of the area of blood vessels. Therefore VM occurs by the migration of tumor cells through the wall of endothelium-dependent vessels or tumor cells are exposed because of the destruction of walls of blood vessels [10]. However several studies have demonstrated the importance of this phenomenon mainly due to the plasticity of melanoma cells. Notably Spinella et al. [12] have recently characterized the cross-signaling between the VEGFR-3 and ET-$_B$R pathways and their implication in cell plasticity with consequences on angiogenesis and lymphangiogenesis.

2.) Intravasation and Survival in the Blood Circulation

New blood vessels provide to tumor cells a pathway in the bloodstream. To do this, they need to pass through the layer of pericytes, degrade the components of the basal membrane and destabilize tight junctions between the endothelial cells. However, the neo-blood vessels, because of their imperfect constitution, are considered more permeable than normal vessels, thereby facilitating access of tumor cells to the bloodstream [13].

Several molecules and events are required for the degradation of matrix membranes, the migration and the entry of the tumor cells into the circulation. Among these, the most studied are MCAM/MUC18 [14], the downregulation of E-cadherin (CDH1) and the upregulation of N-cadherin (CDH2) under the control of the PI3K/PTEN pathway [15] and MMP-9 [16]. Notably, the two molecules CDH1 and CDH2 are important markers of Epithelial-Mesenchymal Transition (EMT), a complex process by which epithelial cells lose their epithelial characteristic and acquire a mesenchymal-like phenotype. Indeed, downregulation of E-cadherin, one of the essential hallmarks for EMT [17], is triggered in melanoma by the activation of SNAI which physically contacts the promoter [18].

Once inside the vessel lumen, it is estimated that only 0.01% of tumor cells reaching the bloodstream survive. This low survival rate is due to the altered physical conditions such as the pressure of the flow of blood cells or elongation and wall friction in the capillaries. But these constraints are not the only obstacles encountered by tumor cells, indeed they need to escape the immune system, and notably the NK cells [19]. Several types of cancer cells, including melanoma, are able to adhere to platelets, which partially mask them from the immune cells and help them to withstand physical constraints encountered [20].

In addition to invading the blood vessels another mechanism of cancer cell dissemination has been described: angiotropism, also known as extravascular migratory metastasis (EVMM). Angiotropism has been defined as "*the presence of tumor cells closely apposed to the abluminal surfaces of blood and lymphatic vessels without intravasation*" [21]. Different studies have strongly suggested that angiotropism in melanoma could be a marker for extravascular migratory metastasis and an angio-tumoral complex has been identified in which tumor cells are linked to endothelium by a matrix containing laminin without evidence of intravasation [22]–[24]. This phenomenon is increasingly recognized as an important mechanism of melanoma metastasis [25].

3.) Adhesion and Transmigration

Extravasation is a controlled process involving the multistep action of traffic signals and adhesion molecules that mediate rolling, adhesion and transendothelial migration of the cells, mainly represented by leukocytes. Extravasation of most cancer cells largely mimics leukocyte transendothelial migration from the blood circulation into sites of tissue inflammation [26] and this is the point which will be developed here. Flow experiments showed that melanoma cell line A375M is able to adhere strongly to endothelial cells Human Umbilical Vein Endothelial Cells (HUVEC) activated with interleukin IL-1, in VCAM-1-dependant way [27]. In the case of melanoma, it was shown that the cells express molecules typically involved in the adhesion and transmigration of immune cells. In fact, melanomas possess on their surface CXCL8 chemokine receptors, CXCR1 and CXCR2 (inhibition of these molecules reduces migration of melanoma in vitro) [28] and SDF-1 receptor, CXCR4 [29]. They are also able to express adhesion molecules such as ICAM-1 whose expression increases during melanoma progression [30], as well as integrins as VLA4 [31]. The latter may promote metastasis by interaction with VCAM-1 (present on the surface of endothelial cells) [32]–[34]. The role of cell adhesion molecules such as E-selectin and P-selectin has also been studied extensively in the process of inflammation [35].

Indeed, leukocyte adhesion during inflammation is thought to proceed in a cascade-like fashion, in which selectins are responsible for leukocyte capture and rolling, and integrins for mediating firm adhesion and transmigration [36], [37]. Among these integrins, Leukocyte Function-Associated antigen-1 (LFA-1; αLβ2) composed of two chains, CD11a and CD18, has been extensively described for its essential role in leukocyte extravasation [26], [38]. It functions as a receptor for ICAM-1 (CD54) [39]–[41]. Besides its role in the firm adhesion of leukocytes to the endothelium, it appears to be a major player in transendothelial migration [38], [42]. LFA-1 has been studied in different tumors. It has been shown for example that expression of LFA-1 correlates with the aggressiveness of myeloma [43] and is present in metastatic gastrointestinal carcinomas [44]. LFA-1 has been shown to promote melanoma cell transmigration in vitro LFA-1 also seems to be responsible for formation of clumps (small cell aggregates), which could enhance further their extravasation capacities [45]. This is consistent with previous reports examining the migration of dendritic cells [46]or extravasation of some tumors [27], [47].

Junctional Adhesion Molecule A (JAM-A) can also interact with LFA-1 via its second membrane-proximal Ig domain [48], [49]. During leukocyte transendothelial migration, the homophilic transendothelial interactions between two molecules of JAM-A must be disrupted to enable a migrating leukocyte to pass through junctions [50] and it has been shown that LFA-1 binding to JAM-A destabilizes the JAM-A homophilic interaction, thus allowing transendothelial migration to proceed [51].

The JAM family is composed of three classical members, JAM-A [50], [52], JAM-B [53], [54] and JAM-C [55], [56]. The role of the JAM proteins has been studied in some cancer cells [57]. It has been demonstrated that JAM-C promotes metastasis by enhancing the adhesion of fibrosarcoma to extracellular matrices [58] and mediating lung carcinoma–endothelial cell interactions [59]. In melanoma, there is evidence in vitro for a differential role of the JAM proteins in melanoma transendothelial migration, where JAM-C promotes their transendothelial migration but JAM-A inhibits this phenomenon [60]. The role of Jam-C has been confirmed in vivo by Langer et al [61]. Moreover, a recent study demonstrated that JAM-B expressed by endothelial cells contributes to murine B16 melanoma cell metastasis through its interaction with JAM-C on tumor cells and might mediate melanoma cell adhesion to primary Lung Microvascular Endothelial Cells [62].

The expression in melanoma cell lines of such molecules which are normally found in immune cells might appear unexpected. However other immune cell specific molecules have already been shown to be expressed on these tumors as for example MHCII (major histocompatibility complex, Class II) [63].

Moreover it should be mentioned that melanoma transendothelial migration was also shown to involve nitric oxide [64], N-cadherin and beta-catenin signaling pathway [65], phospholipase C, integrin alpha(v)beta(3) and cell adhesion molecule L1[66] and neutrophils [67].

4.) Neo-Colonization

Site of metastasis do not seem to be random. In fact, different types of tumors show different preferential localizations. In the case of melanoma, metastases occur preferentially in the brain, lungs and liver. This observation has led Stephen Paget as early as 1889 to propose the hypothesis of "Seed and Soil". According this theory, a secondary tumor can only be established if the seed (the tumor cell) can grow in the ground (soil), that is to say if the microenvironment is compatible with the properties and needs of the cell [68]. This affinity involves different mechanisms, first being the expression of different adhesion molecules on blood vessels according to the tissue. It also seems that a chemotactic axis attract cells having different chemokine receptors specific for an organ. For example, melanomas expressing CXCR4 preferentially metastasize to the lungs and liver, bone and lymph nodes as these organs produce SDF-1 [69]. Melanomas can also express the receptor CXCR1 (whose ligand is CXCL8) which plays an important role in transendothelial migration, and CXCR2 (receptor of CXCL1 and CXCL8), which will promote the development of metastases lung [28], [70], [71]. The expression of CCR10 will promote skin metastasis while expression of CCR9 will favor small intestine metastasis [72].

However, the microenvironment of the metastatic organ may also facilitate metastatic growth of disseminated tumor cells at that site including the creation of a pre-metastatic niche [73]. A recent study has shown that the metastatic microenvironment (brain in this case) also takes part in shaping the malignancy phenotype of melanoma cells both before such tumor cells reach this microenvironment as well as during their residence at that microenvironment, here through CCR4 [74]. Moreover, Han et al. have shown that in the premetastatic phase, the melanoma induces pulmonary inflammation response, changes the lung environment and then facilitates lung metastasis [75]. The microenvironment also seems to be a source of site-specific chemo attractants for tumor cells and the formation of offer a favorable milieu to sustain metastatic cells and promote their propagation by providing survival and proliferation signals.

Finally, the tumor cells must have an intrinsic ability to develop effectively at the new site.

III. Melanoma Plasticity: Involvement in Development of Metastatic Cells

Modification of melanoma properties is essential for the appearance of the metastatic phenotype. Many studies have shown the influence of the tumor microenvironment in this phenomenon, and have associated the appearance of metastatic cells with genetic mutations. These observations do not well explain the adaptive capacity of metastatic cells to new “soil” in neo-colonization and the high frequency of tumor relapse. Recently different studies have suggested the existence of a large adaptability of melanoma cells, suggesting a cellular plasticity.

1.) Melanoma Tumor Cell Plasticity: Influence of the Tumor Microenvironment

A tumor is not a collection of relatively homogeneous cancer cells; it is composed of cancer cells with heterogeneous phenotypes and several other cell types such as fibroblasts and immune cells. Thus it could be considered a type of “organ” whose complexity approaches and may even exceed that of normal healthy tissues, where the different cell types interact and produce factors leading to the creation of a tumor microenvironment [76]. For example, inflammatory immune cells will produce factors promoting proliferation, angiogenesis and invasion such as EGF, VEGF, bFGF and MMPs. Fibroblasts can interact with cancer cells; co-culture experiments show that normal fibroblasts are capable of directing the cancer cells to a more benign phenotype, while fibroblasts activated by tumor cells can stimulate tumor growth [77], [78]. In some cases, genetic alterations of stromal cells precede genotypic changes in epithelial cells [79].

In addition to the influence of the different cell types, hypoxia is another important factor which influences the tumor microenvironment. As we have seen earlier, hypoxia induces the production of pro-angiogenic factors and promotes the selection of the most aggressive cells. Interestingly hypoxia is essential for maintaining the undifferentiated state of human embryonic stem cells [80], [81] and promotes the development of a dedifferentiated phenotype in neuroblastoma cells and breast cancer [82]. More recently it has been shown that hypoxia inhibits the expression of the transcription factor MITF, which seems to be a central player in melanoma plasticity, and increases the tumorigenic and metastatic potential of melanoma cells [83].

These data showed the importance of tumor microenvironment in cancer cell fate and suggested the existence of cellular plasticity. In the case of melanoma, the first observations of the existence of a phenotypic reversibility were made in 1983 on mouse melanoma cells (B16.C3). The differentiation of these cells, induced by culturing in defined medium, led to the appearance of pigmentation, proliferation arrest and melanocyte morphology. When these differentiated cells were cultivated in proliferative medium, some of them were able to return to their initial phenotype, with loss of some pigmentation and a recovery of their growth capacities [84]. These early experiments thus showed the ability of some melanoma cells to change their phenotype depending on environmental conditions.

In agreement with these observations, other studies have shown the influence of the microenvironment on tumor development. Experiments of injection of melanoma cells into chicken and zebra fish embryos have revealed the ability of these cells to reprogram. Injected cells followed the neural crest cell (NCC) migratory pathways (since melanocytes originate from embryonic NCC), colonized the host regions of NCC and re-expressed melanocyte markers which were not expressed before the injection [85], [86].

These experiments showed that melanoma cells were able to be reprogrammed into cells with less aggressive phonotype. Moreover culturing melanoma cells in a medium pre-conditioned with aggressive melanoma cells induced reprogramming in aggressive phenotype. These reprogramming cells showed an increase of expression of gene imply in extracellular matrix modification and an increase of invasive capability [87].

All these data highlight the capability of melanoma cells to adapt to a new microenvironment, and thus highlight the plasticity of melanoma cells.

2.) Phenotype-Switching: Implication in the Metastatic Cells Emergence and in Neo-Colonization

As previously described, microenvironment can influence the behavior of melanoma cells and can induce aggressive phenotype that implies plasticity of cells. Another aspect of tumor development to consider is the existence of heterogeneity. Tumors are not composed of a single cell population but several sub-populations which have different metastatic potential, different proliferative potential and different sensitivity to drugs, as well as variable morphologic phenotype and variable expression of surface markers [88]. As heterogeneity and plasticity make it difficult to develop treatments targeting all subpopulations of a tumor, it is important to understand how this heterogeneity arises and how to regulate plasticity to develop new treatments. For this purpose, several models of cancer cell invasion have been proposed, each providing an explanation for the existence of this observed functional and phenotypic heterogeneity (i.e. clonal evolution, cancer stem cell and phenotype switching). Among these theories only phenotype-switching theory takes into account melanoma cell plasticity and offers an explanation for appearance of metastatic cells. Here we will present the different aspects of this new theory and its involvement in development of new treatments.

a.) The Phenotype-Switching Model: Central Role of MITF

The transcription factor MITF is involved in several cellular functions such as differentiation, proliferation, senescence, cell survival [89]. MITF siRNA experiments have highlighted its dual function in the development of melanoma. Decrease of MITF expression induces cell cycle arrest in G0/G1 depending on stabilization of p27 inhibitor, accompanied by a reorganization of the actin cytoskeleton and an increase in capacity of invasion [90]. Carreira *et al* proposed a model to explain MITF's role in melanoma progression, in melanocyte development and to reconcile its pro-and anti-proliferative functions. They suggested that MITF has a dose effect; the absence of MITF induces apoptosis, low levels of MITF induce cell cycle arrest and increase of invasive capacity, an intermediary level induced proliferation and an important quantity of MITF induces differentiation (Figure 3). In conclusion, this model proposes a central role for MITF in the regulation of invasive and proliferative functions. In this model, final differentiation and apoptosis are the two extreme MITF functions and are not reversible, whereas the intermediate events are reversible and dynamic [90]. It also indicates a precise regulation of MITF expression and its activity, involving several signaling pathways affected by mutations or by tumor micro-environment as we have seen previously.

In agreement with these results, microarray analysis of different cell lines (melanocytes, primary melanoma and metastatic melanoma), performed by Hoek *et al* [91] helped to distinguish two gene expression profiles: a proliferative profile and an invasive profile. Cells with proliferative profile expressed a high level of MITF, and were sensitive to proliferative inhibition by TGFβ. Cells with invasive profile expressed low levels of MITF, and were less sensitive to TGFβ [91]. Following these first data, in vitro experiments showed that cells with the proliferative gene expression profile are more proliferative and less invasive than cells with invasive gene expression profile (Figure 4) [92]. In accordance with the difference of proliferative capacity of melanoma cells observed, in vivo experiments have shown a delay in appearance of tumors when injected cells have an invasive phenotype compared to the cells with a proliferative phenotype (14 +/- 3 days for proliferative phenotype vs 59 +/- 11 days for invasive phenotype). However, although the injected cells were initially "proliferative" or "invasive" and had a homogeneous phenotype, tumors were indistinguishable with immunohistochemistry analyses with MITF or Ki67 markers. In these two cases, the two markers were detected on the periphery of the tumor, suggesting the influence of the micro-environment in the MITF gene expression regulation, according with the level of hypoxia as previously seen [92].

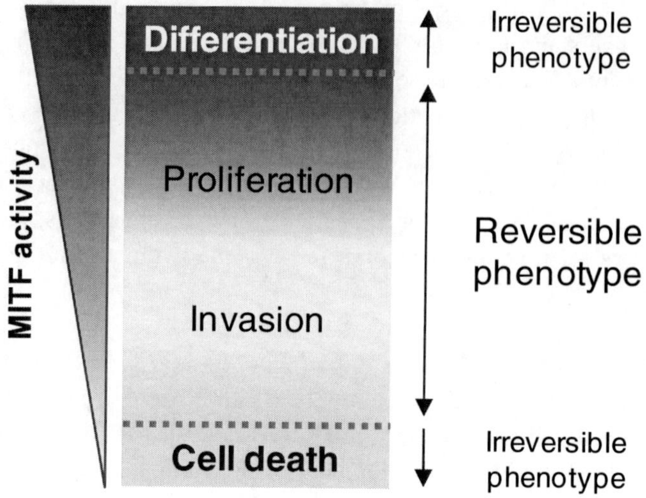

Figure 3. The transcription factor MITF contributes to tumor development and involves epigenetic phenomena. MITF activity is important in the control of cell proliferation, migration, apoptosis and differentiation. These last two phenomena are irreversible in contrast to the proliferation and migration, while involving epigenetic phenomena.

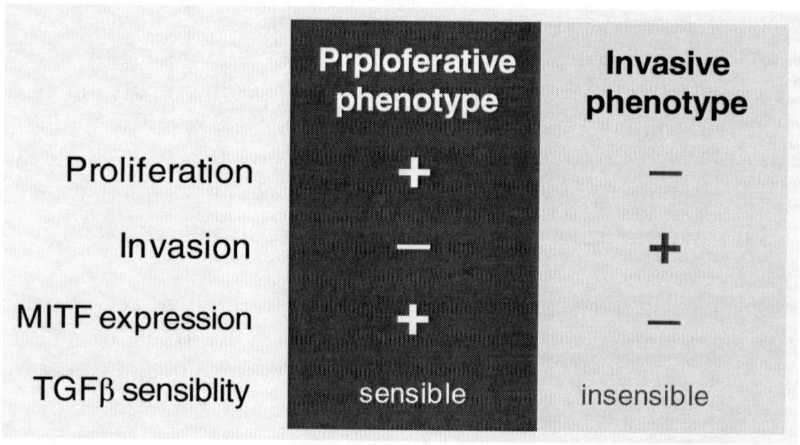

Figure 4. Characteristics and reversibility of invasive and proliferative phenotypes described by Hoek et al. Summary of the different characteristics of the two phenotypes described by Hoek et al.

Globally, these results suggest a capacity of reversion of melanoma cells notably in the case of MITF expression and also show the cellular plasticity of melanoma. In addition all these data highlight the importance of MITF in the phenotype switching of melanoma cells [90], [92].

All the more Carreira *et al* and Hoek *et al* proposed a developmental model which include cell plasticity and therefore could explain tumor heterogeneity and metastatic cells emergence. This model suggests the existence of at least two sub-population (i.e. proliferative population and invasive population), whose phenotypes are interchangeable during tumor development in response to changes in the microenvironment. Phenotypic changes will be occurring by progressive transition of gene expression with or without cell division, thus explaining the observed heterogeneity. Proliferative and invasive phenotypes are the extreme phenotypes in this model in which invasive cells present a decrease of proliferative potential (Figure 5).

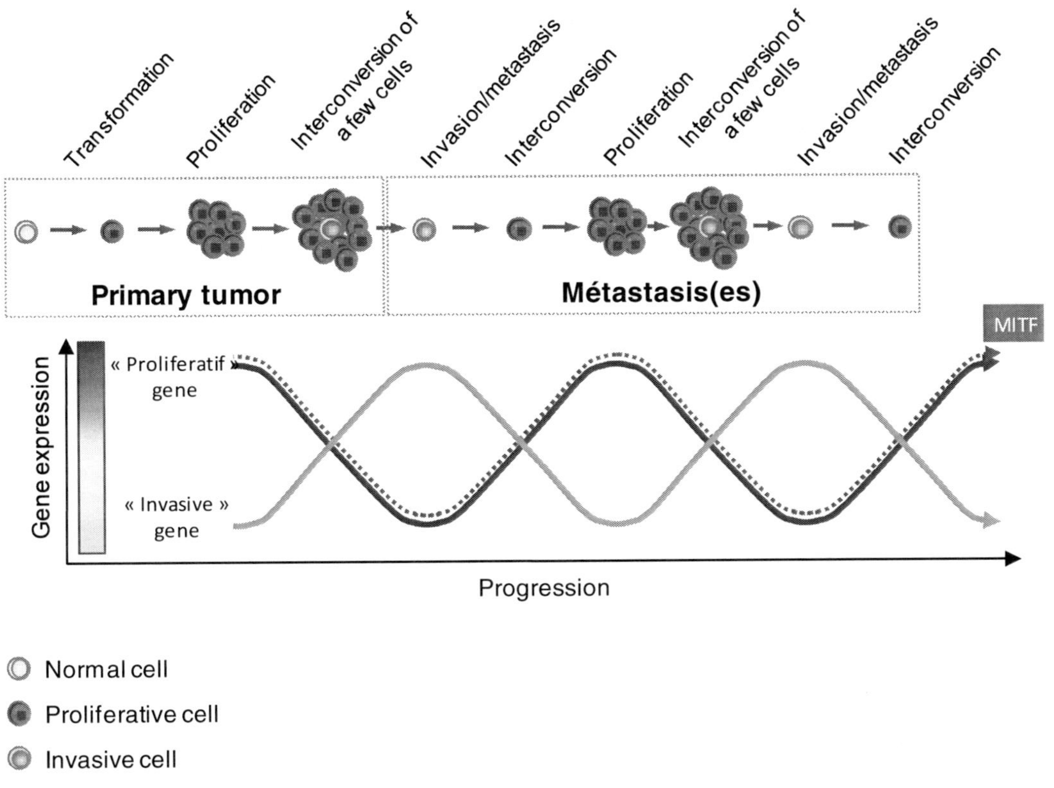

Figure 5. Melanoma progression depending on the phenotype-switching model described by Hoek et al. Gene expression panel varies gradually in response to microenvironment modification leading to change in invasive and proliferative capaticy. MTIF gene expression follows proliferative genes expression panel.

Accordingly to this model, recent publications by Cheli et al have confirmed the central role of MITF [83], [93]. Firstly, they showed that transient depletion of MITF by siRNA in B16 cell line favors the development of tumor in mice. Indeed if MITF is constitutively silenced by shRNA they do not observe tumor. These results evidenced the necessity of MITF re-expression for tumor development. Secondly, in agreement with the phenotype-switching model, they observed cell dedifferentiation of cells in absence of MITF and they observed increase of Oct4 and Nanog (two stem cell marker) [93]. And finally, they observed a significant increased in the number of visceral metastases (ovaries, kidneys, intestine and heart) in mice that received siMITF-transfected B16 cells, regardless the number of injected cells [83].

All this data suggest the importance of the transcription factor MITF in the regulation of phenotype-switching in melanoma. However some recent studies also suggest the involvement of new other factors involved of the regulation of this phenomenon.

b.) Other Molecular Aspect of the Model

Influence of Hypoxia on MITF Expression

As describe above, hypoxia is associated with poor prognostic in the case of melanoma and Bedogni et al have evidence that hypoxia (in association with Akt/mTOR pathway) is an essential factor in development of this cancer [7]. More recently Widmer et al have evidenced that hypoxia induced metastatic phenotype transition [94]. In agreement with these data and with phenotype switching theory, Cheli et al observed a decrease of MITF expression in melanoma cell lines grown in hypoxic conditions, in association with a stabilization of the transcription faction HIF1α, suggesting that hypoxic conditions repress MITF expression in melanoma cell lines. According to these data they observed an inverse correlation between MITF and HIF1α when they performed immunostaining of human tumors, i.e. they observed increase of HIF1α labeling with distance from the blood vessel while MITF labeling was stronger around the blood vessel. But at the molecular level they showed that HIF1α does not regulated directly MITF [95] [83]. These data suggest that hypoxia is important in regulation of the phenotype switching.

Influence of the Wnt Pathway in Phenotype Switching

Hypoxia seems to be an important factor in regulation of MITF, but it seems not to be the only one. Indeed, MITF expression was regulated by over cellular signaling pathway such as Wnt/β-catenin, Akt; and MITF activity was regulated by Akt and MAPK-Erk pathways. Interestingly these pathways have been involved in melanoma development.

Wnt/β-catenin pathway seems to be implicated in phenotype switching. Interestingly, DNA microarray analyses on 86 cultures of melanoma have conducted authors to identify gene expression co-regulation suggesting the influence of TGF-β and Wnt/β-catenin in the changing of phenotype of melanoma cells. Following these results they suggested that Wnt/β-catenin was activated in proliferative, non metastatic melanoma cells (which conduct to increase expression of MITF notably). On the opposite, they proposed that Wnt5A secretion by melanoma cells in response to inflammatory signaling or hypoxia induced invasive phenotype [91]. Immunostaining on melanoma tumors from patient have allowed to show an inverse correlation between MITF and Glut-1 (a hypoxia marker)/Wnt5A [96]. In this model β-catenin seems to be important for the control of the phenotype switching, though its nuclear distribution and activity did not vary between the two phenotypes. Results obtain by Eichhof et al suggest that β-catenin effects were regulated by two of its co-factor, LEF1 which expression is correlated with proliferative phenotype and TCF4 which expression is correlated with invasive phenotype [97]. Interestingly they observed, in accordance with Hoek model proposed in 2006, that LEF1 repressed TCF4 and Wnt5A and that exogenous Wnt5A suppressed proliferative phenotype of melanoma cells.

These last results increase the complexity of the molecular model of phenotype switching and evidence a multifactorial control.

Influence of Chromatin Remodeling Protein in Phenotype Switching and Akt Pathway

All the previous data involved directly or indirectly MITF in the control of phenotype switching and therefore metastasis. Another publication has also raised the possibility of a regulator in chromatin remodeling in the control of phenotype switching. A comparison between a transcriptome of melanoma cells line in bi-dimensional culture condition (mimicking proliferative phenotype) with melanoma cells line in three dimensional (invasive phenotype) allowed to identify PHF19 (PHD Finger protein 19, a member of PRC2 complex [98]) as an important factor in phenotype switching [99], [100]. Indeed PHF19 siRNA transfected cells present a decrease of proliferative capacity and an increase of invasive capacity. Interestingly PHF19 seems to be implicated in cellular differentiation during development, as it allows gene silencing in association with PRC2 complex [101]. But PHF19 does not seem the central player of the control of the phenotype switching, as the study evidenced that Akt pathway is involved in this phenomenon. The inhibition of this pathway induced the decrease of PHF19 gene expression and increase the expression of pluripotency genes Oct4 and Nanog [100] (these last two genes were upregulated in siRNA MITF transfected cells [90]). These last data suggest a complex function of Akt pathway melanoma development where the three isoforms of Akt could have different functions as it has been described for breast cancer [102], [103].

Conclusion: Implication in Therapeutic Approaches

Since the discovery of dacarbazine 30 years ago, little progress has been made in the treatment of metastatic melanoma where the 10 years survival rate for patients with metastatic dissemination is less than 10%, and the frequency of skin cancers is constantly increasing. New alternatives are therefore urgently required.

All these new results provide an interesting approach using for example blocking antibodies against adherent molecules as JAM-C or LFA-1 to control melanoma metastasis, with a thorough analysis of their specific roles depending on the cell types analyzed.

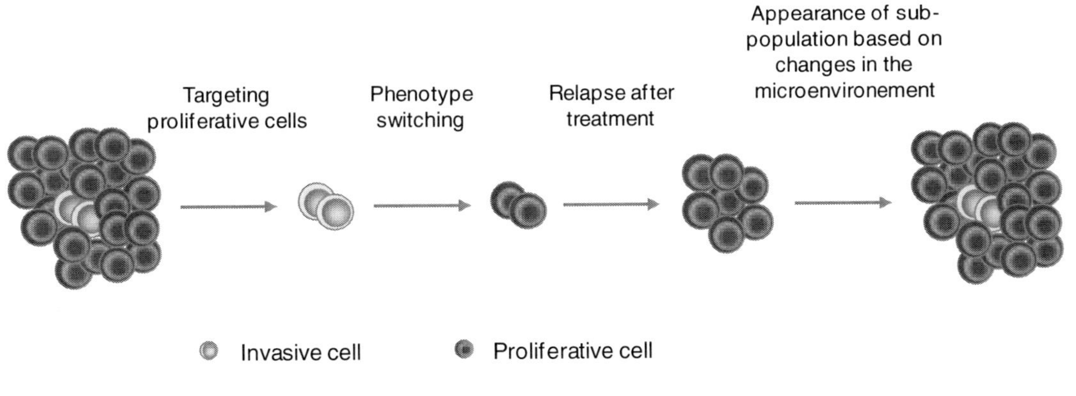

Figure 6. Consequences of the use of conventional therapies based on the phenotype switching model. Use of conventional treatment only proliferative cells and targeted. After stopping treatment non-proliferative cells will change their phenotype and forming new tumor.

Taking account the phenotype switching theory, it can be assumed that cells will resist to treatment thanks to phenotype changes. Most existing treatments targeting only proliferating cells, only this population will be affected. The less proliferative cells (invasive in the model of Hoek et al) will be set apart and upon discontinuation of treatment may grow by changing their phenotype (Figure 6). Hence the development of new therapies is made more difficult by the adaptability of these tumor cells. It is therefore necessary to understand how the phenotypic changes take place in order to control and direct the sub-populations in order to identify specific markers of these sub-populations and develop new targeted therapies.

References

[1] A. J. Miller et M. C. Mihm Jr, « Melanoma », *N. Engl. J. Med.*, vol. 355, n° 1, p. 51-65, juill. 2006.

[2] A. Jemal, R. Siegel, J. Xu, et E. Ward, « Cancer statistics, 2010 », *CA. Cancer J. Clin.*, vol. 60, n° 5, p. 277-300, oct. 2010.

[3] S. Bhatia, S. S. Tykodi, et J. A. Thompson, « Treatment of metastatic melanoma: an overview », *Oncol. Williston Park N*, vol. 23, n° 6, p. 488-496, mai 2009.

[4] Y. Hegerfeldt, M. Tusch, E.-B. Bröcker, et P. Friedl, « Collective cell movement in primary melanoma explants: plasticity of cell-cell interaction, beta1-integrin function, and migration strategies », *Cancer Res.*, vol. 62, n° 7, p. 2125-2130, avr. 2002.

[5] R. Sullivan et C. H. Graham, « Hypoxia-driven selection of the metastatic phenotype », *Cancer Metastasis Rev.*, vol. 26, n° 2, p. 319-331, juin 2007.

[6] P. Vaupel, D. K. Kelleher, et M. Höckel, « Oxygen status of malignant tumors: pathogenesis of hypoxia and significance for tumor therapy », *Semin. Oncol.*, vol. 28, n° 2 Suppl 8, p. 29-35, avr. 2001.

[7] B. Bedogni, S. M. Welford, D. S. Cassarino, B. J. Nickoloff, A. J. Giaccia, et M. B. Powell, « The hypoxic microenvironment of the skin contributes to Akt-mediated melanocyte transformation », *Cancer Cell*, vol. 8, n° 6, p. 443-454, déc. 2005.

[8] M. A. Gimbrone Jr, S. B. Leapman, R. S. Cotran, et J. Folkman, « Tumor dormancy in vivo by prevention of neovascularization », *J. Exp. Med.*, vol. 136, n° 2, p. 261-276, août 1972.

[9] A. J. Maniotis, R. Folberg, A. Hess, E. A. Seftor, L. M. Gardner, J. Pe'er, J. M. Trent, P. S. Meltzer, et M. J. Hendrix, « Vascular channel formation by human melanoma cells in vivo and in vitro: vasculogenic mimicry », *Am. J. Pathol.*, vol. 155, n° 3, p. 739-752, sept. 1999.

[10] S. Zhang, D. Zhang, Y. Wang, W. Zhao, H. Guo, X. Zhao, et B. Sun, « Morphologic research of microcirculation patterns in human and animal melanoma », *Med. Oncol. Northwood Lond. Engl.*, vol. 23, n° 3, p. 403-409, 2006.

[11] D. M. McDonald, L. Munn, et R. K. Jain, « Vasculogenic mimicry: how convincing, how novel, and how significant? », *Am. J. Pathol.*, vol. 156, n° 2, p. 383-388, févr. 2000.

[12] F. Spinella, V. Caprara, V. Di Castro, L. Rosanò, R. Cianfrocca, P. G. Natali, et A. Bagnato, « Endothelin-1 induces the transactivation of vascular endothelial growth

factor receptor-3 and modulates cell migration and vasculogenic mimicry in melanoma cells », *J. Mol. Med. Berl. Ger.*, vol. 91, n° 3, p. 395-405, mars 2013.

[13] K. De Bock, M. Mazzone, et P. Carmeliet, « Antiangiogenic therapy, hypoxia, and metastasis: risky liaisons, or not? », *Nat. Rev. Clin. Oncol.*, vol. 8, n° 7, p. 393-404, 2011.

[14] J. M. Lehmann, G. Riethmüller, et J. P. Johnson, « MUC18, a marker of tumor progression in human melanoma, shows sequence similarity to the neural cell adhesion molecules of the immunoglobulin superfamily », *Proc. Natl. Acad. Sci. U. S. A.*, vol. 86, n° 24, p. 9891-9895, déc. 1989.

[15] L. Hao, J. R. Ha, P. Kuzel, E. Garcia, et S. Persad, « Cadherin switch from E- to N-cadherin in melanoma progression is regulated by the PI3K/PTEN pathway through Twist and Snail », *Br. J. Dermatol.*, vol. 166, n° 6, p. 1184-1197, juin 2012.

[16] E. Candrea, S. Senila, C. Tatomir, et R. Cosgarea, « Active and inactive forms of matrix metalloproteinases 2 and 9 in cutaneous melanoma », *Int. J. Dermatol.*, oct. 2012.

[17] M. Nakamura et Y. Tokura, « Epithelial-mesenchymal transition in the skin », *J. Dermatol. Sci.*, vol. 61, n° 1, p. 7-13, janv. 2011.

[18] M. B. Palmer, P. Majumder, M. R. Green, P. A. Wade, et J. M. Boss, « A 3' enhancer controls snail expression in melanoma cells », *Cancer Res.*, vol. 67, n° 13, p. 6113-6120, juill. 2007.

[19] J. A. Joyce et J. W. Pollard, « Microenvironmental regulation of metastasis », *Nat. Rev. Cancer*, vol. 9, n° 4, p. 239-252, avr. 2009.

[20] B. Nieswandt, M. Hafner, B. Echtenacher, et D. N. Männel, « Lysis of tumor cells by natural killer cells in mice is impeded by platelets », *Cancer Res.*, vol. 59, n° 6, p. 1295-1300, mars 1999.

[21] R. L. Barnhill, P. J. Benson, et C. Lugassy, « Conspicuous angiotropism of malignant melanoma involving the brain: implications for extravascular migratory metastasis », *Am. J. Dermatopathol.*, vol. 31, n° 2, p. 205-208, avr. 2009.

[22] R. Barnhill, K. Dy, et C. Lugassy, « Angiotropism in cutaneous melanoma: a prognostic factor strongly predicting risk for metastasis », *J. Invest. Dermatol.*, vol. 119, n° 3, p. 705-706, sept. 2002.

[23] R. L. Barnhill et C. Lugassy, «Angiotropic malignant melanoma and extravascular migratory metastasis: description of 36 cases with emphasis on a new mechanism of tumour spread», *Pathology (Phila.)*, vol. 36, n° 5, p. 485-490, oct. 2004.

[24] C. Lugassy, H. K. Kleinman, J. A. Engbring, D. R. Welch, J. F. Harms, R. Rufner, G. Ghanem, S. R. Patierno, et R. L. Barnhill, « Pericyte-like location of GFP-tagged melanoma cells: ex vivo and in vivo studies of extravascular migratory metastasis«, *Am. J. Pathol.*, vol. 164, n° 4, p. 1191-1198, avr. 2004.

[25] R. L. Barnhill, H. Kutzner, B. Schmidt, L. Ali, M. Bagot, A. Janin, et C. Lugassy, «Atypical spitzoid melanocytic neoplasms with angiotropism: a potential mechanism of locoregional involvement», *Am. J. Dermatopathol.*, vol. 33, n° 3, p. 236-243, mai 2011.

[26] C. Strell et F. Entschladen, « Extravasation of leukocytes in comparison to tumor cells», *Cell Commun. Signal. Ccs*, vol. 6, p. 10, 2008.

[27] R. Giavazzi, M. Foppolo, R. Dossi, et A. Remuzzi, « Rolling and adhesion of human tumor cells on vascular endothelium under physiological flow conditions», *J. Clin. Invest.*, vol. 92, n° 6, p. 3038-3044, déc. 1993.

[28] M. L. Varney, A. Li, B. J. Dave, C. D. Bucana, S. L. Johansson, et R. K. Singh, « Expression of CXCR1 and CXCR2 receptors in malignant melanoma with different metastatic potential and their role in interleukin-8 (CXCL-8)-mediated modulation of metastatic phenotype«, *Clin. Exp. Metastasis*, vol. 20, n° 8, p. 723-731, 2003.

[29] M. M. Robledo, R. A. Bartolome, N. Longo, J. M. Rodríguez-Frade, M. Mellado, I. Longo, G. N. van Muijen, P. Sánchez-Mateos, et J. Teixidó, « Expression of functional chemokine receptors CXCR3 and CXCR4 on human melanoma cells«, *J. Biol. Chem.*, vol. 276, n° 48, p. 45098-45105, nov. 2001.

[30] J. P. Johnson, « Cell adhesion molecules in the development and progression of malignant melanoma«, *Cancer Metastasis Rev.*, vol. 18, n° 3, p. 345-357, 1999.

[31] D. Schadendorf, J. Heidel, C. Gawlik, L. Suter, et B. M. Czarnetzki, « Association with clinical outcome of expression of VLA-4 in primary cutaneous malignant melanoma as well as P-selectin and E-selectin on intratumoral vessels«, *J. Natl. Cancer Inst.*, vol. 87, n° 5, p. 366-371, mars 1995.

[32] H. Okahara, H. Yagita, K. Miyake, et K. Okumura, « Involvement of very late activation antigen 4 (VLA-4) and vascular cell adhesion molecule 1 (VCAM-1) in tumor necrosis factor alpha enhancement of experimental metastasis«, *Cancer Res.*, vol. 54, n° 12, p. 3233-3236, juin 1994.

[33] A. Garofalo, R. G. Chirivi, C. Foglieni, R. Pigott, R. Mortarini, I. Martin-Padura, A. Anichini, A. J. Gearing, F. Sanchez-Madrid, et E. Dejana, « Involvement of the very late antigen 4 integrin on melanoma in interleukin 1-augmented experimental metastases», *Cancer Res.*, vol. 55, n° 2, p. 414-419, janv. 1995.

[34] E. H. Danen, C. Marcinkiewicz, I. M. Cornelissen, A. A. van Kraats, J. A. Pachter, D. J. Ruiter, S. Niewiarowski, et G. N. van Muijen, « The disintegrin eristostatin interferes with integrin alpha 4 beta 1 function and with experimental metastasis of human melanoma cells«, *Exp. Cell Res.*, vol. 238, n° 1, p. 188-196, janv. 1998.

[35] H. Kobayashi, K. C. Boelte, et P. C. Lin, « Endothelial cell adhesion molecules and cancer progression«, *Curr. Med. Chem.*, vol. 14, n° 4, p. 377-386, 2007.

[36] E. C. Butcher, « Leukocyte-endothelial cell recognition: three (or more) steps to specificity and diversity«, *Cell*, vol. 67, n° 6, p. 1033-1036, déc. 1991.

[37] U. Jung, K. E. Norman, K. Scharffetter-Kochanek, A. L. Beaudet, et K. Ley, « Transit time of leukocytes rolling through venules controls cytokine-induced inflammatory cell recruitment in vivo«, *J. Clin. Invest.*, vol. 102, n° 8, p. 1526-1533, oct. 1998.

[38] J. L. Dunne, C. M. Ballantyne, A. L. Beaudet, et K. Ley, « Control of leukocyte rolling velocity in TNF-alpha-induced inflammation by LFA-1 and Mac-1», *Blood*, vol. 99, n° 1, p. 336-341, janv. 2002.

[39] M. L. Dustin, R. Rothlein, A. K. Bhan, C. A. Dinarello, et T. A. Springer, « Induction by IL 1 and interferon-gamma: tissue distribution, biochemistry, and function of a natural adherence molecule (ICAM-1)», *J. Immunol. Baltim. Md 1950*, vol. 137, n° 1, p. 245-254, juill. 1986.

[40] K. A. Roebuck et A. Finnegan, « Regulation of intercellular adhesion molecule-1 (CD54) gene expression«, *J. Leukoc. Biol.*, vol. 66, n° 6, p. 876-888, déc. 1999.

[41] R. Rothlein, M. L. Dustin, S. D. Marlin, et T. A. Springer, « A human intercellular adhesion molecule (ICAM-1) distinct from LFA-1», *J. Immunol. Baltim. Md 1950*, vol. 137, n° 4, p. 1270-1274, août 1986.

[42] Z. M. Ding, J. E. Babensee, S. I. Simon, H. Lu, J. L. Perrard, D. C. Bullard, X. Y. Dai, S. K. Bromley, M. L. Dustin, M. L. Entman, C. W. Smith, et C. M. Ballantyne, «Relative contribution of LFA-1 and Mac-1 to neutrophil adhesion and migration», *J. Immunol. Baltim. Md 1950*, vol. 163, n° 9, p. 5029-5038, nov. 1999.

[43] T. Tatsumi, C. Shimazaki, H. Goto, S. Araki, Y. Sudo, N. Yamagata, E. Ashihara, T. Inaba, N. Fujita, et M. Nakagawa, « Expression of adhesion molecules on myeloma cells», *Jpn. J. Cancer Res. Gann*, vol. 87, n° 8, p. 837-842, août 1996.

[44] M. V. Gulubova, «Expression of cell adhesion molecules, their ligands and tumour necrosis factor alpha in the liver of patients with metastatic gastrointestinal carcinomas», *Histochem. J.*, vol. 34, n° 1-2, p. 67-77, févr. 2002.

[45] S. Ghislin, D. Obino, S. Middendorp, N. Boggetto, C. Alcaide-Loridan, et F. Deshayes, « LFA-1 and ICAM-1 expression induced during melanoma-endothelial cell co-culture favors the transendothelial migration of melanoma cell lines in vitro », *Bmc Cancer*, vol. 12, p. 455, 2012.

[46] A. M. Witkowska et M. H. Borawska, « Soluble intercellular adhesion molecule-1 (sICAM-1): an overview», *Eur. Cytokine Netw.*, vol. 15, n° 2, p. 91-98, juin 2004.

[47] M. Yamada, K. Yanaba, K. Takehara, et S. Sato, « Clinical significance of serum levels of soluble intercellular adhesion molecule-1 and soluble L-selectin in malignant melanoma », *Arch. Dermatol. Res.*, vol. 297, n° 6, p. 256-260, déc. 2005.

[48] L. Fraemohs, R. R. Koenen, G. Ostermann, B. Heinemann, et C. Weber, « The functional interaction of the beta 2 integrin lymphocyte function-associated antigen-1 with junctional adhesion molecule-A is mediated by the I domain », *J. Immunol. Baltim. Md 1950*, vol. 173, n° 10, p. 6259-6264, nov. 2004.

[49] G. Ostermann, K. S. C. Weber, A. Zernecke, A. Schröder, et C. Weber, « JAM-1 is a ligand of the beta(2) integrin LFA-1 involved in transendothelial migration of leukocytes », *Nat. Immunol.*, vol. 3, n° 2, p. 151-158, févr. 2002.

[50] L. A. Williams, I. Martin-Padura, E. Dejana, N. Hogg, et D. L. Simmons, « Identification and characterisation of human Junctional Adhesion Molecule (JAM) », *Mol. Immunol.*, vol. 36, n° 17, p. 1175-1188, déc. 1999.

[51] E. P. Wojcikiewicz, R. R. Koenen, L. Fraemohs, J. Minkiewicz, H. Azad, C. Weber, et V. T. Moy, « LFA-1 binding destabilizes the JAM-A homophilic interaction during leukocyte transmigration », *Biophys. J.*, vol. 96, n° 1, p. 285-293, janv. 2009.

[52] I. Martìn-Padura, S. Lostaglio, M. Schneemann, L. Williams, M. Romano, P. Fruscella, C. Panzeri, A. Stoppacciaro, L. Ruco, A. Villa, D. Simmons, et E. Dejana, « Junctional adhesion molecule, a novel member of the immunoglobulin superfamily that distributes at intercellular junctions and modulates monocyte transmigration », *J. Cell Biol.*, vol. 142, n° 1, p. 117-127, juill. 1998.

[53] S. A. Cunningham, M. P. Arrate, J. M. Rodriguez, R. J. Bjercke, P. Vanderslice, A. P. Morris, et T. A. Brock, « A novel protein with homology to the junctional adhesion

molecule. Characterization of leukocyte interactions », *J. Biol. Chem.*, vol. 275, n° 44, p. 34750-34756, nov. 2000.

[54] D. Palmeri, A. van Zante, C. C. Huang, S. Hemmerich, et S. D. Rosen, « Vascular endothelial junction-associated molecule, a novel member of the immunoglobulin superfamily, is localized to intercellular boundaries of endothelial cells », *J. Biol. Chem.*, vol. 275, n° 25, p. 19139-19145, juin 2000.

[55] M. P. Arrate, J. M. Rodriguez, T. M. Tran, T. A. Brock, et S. A. Cunningham, « Cloning of human junctional adhesion molecule 3 (JAM3) and its identification as the JAM2 counter-receptor », *J. Biol. Chem.*, vol. 276, n° 49, p. 45826-45832, déc. 2001.

[56] M. Aurrand-Lions, L. Duncan, C. Ballestrem, et B. A. Imhof, « JAM-2, a novel immunoglobulin superfamily molecule, expressed by endothelial and lymphatic cells », *J. Biol. Chem.*, vol. 276, n° 4, p. 2733-2741, janv. 2001.

[57] E. A. McSherry, S. F. McGee, K. Jirstrom, E. M. Doyle, D. J. Brennan, G. Landberg, P. A. Dervan, A. M. Hopkins, et W. M. Gallagher, « JAM-A expression positively correlates with poor prognosis in breast cancer patients », *Int. J. Cancer J. Int. Cancer*, vol. 125, n° 6, p. 1343-1351, sept. 2009.

[58] C. Fuse, Y. Ishida, T. Hikita, T. Asai, et N. Oku, « Junctional adhesion molecule-C promotes metastatic potential of HT1080 human fibrosarcoma », *J. Biol. Chem.*, vol. 282, n° 11, p. 8276-8283, mars 2007.

[59] S. Santoso, U. J. H. Sachs, H. Kroll, M. Linder, A. Ruf, K. T. Preissner, et T. Chavakis, « The junctional adhesion molecule 3 (JAM-3) on human platelets is a counterreceptor for the leukocyte integrin Mac-1 », *J. Exp. Med.*, vol. 196, n° 5, p. 679-691, sept. 2002.

[60] S. Ghislin, D. Obino, S. Middendorp, N. Boggetto, C. Alcaide-Loridan, et F. Deshayes, « Junctional adhesion molecules are required for melanoma cell lines transendothelial migration in vitro », *Pigment Cell Melanoma Res.*, avr. 2011.

[61] H. F. Langer, V. V. Orlova, C. Xie, S. Kaul, D. Schneider, A. S. Lonsdorf, M. Fahrleitner, E. Y. Choi, V. Dutoit, M. Pellegrini, S. Grossklaus, P. P. Nawroth, G. Baretton, S. Santoso, S. T. Hwang, B. Arnold, et T. Chavakis, « A novel function of junctional adhesion molecule-C in mediating melanoma cell metastasis », *Cancer Res.*, vol. 71, n° 12, p. 4096-4105, juin 2011.

[62] M.-L. Arcangeli, V. Frontera, F. Bardin, J. Thomassin, B. Chetaille, S. Adams, R. H. Adams, et M. Aurrand-Lions, « The Junctional Adhesion Molecule-B regulates JAM-C-dependent melanoma cell metastasis », *Febs Lett.*, vol. 586, n° 22, p. 4046-4051, nov. 2012.

[63] I. Martins, F. Deshayes, F. Baton, A. Forget, I. Ciechomska, K. Sylla, F. Aoudjit, D. Charron, R. Al-Daccak, et C. Alcaide-Loridan, « Pathologic expression of MHC class II is driven by mitogen-activated protein kinases », *Eur. J. Immunol.*, vol. 37, n° 3, p. 788-797, mars 2007.

[64] A. Carreau, C. Kieda, et C. Grillon, « Nitric oxide modulates the expression of endothelial cell adhesion molecules involved in angiogenesis and leukocyte recruitment », *Exp. Cell Res.*, vol. 317, n° 1, p. 29-41, janv. 2011.

[65] J. Qi, J. Wang, O. Romanyuk, et C.-H. Siu, « Involvement of Src family kinases in N-cadherin phosphorylation and beta-catenin dissociation during transendothelial migration of melanoma cells », *Mol. Biol. Cell*, vol. 17, n° 3, p. 1261-1272, mars 2006.

[66] E. B. Voura, R. A. Ramjeesingh, A. M. Montgomery, et C. H. Siu, « Involvement of integrin alpha(v)beta(3) and cell adhesion molecule L1 in transendothelial migration of melanoma cells », *Mol. Biol. Cell*, vol. 12, n° 9, p. 2699-2710, sept. 2001.

[67] C. Dong, M. J. Slattery, S. Liang, et H.-H. Peng, « Melanoma cell extravasation under flow conditions is modulated by leukocytes and endogenously produced interleukin 8 », *Mol. Cell. Biomech. Mcb*, vol. 2, n° 3, p. 145-159, sept. 2005.

[68] T. R. Geiger et D. S. Peeper, « Metastasis mechanisms », *Biochim. Biophys. Acta*, vol. 1796, n° 2, p. 293-308, déc. 2009.

[69] J. Kim, T. Mori, S. L. Chen, F. F. Amersi, S. R. Martinez, C. Kuo, R. R. Turner, X. Ye, A. J. Bilchik, D. L. Morton, et D. S. B. Hoon, « Chemokine receptor CXCR4 expression in patients with melanoma and colorectal cancer liver metastases and the association with disease outcome », *Ann. Surg.*, vol. 244, n° 1, p. 113-120, juill. 2006.

[70] S. Singh, M. Varney, et R. K. Singh, « Host CXCR2-dependent regulation of melanoma growth, angiogenesis, and experimental lung metastasis », *Cancer Res.*, vol. 69, n° 2, p. 411-415, janv. 2009.

[71] R. Ramjeesingh, R. Leung, et C.-H. Siu, « Interleukin-8 secreted by endothelial cells induces chemotaxis of melanoma cells through the chemokine receptor CXCR1 », *Faseb J. Off. Publ. Fed. Am. Soc. Exp. Biol.*, vol. 17, n° 10, p. 1292-1294, juill. 2003.

[72] H. Seidl, E. Richtig, H. Tilz, M. Stefan, U. Schmidbauer, M. Asslaber, K. Zatloukal, M. Herlyn, et H. Schaider, « Profiles of chemokine receptors in melanocytic lesions: de novo expression of CXCR6 in melanoma », *Hum. Pathol.*, vol. 38, n° 5, p. 768-780, mai 2007.

[73] H. Peinado, S. Lavotshkin, et D. Lyden, « The secreted factors responsible for pre-metastatic niche formation: old sayings and new thoughts », *Semin. Cancer Biol.*, vol. 21, n° 2, p. 139-146, avr. 2011.

[74] A. Klein, O. Sagi-Assif, S. Izraely, T. Meshel, M. Pasmanik-Chor, C. Nahmias, P.-O. Couraud, N. Erez, D. S. B. Hoon, et I. P. Witz, « The metastatic microenvironment: Brain-derived soluble factors alter the malignant phenotype of cutaneous and brain-metastasizing melanoma cells », *Int. J. Cancer J. Int. Cancer*, vol. 131, n° 11, p. 2509-2518, déc. 2012.

[75] M. Han, J. Xu, Y. Bi, M. Jiang, X. Xu, Q. Liu, et J. Jia, « Primary tumor regulates the pulmonary microenvironment in melanoma carcinoma model and facilitates lung metastasis », *J. Cancer Res. Clin. Oncol.*, vol. 139, n° 1, p. 57-65, janv. 2013.

[76] D. Hanahan et R. A. Weinberg, « Hallmarks of cancer: the next generation », *Cell*, vol. 144, n° 5, p. 646-674, mars 2011.

[77] S. Atula, R. Grenman, et S. Syrjänen, « Fibroblasts can modulate the phenotype of malignant epithelial cells in vitro », *Exp. Cell Res.*, vol. 235, n° 1, p. 180-187, août 1997.

[78] A. F. Olumi, G. D. Grossfeld, S. W. Hayward, P. R. Carroll, T. D. Tlsty, et G. R. Cunha, « Carcinoma-associated fibroblasts direct tumor progression of initiated human prostatic epithelium », *Cancer Res.*, vol. 59, n° 19, p. 5002-5011, oct. 1999.

[79] F. Moinfar, Y. G. Man, L. Arnould, G. L. Bratthauer, M. Ratschek, et F. A. Tavassoli, « Concurrent and independent genetic alterations in the stromal and epithelial cells of

mammary carcinoma: implications for tumorigenesis », *Cancer Res.*, vol. 60, n° 9, p. 2562-2566, mai 2000.

[80] T. Ezashi, P. Das, et R. M. Roberts, « Low O2 tensions and the prevention of differentiation of hES cells », *Proc. Natl. Acad. Sci. U. S. A.*, vol. 102, n° 13, p. 4783-4788, mars 2005.

[81] S. M. Prasad, M. Czepiel, C. Cetinkaya, K. Smigielska, S. C. Weli, H. Lysdahl, A. Gabrielsen, K. Petersen, N. Ehlers, T. Fink, S. L. Minger, et V. Zachar, « Continuous hypoxic culturing maintains activation of Notch and allows long-term propagation of human embryonic stem cells without spontaneous differentiation », *Cell Prolif.*, vol. 42, n° 1, p. 63-74, févr. 2009.

[82] H. Axelson, E. Fredlund, M. Ovenberger, G. Landberg, et S. Påhlman, « Hypoxia-induced dedifferentiation of tumor cells--a mechanism behind heterogeneity and aggressiveness of solid tumors », *Semin. Cell Dev. Biol.*, vol. 16, n° 4-5, p. 554-563, oct. 2005.

[83] Y. Cheli, S. Giuliano, N. Fenouille, M. Allegra, V. Hofman, P. Hofman, P. Bahadoran, J.-P. Lacour, S. Tartare-Deckert, C. Bertolotto, et R. Ballotti, « Hypoxia and MITF control metastatic behaviour in mouse and human melanoma cells », *Oncogene*, vol. 31, n° 19, p. 2461-2470, mai 2012.

[84] D. C. Bennett, « Differentiation in mouse melanoma cells: initial reversibility and an on-off stochastic model », *Cell*, vol. 34, n° 2, p. 445-453, sept. 1983.

[85] P. M. Kulesa, J. C. Kasemeier-Kulesa, J. M. Teddy, N. V. Margaryan, E. A. Seftor, R. E. B. Seftor, et M. J. C. Hendrix, « Reprogramming metastatic melanoma cells to assume a neural crest cell-like phenotype in an embryonic microenvironment », *Proc. Natl. Acad. Sci. U. S. A.*, vol. 103, n° 10, p. 3752-3757, mars 2006.

[86] L. M. J. Lee, E. A. Seftor, G. Bonde, R. A. Cornell, et M. J. C. Hendrix, « The fate of human malignant melanoma cells transplanted into zebrafish embryos: assessment of migration and cell division in the absence of tumor formation », *Dev. Dyn. Off. Publ. Am. Assoc. Anat.*, vol. 233, n° 4, p. 1560-1570, août 2005.

[87] E. A. Seftor, P. S. Meltzer, D. A. Kirschmann, N. V. Margaryan, R. E. B. Seftor, et M. J. C. Hendrix, « The epigenetic reprogramming of poorly aggressive melanoma cells by a metastatic microenvironment », *J. Cell. Mol. Med.*, vol. 10, n° 1, p. 174-196, mars 2006.

[88] G. H. Heppner, « Tumor heterogeneity », *Cancer Res.*, vol. 44, n° 6, p. 2259-2265, juin 1984.

[89] L. Denat et L. Larue, « [Malignant melanoma and the role of the paradoxal protein Microphthalmia transcription factor] », *Bull. Cancer (Paris)*, vol. 94, n° 1, p. 81-92, janv. 2007.

[90] S. Carreira, J. Goodall, L. Denat, M. Rodriguez, P. Nuciforo, K. S. Hoek, A. Testori, L. Larue, et C. R. Goding, « Mitf regulation of Dia1 controls melanoma proliferation and invasiveness », *Genes Dev.*, vol. 20, n° 24, p. 3426-3439, déc. 2006.

[91] K. S. Hoek, N. C. Schlegel, P. Brafford, A. Sucker, S. Ugurel, R. Kumar, B. L. Weber, K. L. Nathanson, D. J. Phillips, M. Herlyn, D. Schadendorf, et R. Dummer, « Metastatic potential of melanomas defined by specific gene expression profiles with

no BRAF signature », *Pigment Cell Res. Spons. Eur. Soc. Pigment Cell Res. Int. Pigment Cell Soc.*, vol. 19, n° 4, p. 290-302, août 2006.

[92] K. S. Hoek, O. M. Eichhoff, N. C. Schlegel, U. Döbbeling, N. Kobert, L. Schaerer, S. Hemmi, et R. Dummer, « In vivo switching of human melanoma cells between proliferative and invasive states », *Cancer Res.*, vol. 68, n° 3, p. 650-656, févr. 2008.

[93] Y. Cheli, S. Giuliano, T. Botton, S. Rocchi, V. Hofman, P. Hofman, P. Bahadoran, C. Bertolotto, et R. Ballotti, « Mitf is the key molecular switch between mouse or human melanoma initiating cells and their differentiated progeny », *Oncogene*, vol. 30, n° 20, p. 2390, mai 2011.

[94] D. S. Widmer, K. S. Hoek, P. F. Cheng, O. M. Eichhoff, T. Biedermann, M. I. G. Raaijmakers, S. Hemmi, R. Dummer, et M. P. Levesque, « Hypoxia Contributes to Melanoma Heterogeneity by Triggering HIF1α-Dependent Phenotype Switching », *J. Invest. Dermatol.*, mars 2013.

[95] M. Olbryt, M. Jarzab, J. Jazowiecka-Rakus, K. Simek, S. Szala, et A. Sochanik, « Gene expression profile of B 16(F10) murine melanoma cells exposed to hypoxic conditions in vitro », *Gene Expr.*, vol. 13, n° 3, p. 191-203, 2006.

[96] O. M. Eichhoff, M. C. Zipser, M. Xu, A. T. Weeraratna, D. Mihic, R. Dummer, et K. S. Hoek, « The immunohistochemistry of invasive and proliferative phenotype switching in melanoma: a case report », *Melanoma Res.*, vol. 20, n° 4, p. 349-355, août 2010.

[97] O. M. Eichhoff, A. Weeraratna, M. C. Zipser, L. Denat, D. S. Widmer, M. Xu, L. Kriegl, T. Kirchner, L. Larue, R. Dummer, et K. S. Hoek, « Differential LEF1 and TCF4 expression is involved in melanoma cell phenotype switching », *Pigment Cell Melanoma Res.*, vol. 24, n° 4, p. 631-642, août 2011.

[98] G. Boulay, C. Rosnoblet, C. Guérardel, P.-O. Angrand, et D. Leprince, « Functional characterization of human Polycomb-like 3 isoforms identifies them as components of distinct EZH2 protein complexes », *Biochem. J.*, vol. 434, n° 2, p. 333-342, mars 2011.

[99] S. Ghislin, F. Deshayes, J. Lauriol, S. Middendorp, I. Martins, R. Al-Daccak, et C. Alcaide-Loridan, « Plasticity of melanoma cells induced by neural cell crest conditions and three-dimensional growth », *Melanoma Res.*, vol. 22, n° 3, p. 184-194, juin 2012.

[100] S. Ghislin, F. Deshayes, S. Middendorp, N. Boggetto, et C. Alcaide-Loridan, « PHF19 and Akt control the switch between proliferative and invasive states in melanoma », *Cell Cycle Georget. Tex*, vol. 11, n° 8, p. 1634-1645, avr. 2012.

[101] G. L. Brien, G. Gambero, D. J. O'Connell, E. Jerman, S. A. Turner, C. M. Egan, E. J. Dunne, M. C. Jurgens, K. Wynne, L. Piao, A. J. Lohan, N. Ferguson, X. Shi, K. M. Sinha, B. J. Loftus, G. Cagney, et A. P. Bracken, « Polycomb PHF19 binds H3K36me3 and recruits PRC2 and demethylase NO66 to embryonic stem cell genes during differentiation », *Nat. Struct. Mol. Biol.*, vol. 19, n° 12, p. 1273-1281, déc. 2012.

[102] M. Yoeli-Lerner, G. K. Yiu, I. Rabinovitz, P. Erhardt, S. Jauliac, et A. Toker, « Akt blocks breast cancer cell motility and invasion through the transcription factor NFAT », *Mol. Cell*, vol. 20, n° 4, p. 539-550, nov. 2005.

[103] M. Yoeli-Lerner, Y. R. Chin, C. K. Hansen, et A. Toker, « Akt/protein kinase b and glycogen synthase kinase-3beta signaling pathway regulates cell migration through the NFAT1 transcription factor », *Mol. Cancer Res. Mcr*, vol. 7, n° 3, p. 425- 432, mars 2009.

In: Melanoma
Editor: Alexander C. Jones

ISBN: 978-1-62808-608-9

Chapter 5

THE SURGICAL EXTENT OF REGIONAL LYMPH NODE DISSECTION FOR CUTANEOUS MELANOMA AND ITS NOVEL TECHNIQUES AND MODIFICATIONS

Yasuhiro Nakamura**, *Yukiko Teramoto and Akifumi Yamamoto
Department of Skin Oncology/Dermatology, Comprehensive Cancer Center
International Medical Center, Saitama Medical University, Saitama, Japan

ABSTRACT

With the advent of the sentinel lymph node biopsy technique, the rate of patients with melanoma who have microscopic nodal metastases has increased. However, patients with clinical nodal disease are still encountered despite the development of sentinel lymph node biopsy. Although surgery is still the most important staging tool and treatment option for patients with microscopic or clinical nodal metastases and because surgery offers the chance for regional control and cure, the therapeutic value and the appropriate surgical extent of lymph node dissection and the appropriate selection of patients for lymph node dissection remain unclear. There are few specific recommendations available in the published guidelines, and there are reports with only low levels of evidence supporting the appropriate surgical extent of lymph node dissection of the cervical, axillary, and ilioinguinal regions. Ultimately, the individual surgeon decides the extent of lymph node dissection that is appropriate for each patient.

The indications for regional lymph node dissection for patients with melanoma continue to evolve. Several studies regarding the extent of dissection, its novel techniques, and modifications of the procedure to reduce postoperative morbidity have been reported. In this chapter, we will review the currently available information on regional lymph node dissection for cutaneous melanoma, assess the current strategies of lymph node dissection, discuss relevant controversial issues, and examine future steps required to improve the regional control of metastasis.

* Corresponding author: Yasuhiro Nakamura, M.D., Ph.D., E-mail: ynakamur@saitama-med. ac.jp.

INTRODUCTION

Regional lymph node metastases from cutaneous melanoma often involve the cervical, axillary, or inguinal lymph nodes, depending on the site of the primary lesion. Lymph node dissection (LND) for regional lymph node metastasis in melanoma patients has substantially changed over the past 15 years with the advent of the sentinel lymph node biopsy (SLNB) technique. Before the advent of SLNB, some surgeons had advocated wide excision of the primary tumor with elective lymph node dissection (ELND), while others had recommended excision of the primary site alone with therapeutic lymph node dissection (TLND) only when clinical nodal disease was evident. Because several studies conducted in the 1970s demonstrated no overall survival advantage for ELND [1, 2], the procedure was contested and largely abandoned. At present, SLNB-guided LND is widely accepted in place of ELND.

The therapeutic value of LND and the appropriate selection of patients for LND remain questionable. It is still controversial whether patients who undergo regional LND after confirmation of a positive SLN have a better prognosis than patients who undergo TLND after occurrence of clinical nodal disease. The third interim analysis of the Multicenter Selective Lymphadenectomy Trial 1 (MLST-1), the only randomized controlled trial with available results, failed to demonstrate a 5-year survival advantage for the SLNB group when compared with the observation group and only a disease-free survival benefit for the SLNB group [3]. In a subgroup analysis, patients who underwent SLNB-guided LND showed an improvement in 5-year survival of approximately 20% when compared with patients who underwent TLND after nodal observation and subsequently occurring clinical nodal disease (72.3% vs. 52.4%; P = .004). What is currently clear is that SLNB can provide staging information that is helpful in predicting prognosis and may impact clinical management. In addition, patients with bulky nodal disease still exist despite the availability of SLNB. These patients require LND for regional control of metastasis.

As for the extent of LND, few specific recommendations are available across several guidelines [4-6], with the common description being "a thorough dissection." Although evidence levels are not high in all studies, an increasing number of studies have described the appropriate surgical extent of LND of the cervical, axillary, and inguinal regions. Furthermore, the role of LND in patients with microscopic nodal disease is also a clinically important question because only 10%–25% patients with positive SLNs will have additional microscopic metastasis in non-SLNs [7-9]. Thus, many patients with microscopic SLN metastasis may undergo unnecessary LND. To address this problem, many authors have attempted to precisely categorized SLN by assigning several variables in an effort to find a reliable indicator of non-SLN status [10, 11]. However, it remains unclear what size and histopathological location of a microscopic metastasis identified by SLN should indicate SLN vs. non-SLN status [11]. Thus, the application of LND and the extent of LND are ultimately decided by the individual surgeon [12].

There are still no satisfactory adjuvant treatment options for patients with melanoma, and surgery is the only effective form of management. When regional lymph node metastasis occurs, LND is still the primary treatment modality and is curative in a quarter to half of all melanoma patients, whether nodal metastases are diagnosed clinically or histologically in clinically negative nodes.

Neck Dissection

Extent of Dissection

The main purpose of neck dissection is regional control of metastasis, and it has little impact on overall survival. The cervical nodes are designated as level I to level V nodes (Figure 1).

Although many surgeons have advocated various extents of neck dissection, the appropriate extent of neck dissection is still controversial. However, preoperative lymphoscintigraphy has often predicted drainage outside the cervical region, such as the preauricular, postauricular, parotid, occipital, and buccal nodes. Radical neck dissection (RND) has been the gold standard for neck dissection for melanoma and includes removal of level I to V nodes as well as nonlymphatic tissue such as the sternocleidomastoid muscle, the internal jugular vein, and the spinal accessory nerve.[13] However, O'Brien et al. reported that regional control with RND was unsatisfactory, with a 28% regional recurrence observed in patients with all nodal diseases and a 34% recurrence observed in patients with clinical nodal disease, despite extensive boundaries of dissection [13]. Because RND generally increases postoperative morbidity, some authors have recommended a modified RND (MRND) or functional neck dissection, including preservation of any or all of the sternocleidomastoid, the internal jugular vein, and the spinal accessory nerve [14, 15]. With this procedure, Byers reported a 16% recurrence rate [16], which is lower than that with RND. Furthermore, in retrospective studies of patients with clinical nodal disease, several authors demonstrated that regional recurrence rates were 14%–32% in patients receiving RND, 0% in patients receiving MRND, and 23%–29% in those undergoing selective neck dissection (SND), with no statistically significant differences noted among groups [17-19]. Based on these studies, MRND has been advocated even in the setting of clinical nodal disease. In addition, as an even more selective approach, the lymphatic drainage patterns of head and neck melanoma and recommended surgical extent of dissection have been described by some authors, although dissection of all levels of cervical region and parotid nodes are recommended in some primary sites [18, 20, 21] (Table 1).

Several authors have reported relatively high regional recurrence rates of 23%–29% in patients receiving SND; these studies include clinical N2–N3 disease, which will have a higher risk of recurrence than N1 disease [17, 18]. In a study of 37 consecutive patients with N1 neck disease, 6 patients underwent RND, 24 patients underwent MRND, and 7 patients underwent SND. There were no reported cases of local recurrence among the 3 groups during a mean follow-up period of 46 months, indicating that SND may be an alternative to RND or MRND for clinical N1 disease [22].

The appropriate extent of dissection in patients with microscopic SLN metastasis is also controversial. Pu et al. described 23 consecutive patients with positive SLNs who underwent MRND or superficial parotidectomy, and 21 patients (91.3%) had no additional positive non-SLNs and only 2 (8.7%) had 1 additional positive non-SLN [23]. No patient developed regional local recurrence during the mean follow-up period of 23.7 months. These results indicate that when microscopic SLN metastasis exists, nodal disease is confined to the SLN alone in most patients and SND may be selected in such cases.

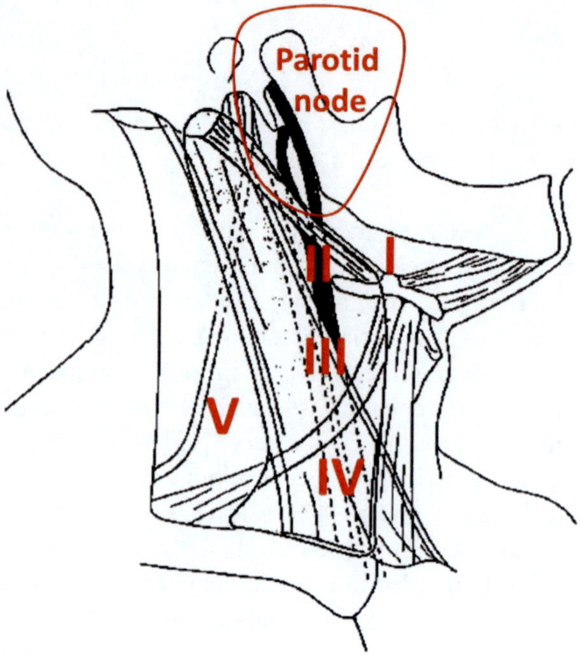

Figure 1. Lymphatic anatomy of the head and neck showing 5 major lymph node levels and parotid nodes (right neck).

Table 1. Predicted lymphatic drainage and extent of neck dissection recommended by O'Brien et al. and The Netherlands Cancer Institute (NKI-AvL) Treatment Protocol [18, 20, 21]

Location of primary tumor	Predicted lymphatic drainage (O'Brien)	NKI-AvL treatment protocol
Anterior scalp	I–III or IV, parotid	I–V, parotid
Coronal scalp	I–V, parotid	I–V, parotid
Posterior scalp	II–V, occitital nodes	II–V, occital nodes
Preauricular	I–III or IV	I–V, parotid
Ear	II–V, occipital nodes	I–V, parotid
Upper face	I–III or IV, parotid	I–V, parotid
Nose	I–III or IV, parotid	I–V, parotid
Lower face	I–III or IV, parotid	I–V, parotid
Anterior upper neck	I–III or IV, parotid	I–V
Anterior lower neck	II–V	II–V
Coronal upper neck	I–V, parotid	I–V, parotid
Coronal lower neck	III–V	II–V
Posterior upper neck	II–V, occipital nodes	II–V, occipital nodes
Posterior lower neck	III–V	II–V, occipital nodes

As for parotid gland nodes, patients with clinically palpable parotid nodes have a 28%–58% risk of microscopic metastasis in the cervical nodes [24-26]. Although neck dissection should be included when clinical parotid disease is present, the appropriate extent of neck dissection is still unclear. Ch'ng et al. reviewed their experience of lymphoscintigraphy and single-photon emission CT (SPECT) in patients with melanoma who had a sentinel node in the parotid to determine involvement of the second-tier cervical lymph nodes because level II and level III nodes make up 82% of second-tier nodes for the parotid. They concluded that SND of level II and level III nodes is likely to be an effective staging procedure in patients with isolated parotid metastases [27]. The need to treat parotid nodes in cases where clinical nodal disease of the neck is present is also controversial. In such cases, many surgeons selectively perform superficial parotidectomy combined with a neck dissection according to O'Brien's lymphatic map or the protocol or guideline of the individual institute [18, 20, 21].

As a result, lymphatic drainage in the head and neck is generally complex, and 8%–43% patients have unexpected drainage patterns in the occipital, postauricular, and contralateral nodes [20, 28-31]. As a result, there is an emerging trend to perform SND that is tailored to the individual patient according to the location of the SLN and second-tier nodes.

Technical Advances and Modification

Significant postoperative morbidity associated with RND may include hematomas, facial and spinal accessory nerve injuries, chylous fistulae, and skin flap necrosis [32]. The rate of morbidity depends on the extent of dissection and is considered to be reduced by MRND and further reduced by SND. However, detailed morbidity rates of neck dissection for melanoma have not been reported. It is generally accepted that neck dissection and parotidectomy is safe when surgery is appropriately planned preoperatively and is performed by well-experienced surgeons.

Accordingly, there are few technical advances and modifications established for neck dissection. The only technical variables in neck dissection are related to the types of skin incisions. Single Y, triradiate [33], single T, or double Y-type incisions are commonly used, which provide excellent exposure to the entire neck (Figure 2a–2d). However, the edge of the flap often has a poor blood supply at the point where the three flaps interdigitate, and wound dehiscence may occur subsequently. This can lead to exposure of the underlying carotid artery and internal jugular vein as well as life-threatening risk of rupture of these vessels. The three-point suture line gives a high incidence rate of postoperative scar contracture [34, 35]. A (modified) Macfee's transverse incision [36] was designed to eliminate the three-point exposure line that gives a good cosmetic result and reduces the incidence of scar contracture (Figure 3a). In contrast, optimal exposure is difficult with this incision, particularly in a short fat neck, and excessive traction of the skin flaps can result in damaged skin edges.[35] In our experience, preservation of the sternocleidomastoid is also difficult because of the limited surgical exposure associated with this incision. Alternative incisions may be used, including large, single incisions such as the U-flap [37], apron flap [37], and (modified) hockey stick incision [38]. The U-flap and apron flap incisions lie within the relaxed skin tension lines of the neck, and the modified hockey stick incision offers a rich blood supply to the flap (Figure 3b–3d).

The choice of incision greatly depends on the preference and experience of the individual surgeon. It should be noted that each incision will be independently selected when performing RND or MRND. A short, minimally invasive incision line should be considered in SND, where the extent of dissection is more limited (Figure 4a, 5b). In addition, an extended incision to the preauricular region is required when undergoing parotidectomy (Figure 5a, 5b).

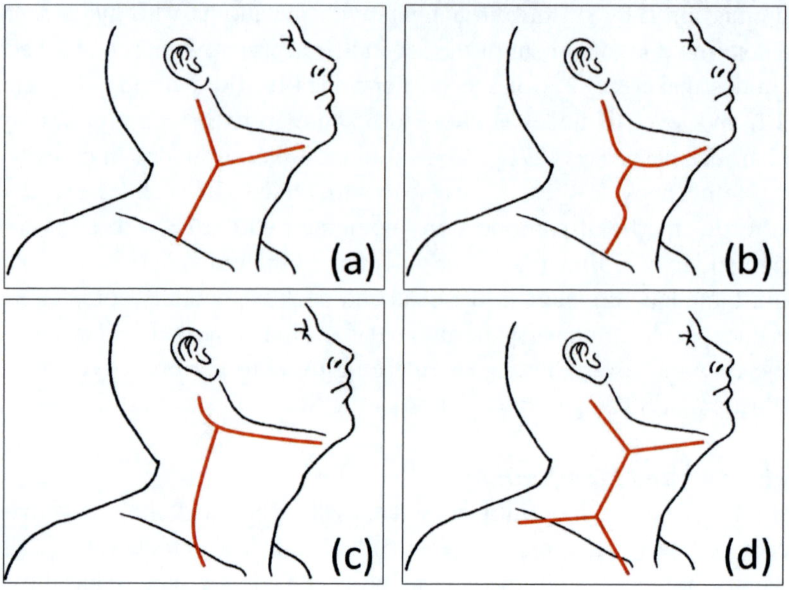

Figure 2. Classical variations of skin incision for neck dissection; (a) single Y incision; (b) triradiate incision; (c) single T incision; (d) double Y incision.

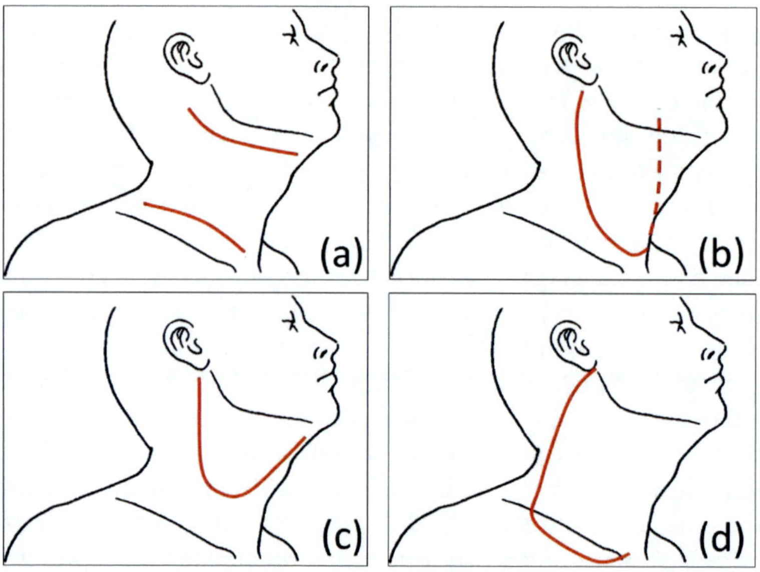

Figure 3. Another variation of skin incision for neck dissection; (a) (modified) Macfee's incision; (b) U-flap incision; (c) apron incision; (d) hockey stick incision.

Axillary Lymph Node Dissection

Extent of Dissection

The purpose of axillary LND for patients with melanoma is mainly for regional control and staging [39], and the therapeutic value is still unclear. The axillary nodes are divided into level I, II, and III nodes. Level I nodes are lateral to the lateral edge of the pectoralis minor muscle. Level II nodes are between the medial and lateral edges of the pectoralis minor. Level III nodes are medial to the medial edge of the pectoralis minor, in the apex of the axilla. Most authors have advocated that the extent of dissection should include level I, II, and III nodes because there are various drainage patterns in this area, which may potentially lead to an increased risk of recurrence with a less extensive dissection [40-44]. Furthermore, several authors recommend a more extensive dissection, including the supra-axillary fatty areolar tissue, because approximately 14% patients will have metastatic nodes in this tissue [39, 45]. However, the removal of supra-axillary fatty tissue is associated with the potential risk for complications such as injury of the brachial plexus. Furthermore, skeletonization of the axillary vein may anatomically increase the incidence of postoperative lymphedema. In contrast, several authors have questioned whether a level III dissection is necessary in all patients with melanoma with a positive SLN and have advocated that level III dissection should be included only when suspicious nodes are present at this level [41, 43, 46]. Namm et al. advocated that level I and II dissections should be applied for positive-SLN patients because of the low regional recurrence rate and low postoperative morbidity and concluded that a level III dissection is not necessary for regional control in patients with microscopic metastasis [47].

Using the approaches described above, regional recurrence was reported in approximately 10%–19% patients during a 30-month median follow-up period [48-50]. However, in most of these studies, all the dissected levels and the extent of dissection was not documented. Veenstra et al. reported a 4% regional recurrence rate and documented the levels of dissection; however, the axillary recurrence rate was not specified [51]. In a study of level I and II dissections for patients with a positive SLN, a low recurrence rate of 4% during a 39-month median follow-up was reported by Namm et al. [47].

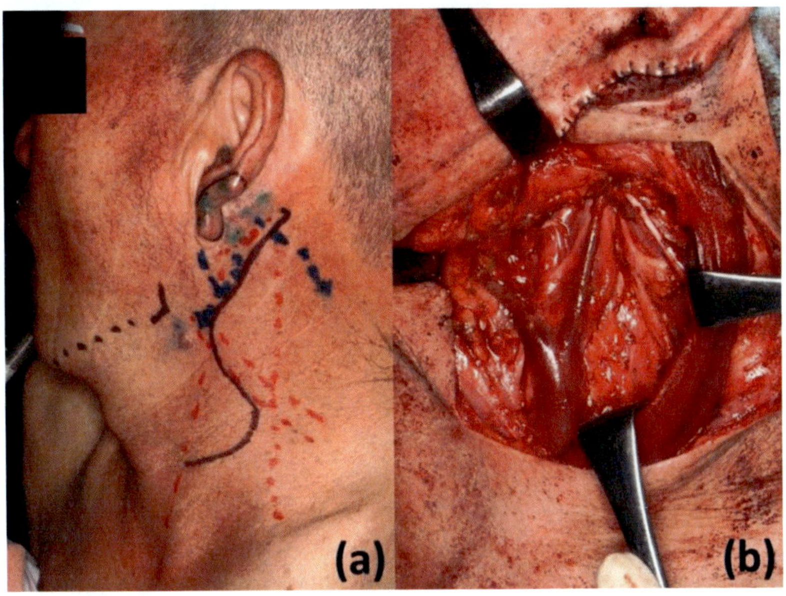

Figure 4. Short "wavy" incision for selective neck dissection; (a) solid black line represents incision line and (b) Surgical field after selective neck dissection of level II, III, and Va.

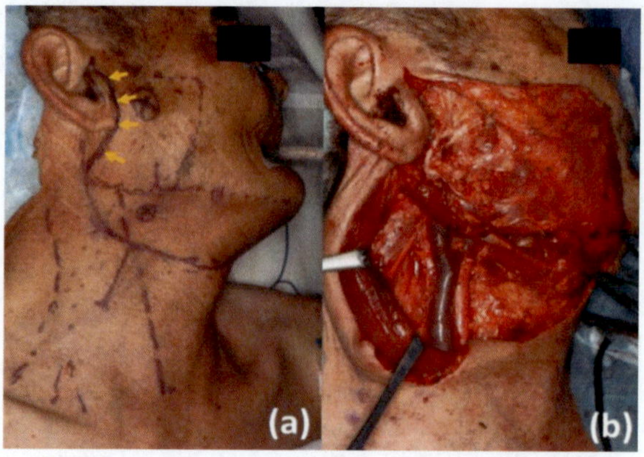

Figure 5. Incision line of parotidectomy and selective neck dissection (levels I, II, III, and Va).

(a) Additional incision line on the preauricular region for parotidectomy (arrows) (b) Surgical field after dissection.

Technical Advances and Modification

An optimal surgical technique for performing axillary LND has not been established. Several types of skin incisions have been technically modified for this procedure and are commonly used (Figure 6). A transverse incision is one of these incision types and extends from the edge of the pectoralis major muscle to the border of the latissimus dorsi muscle, approximately two fingerbreadths below the axillary crease [45]. The extended incision follows the contour of the pectoralis major into the axillary apex and then down to the medial arm [52]. A "lazy-S" incision runs from the superior border of the pectoralis major and extends transversely in a caudal direction across the axilla then longitudinally over the latissimus dorsi, providing optimal access to the entire axilla [53]. The authors usually use a wavy incision over the contour of the pectoralis major. This type of incision is relatively smaller in length and enables us to easily perform level I and II dissections (Figure 7a–7c).

Although variables such as skin necrosis, wound infection, dehiscence, and scar contracture can affect the incidence of complications associated with skin incisions, there is no available data supporting the use of one incision over another in terms of reducing the complication rate.

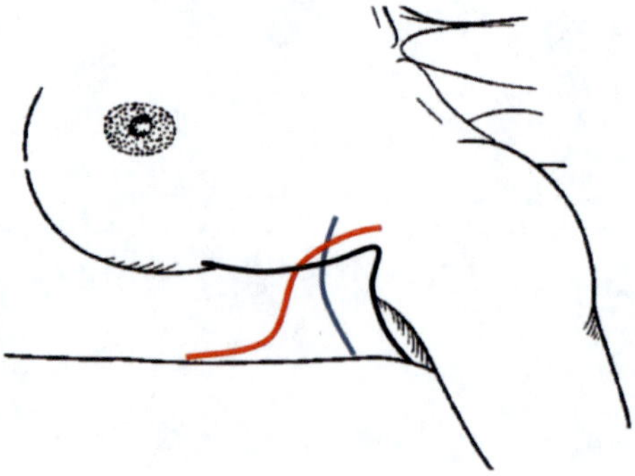

Figure 6. Variations of skin incisions used in axillary dissections.

Transverse incision (blue line), extended incision (black line), and lazy-S incision (red line).

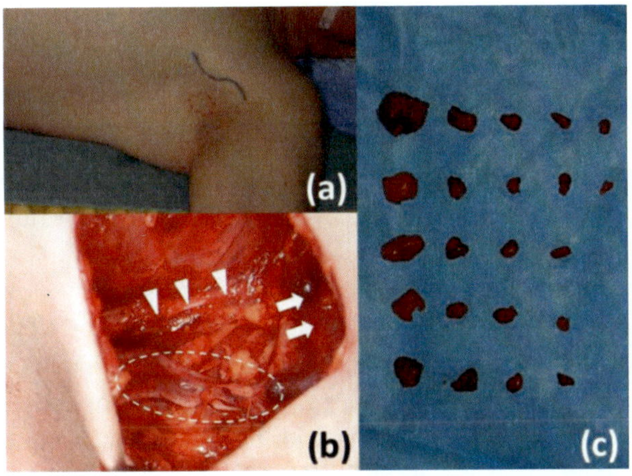

Figure 7. Axillary node dissection with minimally invasive wavy incision; (a) Incision line (black solid line); (b) operating field after dissection; arrowheads, arrows, and dotted line indicate the long thoracic nerve, the axillary vein, and the thoracodorsal neurovascular bundle, respectively; (c) Dissected fatty areolar tissue containing 22 lymph nodes (level I and II nodes).

Optimal surgical exposure for level III dissection sometimes requires transection of the pectoralis minor, and several authors have suggested routine en bloc dissection of the pectoralis minor for TLND [43, 45, 54].

Lawton et al. reported preserving the muscle fascia overlying the pectoralis major, pectoralis minor, serratus, and latissimus dorsi muscles in an effort to reduce lymphedema [55]. Of the 110 patients who underwent fascia-preserving ELNDs and TLNDs, 5% developed long-term lymphedema, which is the same as or slightly lower than the incidence rates reported by other studies described below [43, 45, 56].

The long thoracic and thoracodorsal nerves are routinely preserved, although the intercostobrachial nerves are often sacrificed when performing TLND [40, 43].

As for the complication rate of axillary LND, Wrightson et al. reported that 19.9% of 262 patients undergoing axillary LND had postoperative complications; most of these cases were considered a level I to III dissection for a positive SLN [56]. Other studies were associated with a complication rate of 14%–21% for wound infection and 19%–36% for lymphocele when performing level I to level III dissections [57-59]. Although the definition of lymphedema varies among several studies, the long-term lymphedema rate was reported to be 1%–17% [43, 45, 56, 59]. By contrast, postoperative complications in level I to II dissections occurred in 11% patients and infectious complications occurred in 8%[47], although there are no studies comparing level I to II dissections with level I to III dissections. These data indicate that there are no modifications that clearly reduce the complication rate, and only the extent of dissection may influence the complication rate.

Ilioinguinal Lymph Node Dissection

Extent of Dissection

The inguinal nodes drain the skin of the lower extremity, the lower trunk, and perineum. The standard boundaries of inguinal LND is within the femoral triangle, i.e., the inguinal ligament superiorly, the sartorius laterally, the adductor longus medially, and the point at which the sartorius crosses over the femoral vessels overlapping the underlying adductor longus (i.e., the apex of the femoral triangle) distally. The floor of the dissection was the femoral vessels and the pectineus muscle, with the superficial and deep nodes removed.

The most controversial issue in performing LND in the inguinal area is the choice between performing an inguinal LND alone or an ilioinguinal LND [inguinal + pelvic (iliac and obturator) LND] [41, 43, 46, 60-62]. When an iliac or obturator node metastasis is clinically or radiologically suspected in addition to inguinal node involvement, the addition of a pelvic LND is generally recommended [41, 61, 63, 64]. Pelvic LND has not been widely accepted in patients with clinically palpable inguinal node involvement alone because pelvic LND shows no overall survival benefit [60, 62]. In contrast, some authors have advocated ilioinguinal LND because 30%–50% patients with palpable inguinal nodal disease also have microscopic pelvic lymph node metastasisis [60-62, 65-67]. As for predictive factors for pelvic nodal status, there are no reliable predictive factors for pelvic node metastases. Strobbe et al. reported that the number of positive inguinal nodes is an unreliable predictive factor for pelvic nodal status, with a sensitivity of 41% and a negative predictive value of 78% [67]. Cloquet's node status also has a limited sensitivity of 65% in predicting involvement of the pelvic nodes and has a negative predictive value of 78%. In patients with clinical inguinal nodal disease, a Cloquet node metastasis has a 69% risk of additional pelvic node metastases [67]. In addition to these studies described above, the National Comprehensive Cancer Network (NCCN) guidelines also suggest that ilioinguinal LND may be considered if there are clinically positive inguinal nodes, three positive inguinal nodes, or a positive Cloquet's node. Although pelvic nodes seem unlikely to be involved when an inguinal SLN has only microscopic metastasis [68, 69], there are several reports stating that 9%–17% patients with a positive inguinal SLN also have positive pelvic nodes [70-72]. In addition, a study of lymphatic flow using lymphoscintigraphy and/or SPECT revealed that more than 50% patients with a positive inguinal SLN showed second-tier nodal drainage to the pelvic nodes [73]. This study suggests that pelvic LND should be selectively performed based on confirmation of the location of second-tier nodes lymphoscintigraphy and/or SPECT in positive inguinal SLN patients [73, 74]. Furthermore, the extent to which inguinal LND alone is indicated in positive inguinal SLN patients is also controversial. In a study of lymphatic flow of the inguinal region in patients with a positive SLN, Van der Ploeg et al. [73] reported that there is no lymphatic drainage to the inferior lateral zone, which is just lateral to the femoral artery and inferior to the level of saphenofemoral junction. Therefore, they advocated that dissection of this zone could be spared in such patients.

Rates of regional recurrence reported after inguinal or ilioinguinal LND in patients with clinical nodal involvement is 0%–33.6% (inguinal LND, 11.7%–13%; ilioinguinal LND, 0%–17.9%) [41, 60-64]. In a comparable study, Sterne et al. reported that patients with palpable nodal disease who underwent inguinal LND alone had a regional recurrence rate of 12.5% (2/16 patients), whereas those who underwent ilioinguinal LND had a regional recurrence rate of 0% (0/25 patients) [63]. Pearlman et al. reported performing a modified inguinal LND with limited boundaries of dissection that did not violate the femoral sheath; however, a 16% rate of regional recurrence was reported [75].

Technical Advances and Modifications

Of the three nodal basins, ilioinguinal LND is associated with the greatest postoperative morbidity, in both frequency and severity. Therefore, many technical variables and modifications have been proposed in an effort to reduce morbidity. Of patients who underwent inguinal LND, the following postoperative morbidity occurred in 20%–77%: skin necrosis and wound dehiscence (7%–55%); wound infection (5%–15%); lymphocele/seroma (2%–46%); and lymphedema (5%–64%) [76]. Ilioinguinal LND seems to be associated with a greater risk for postoperative morbidity than inguinal LND alone; however, performing an additional pelvic LND did not significantly increase the risk of postoperative wound complications [61, 77-80]. By contrast, in some studies, lymphedema was more common after inguinal LND alone, although one study specifically evaluating the incidence of lymphedema showed no statistical difference between the two procedures [61, 81, 82]. The lack of consensus regarding complications of an additional pelvic LND may suggest that concerns regarding increased morbidity should not be a reason to avoid ilioinguinal LND.

Common variables related to the development of complications in ilioinguinal LND include the type of skin incision, thickness of the skin flap, preservation of the large saphenous vein, sartorius muscle transposition over the femoral vessels, continuous dissection with or without division of the inguinal ligament, and excision of skin flap edges [40].

Several skin incisions such as a straight vertical incision in the middle of the inguinal region, a lazy-S incision from just medial to the anterior superior iliac spine to the inferior margin of the femoral triangle, paired oblique incisions or an oblique/transverse incision above the inguinal crease with a longitudinal incision below and a skin bridge between are commonly available [46, 55, 75] (Figure 8). Inguinal skin flaps created during and after inguinal LND rely on anastomotic branches and the microcirculation in the flaps to reduce the incidence of flap necrosis. In the inguinal region, the skin creases and the subcutaneous anastomotic plexus tend to parallel the inguinal ligament [83]. Therefore, a straight vertical incision cut across the anastomotic vessels in Camper's fascia is associated with high incidence of flap necrosis, although this incision provides optimal exposure. Lazy-S incisions provide optimal exposure and less subcutaneous lymphatic disruption because most of the incision parallels the inguinal ligament [40]. In contrast, paired oblique incisions or an oblique/transverse incision can avoid an incision in the inguinal crease [55]. Both these incisions run almost parallel to the inguinal ligament; however, it is a little difficult for the surgeon to obtain optimal exposure of surgical field. Recently, Spillane et al. reported use of minimal access 3 to 6 cm long paired oblique incisions above and below the inguinal ligament; however, compared with straight vertical and lazy-S incisions, there were no significant differences observed with use of these paired oblique incisions in terms of wound and lymphedema complications [72]. In contrast, Sabel et al. reported that an incision avoiding the inguinal crease decreased the wound complication rate from 21% to 9%, which was also statistically not significant [82]. Video-assisted endoscopic inguinal LND is currently being investigated as a minimally invasive and less morbid approach; however, it is not widely used [84, 85]. This procedure only requires 3 incisions, 10 to 12 mm in length, around the apex of the femoral triangle. The incidence of wound complications with this technique is low but includes cellulitis without wound dehiscence (13%), seroma (2%), and focal skin necrosis (2%) [84]. This may be an alternative approach to traditional inguinal LND.

The question regarding the use of thin skin flaps with a 2–4 mm thickness of subcutaneous fat had been classically raised [40, 83]; however, an embryological study reported by Micheletti et al. revealed that no lymph nodes were observed above the superficial fascia in the femoral triangle [86]. Currently, thick skin flaps at the level of the superficial fascia (Scarpa's fascia) are commonly used. However, a 26%– 34% rate of skin necrosis and wound infection has still been reported [55, 75].

Saphenous vein removal limits the number and effectiveness of any lymphovenous shunts that may otherwise form in response to a proximal lymphatic obstruction [75]. However, sparing the saphenous vein (Figure 9a, 9b) has the theoretical objective of reducing the rate of lymphedema, wound complications, and the potential for venous thromboembolism. Sabel et al. reported that preservation of the saphenous vein decreased the lymphedema rate from 30% to 13% and the wound complication rate from 20% to 7% [82]. However, this study was relatively small and nonrandomized, and these results were not statistically significant. Pearlman et al. reported no incidence of lymphedema with this procedure [75]. Unfortunately, there are no studies examining the rate of venous thrombosis; however, a reduction of this complication would be another theoretical benefit. There seems to be a role for preserving the saphenous vein in cases of microscopic metastasis only if the saphenous vein is not in close proximity to the positive SLN.

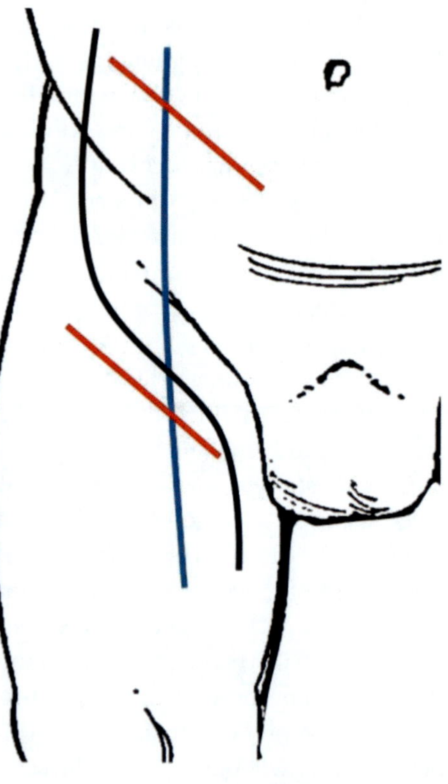

Figure 8. Variables of skin incision for ilioinguinal node dissection; straight vertical incision (blue line), lazy-S incision (black line), and oblique/transverse incision (red line).

The sartorius may be transposed to cover the femoral vessels before closure of the wound during inguinal LND [53, 87] (Figure 9a, 9c), which is useful in patients at risk for wound dehiscence (i.e., obese, elderly, patients who have peripheral vascular disease). Complications with this modification reported by Baas et al. include temporary seroma (17%), wound infection (9%), wound necrosis (3%), and edema (20%) [87]. In nonrandomized retrospective studies, Sabel et al. found no significant difference in wound complication or lymphedema rates in their patients who underwent sartorius transposition vs. those who did not [82].

When performing pelvic LND in addition to inguinal LND, technical variables include a continuous dissection by dividing the inguinal ligament or an abdominal wall incision above and parallel to the inguinal ligament to expose the retroperitoneal space [46, 55, 64] (Figure 10). Although advantages of inguinal ligament division include optimal exposure and possible continuity dissection, the main potential disadvantage is long-term abdominal wall weakness that may lead to an abdominal incisional hernia. As another modification, Lawton et al. advocated fascia-preserving ilioinguinal LND, and the rate of long-term lymphedema was 14% [55].

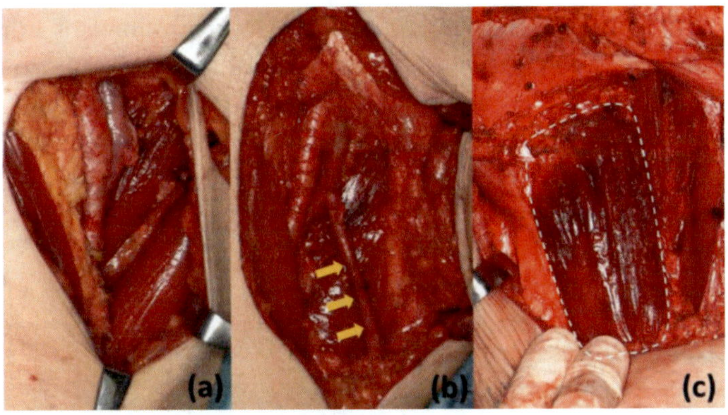

Figure 9. Modification of inguinal lymph node dissection (ILND; right groin); (a) ordinary lymph node dissection; (b) preservation of saphenous vein (arrows); (c) vessel coverage by the sartorius muscle transposition (dotted line).

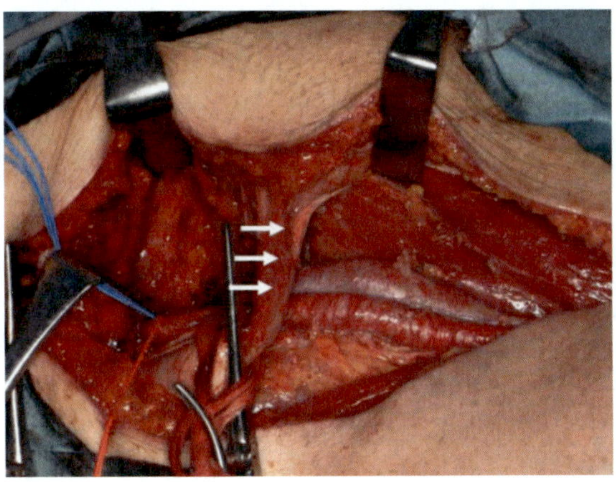

Figure 10. Inguinal ligament-spared ilioinguinal lymph node dissection (right groin); arrows indicate the preserved inguinal ligament.

In an effort to decrease postoperative morbidity, the addition of fibrin sealants has been disappointing in ilioinguinal LND for melanoma [88, 89]. In one randomized controlled trial of 30 melanoma patients, fibrin sealant did not decrease seroma output or time to drain removal following ilioinguinal LND [88]. In another randomized study of 58 melanoma patients who underwent ilioinguinal LND, the intraoperative application of fibrin sealant did not reduce the duration of closed suction drainage or length of postoperative hospital stay [89]. However, in one prospective study, a fibrinogen/thrombin-coated collagen sealant patch was used in 70 melanoma patients who underwent axillary (n = 47) and ilioinguinal (n = 23) LND. The mean duration of drainage was significantly reduced with use of the patch (20.1 ± 5.1 days vs. 23.3 ± 5.1 days; $P = 0.010$). Nakamura et al. reported a simple method using the intraoperative injection of blue dye during inguinal LND without modifications to identify leakage from injured lymphatic vessels for the prevention of lymphocele [90] (Figure 11). There was no incidence of lymphocele after removal of a suction catheter in the blue dye injection group, and the lymphatic drainage output from the inguinal region was less, leading to early removal of the suction catheter (4.3 days vs. 7.7 days; $P < 0.05$).

Despite many technical variables and modifications, it is difficult to evaluate each technique because of different study designs, variable definitions of complications, and different patient populations. Multicenter, randomized prospective trials with a standardized definition of complications are required in the future. As another factor for postoperative morbidity, a patients' inguinal node status is also an important in predicting the incidence rate of postoperative complications. Sabel et al. reported that patients undergoing an inguinal LND for a positive SLN have a significantly lower risk of postoperative morbidity than those undergoing ILND for clinically palpable disease (14% vs. 28%, $P = 0.02$) [82]. One strategy of reducing the risk of morbidity may be performing a selective inguinal LND based on the SLNB, rather than delaying the operation until the nodal disease is clinically evident.

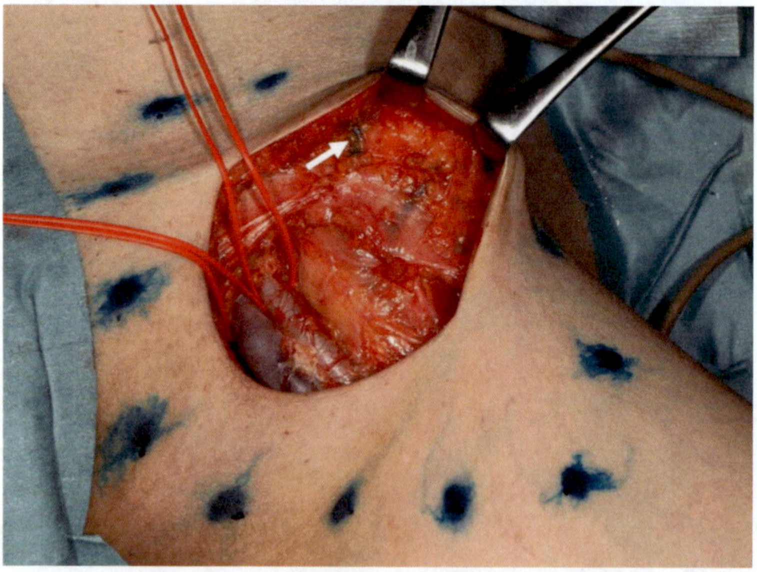

Figure 11. Intraoperative blue dye injection during inguinal lymph node dissection for detection of injured lymphatic vessels; blue-staining lymphatic leak (arrow) is observed in the surgical field.

Adjuvant Radiation Therapy to the Regional Lymph Node Basin after LND

Regional nodal recurrence occurs in 20%–50% patients after TLND. High-risk factors associated with regional recurrence include large lymph nodes, multiple positive lymph nodes, extracapsular extension, and a cervical lymph node basin [91]. Patients who have these risk factors are appropriate candidates for adjuvant radiation therapy [92], and several nonrandomized studies have demonstrated that adjuvant radiation therapy after LND for patients with regional nodal disease can reduce the risk of regional recurrence to between 5% and 20% [92-96]. Recently, in a prospective phase II trial by the Trans Tasman Radiation Oncology Group (TROG Study 96.06), the recurrence of disease was evaluated in patients with regional nodal disease following adjuvant radiation therapy after LND. Regional in-field recurrences were noted in only 7% patients [96]. Although adjuvant radiation therapy can be effective in achieving regional control after TLND, it increases chronic lymphedema, which is the major morbidity associated with TLND [97]. The morbidities associated with adjuvant radiation therapy following RND or MRND is potentially significant and includes hearing loss, ear pain, bone exposure, and wound dehiscence. In the axillary region, morbidities associated with radiation therapy may occur in 30% patients at 5 years, with the most significant being lymphedema. The inguinal region also has the greatest risk for lymphedema after additional radiation therapy [98]. Although there is favorable regional control with adjuvant radiation therapy compared with LND alone, a careful assessment of the risks and benefits of radiation is needed to select the appropriate candidates for adjuvant therapy after LND.

Future Directions

The surgical approach to regional lymph nodal disease of cutaneous melanoma is still challenging. SLNB allows accurate staging of nodal status and prediction of prognosis. A positive SLN should be treated with LND for regional control of metastasis. However, the impact on SLNB on overall survival remains unclear, and the appropriate surgical extent of LND in the cervical, axillary, and inguinal regions is also a point of debate.

Postoperative morbidity after LND still remains problematic; however, technical advances and modifications may reduce the incidence rate of morbidity. The best way to limit the morbidity of LND is to avoid utilizing the procedure. It is possible that patients with microscopic nodal disease may never develop further nodal recurrence after SLNB alone. More research is required to provide evidence-based guidelines for surgeons regarding the extent of LND and sparing LND and also to investigate the factors that may lead to a more patient-tailored approach.

Acknowledgments

This work was partly supported by the National Cancer Center Research and Development Fund (23-A-22).

REFERENCES

[1] Veronesi, U., Adamus, J., Bandiera, D. C., Brennhovd, I. O., Caceres, E., Cascinelli, N., Claudio, F., Ikonopisov, R. L., Javorskj, V. V., Kirov, S., Kulakowski, A., Lacoub, J., Lejeune, F., Mechl, Z., Morabito, A., Rode, I., Sergeev, S., van Slooten, E., Szcygiel, K. & Trapeznikov, N. N. (1977). Inefficacy of immediate node dissection in stage 1 melanoma of the limbs. *N Engl J Med*, *297*, 627-630.

[2] Sim, F. H., Taylor, W. F., Pritchard, D. J. & Soule, E. H. (1986). Lymphadenectomy in the management of stage I malignant melanoma: a prospective randomized study. *Mayo Clin Proc*, *61*, 697-705.

[3] Morton, D. L., Thompson, J. F., Cochran, A. J., Mozzillo, N., Elashoff, R., Essner, R., Nieweg, O. E., Roses, D. F., Hoekstra, H. J., Karakousis, C. P., Reintgen, D. S., Coventry, B. J., Glass, E. C. & Wang, H. J. (2006). Sentinel-node biopsy or nodal observation in melanoma. *N Engl J Med*, *355*, 1307-1317.

[4] Marsden, J. R., Newton-Bishop, J. A., Burrows, L., Cook, M., Corrie, P. G., Cox, N. H., Gore, M. E., Lorigan, P., MacKie, R., Nathan, P., Peach, H., Powell, B. & Walker, C. (2010). Revised U.K. guidelines for the management of cutaneous melanoma 2010. *Br J Dermatol*, *163*, 238-256.

[5] Garbe, C., Peris, K., Hauschild, A., Saiag, P., Middleton, M., Spatz, A., Grob, J. J., Malvehy, J., Newton-Bishop, J., Stratigos, A., Pehamberger, H. & Eggermont, A. (2010). Diagnosis and treatment of melanoma: European consensus-based interdisciplinary guideline. *Eur J Cancer*, *46*, 270-283.

[6] Gershenwald, J. E. & Ross M. I. (2011). Sentinel-lymph-node biopsy for cutaneous melanoma. *N Engl J Med*, *364*, 1738-1745.

[7] Govindarajan, A., Ghazarian, D. M., McCready, D. R. & Leong, W. L. (2007). Histological features of melanoma sentinel lymph node metastases associated with status of the completion lymphadenectomy and rate of subsequent relapse. *Ann Surg Oncol*, *14*, 906-912.

[8] Gershenwald, J. E., Andtbacka, R. H., Prieto, V. G., Johnson, M. M., Diwan, A. H., Lee, J. E., Mansfield, P. F., Cormier, J. N., Schacherer, C. W. & Ross, M. I. (2008). Microscopic tumor burden in sentinel lymph nodes predicts synchronous nonsentinel lymph node involvement in patients with melanoma. *J Clin Oncol*, *26*, 4296-4303.

[9] Vuylsteke, R. J., Borgstein, P. J., van Leeuwen, P. A., Gietema, H. A., Molenkamp, B. G., Statius Muller, M. G., van Diest, P. J., van der Sijp, J. R. & Meijer, S. (2005). Sentinel lymph node tumor load: an independent predictor of additional lymph node involvement and survival in melanoma. *Ann Surg Oncol*, *12*, 440-448.

[10] Francischetto, T., Spector, N., Neto Rezende, J. F., de Azevedo Antunes, M., de Oliveira Romano, S., Small, I. A. & Gil Ferreira, C. (2010). Influence of sentinel lymph node tumor burden on survival in melanoma. *Ann Surg Oncol*, *17*, 1152-1158.

[11] van der Ploeg, A. P., van Akkooi, A. C., Schmitz, P. I., Koljenovic, S., Verhoef, C. & Eggermont, A. M. (2010). EORTC Melanoma Group sentinel node protocol identifies high rate of submicrometastases according to Rotterdam Criteria. *Eur J Cancer*, *46*, 2414-2421.

[12] Pasquali, S., Spillane, A. J., de Wilt, J. H., McCaffery, K., Rossi, C. R., Quinn, M. J., Saw, R. P., Shannon, K. F., Stretch, J. R. & Thompson, J. F. (2012). Surgeons' opinions

on lymphadenectomy in melanoma patients with positive sentinel nodes: a worldwide web-based survey. *Ann Surg Oncol*, *19*, 4322-4329.

[13] O'Brien, C. J., Gianoutsos, M. P. & Morgan, M. J. (1992). Neck dissection for cutaneous malignant melanoma. *World J Surg*, *16*, 222-226.

[14] Calearo, C. V. & Teatini, G. (1983). Functional neck dissection. Anatomical grounds, surgical technique, clinical observations. *Ann Otol Rhinol Laryngol*, *92*, 215-222.

[15] O'Brien, C. J., Coates, A. S., Petersen-Schaefer, K., Shannon, K., Thompson, J. F., Milton, G. W. & McCarthy, W. H. (1991). Experience with 998 cutaneous melanomas of the head and neck over 30 years. *Am J Surg*, *162*, 310-314.

[16] Byers, R. M. (1986). The role of modified neck dissection in the treatment of cutaneous melanoma of the head and neck. *Arch Surg*, *121*, 1338-1341.

[17] Turkula, L. D. & Woods, J. E. (1984). Limited or selective nodal dissection for malignant melanoma of the head and neck. *Am J Surg*, *148*, 446-448.

[18] O'Brien, C. J., Petersen-Schaefer, K., Ruark, D., Coates, A. S., Menzie, S. J. & Harrison, R. I. (1995). Radical, modified, and selective neck dissection for cutaneous malignant melanoma. *Head Neck*, *17*, 232-241.

[19] Jonk, A., Strobbe, L. J., Kroon, B. B., Mooi, W. J., Hart, A. A., Nieweg, O. E. & Balm, A. J. (1998). Cervical lymph-node metastasis from cutaneous melanoma of the head and neck: a search for prognostic factors. *Eur J Surg Oncol*, *24*, 298-302.

[20] Lin, D., Franc, B. L., Kashani-Sabet, M. & Singer, M. I. (2006). Lymphatic drainage patterns of head and neck cutaneous melanoma observed on lymphoscintigraphy and sentinel lymph node biopsy. *Head Neck*, *28*, 249-255.

[21] Klop, W. M., Veenstra, H. J., Vermeeren, L., Nieweg, O. E., Balm, A. J. & Lohuis, P. J. (2011). Assessment of lymphatic drainage patterns and implications for the extent of neck dissection in head and neck melanoma patients. *J Surg Oncol*, *103*, 756-760.

[22] White, N., Yap, L. H. & Srivastava, S. (2009). Lymphadenectomy for melanoma in the clinically N1 neck: radical, modified radical, or selective? *J Craniofac Surg*, *20*, 385-388.

[23] Pu, L. L., Wells, K. E., Cruse, C. W., Shons, A. R. & Reintgen, D. S. (2003). Prevalence of additional positive lymph nodes in complete lymphadenectomy specimens after positive sentinel lymphadenectomy findings for early-stage melanoma of the head and neck. *Plast Reconstr Surg*, *112*, 43-49.

[24] O'Brien, C. J., McNeil, E. B., McMahon, J. D., Pathak, I. & Lauer, C. S. (2001). Incidence of cervical node involvement in metastatic cutaneous malignancy involving the parotid gland. *Head Neck*, *23*, 744-748.

[25] Barr, L. C., Skene, A. I., Fish, S. & Thomas, J. M. (1994). Superficial parotidectomy in the treatment of cutaneous melanoma of the head and neck. *Br J Surg*, *81*, 64-65.

[26] Caldwell, C. B. & Spiro, R. H. (1988). The role of parotidectomy in the treatment of cutaneous head and neck melanoma. *Am J Surg*, *156*, 318-322.

[27] Ch'ng, S., Pinna, A., Ioannou, K., Juszczyk, K., Shannon, K., Clifford, A., Uren, R. & Clark J. R. Assessment of second tier lymph nodes in melanoma and implications for extent of elective neck dissection in metastatic cutaneous malignancy of the parotid. *Head Neck*, *35*, 205-208.

[28] Fincher, T. R., O'Brien, J. C., McCarty, T. M., Fisher, T. L., Preskitt, J. T., Lieberman, Z. H., Stephens, J. F. & Kuhn, J. A. (2004). Patterns of drainage and recurrence

following sentinel lymph node biopsy for cutaneous melanoma of the head and neck. *Arch Otolaryngol Head Neck Surg*, *130*, 844-848.

[29] O'Brien, C. J., Uren, R. F., Thompson, J. F., Howman-Giles, R. B., Petersen-Schaefer, K., Shaw, H. M., Quinn, M. J. & McCarthy, W. H. (1995). Prediction of potential metastatic sites in cutaneous head and neck melanoma using lymphoscintigraphy. *Am J Surg*, *170*, 461-466.

[30] Pathak, I., O'Brien, C. J., Petersen-Schaeffer, K., McNeil, E. B., McMahon, J., Quinn, M. J., Thompson, J. F. & McCarthy, W. H. (2001). Do nodal metastases from cutaneous melanoma of the head and neck follow a clinically predictable pattern? *Head Neck*, *23*, 785-790.

[31] Reynolds, H. M., Smith, N. P., Uren, R. F., Thompson, J. F. & Dunbar, P. R. (2009). Three-dimensional visualization of skin lymphatic drainage patterns of the head and neck. *Head Neck*, *31*, 1316-1325.

[32] Leong, S. P. (2011). Role of selective sentinel lymph node dissection in head and neck melanoma. *J Surg Oncol*, *104*, 361-368.

[33] Yii, N. W., Patel, S. G., Williamson, P. & Breach, N. M. (1999). Use of apron flap incision for neck dissection. *Plast Reconstr Surg*, *103*, 1655-1660.

[34] Attie, J. N. (1957). A single transverse incision for radical neck dissection. *Surgery*, *41*, 498-502.

[35] Macfee, W. F. (1960). Transverse incisions for neck dissection. *Ann Surg*, *151*, 279-284.

[36] Shaw, H. J. (1988). A modification of the MacFee incisions for neck dissection. *J Laryngol Otol*, *102*, 1124-1126.

[37] King, G. D. (1965). Radical Head and Neck Surgery in Irradiated Patients: Complications and Safeguards. *Surg Clin North Am*, *45*, 567-572.

[38] Dancey, A. L. & Srivastava, S. (2006). Experience with the modified hockey stick incision for block dissection of neck. *J Plast Reconstr Aesthet Surg*, *59*, 1276-1279.

[39] Balch, C. M. (1990). Axillary lymph node dissection: differences in goals and techniques when treating melanoma and breast cancer. *Surgery*, *108*, 118-119.

[40] Karakousis, C. P. (1998). Therapeutic node dissections in malignant melanoma. *Semin Surg Oncol*, *14*, 291-301.

[41] Meyer, T., Merkel, S., Gohl, J. & Hohenberger, W. (2002). Lymph node dissection for clinically evident lymph node metastases of malignant melanoma. *Eur J Surg Oncol*, *28*, 424-430.

[42] Essner, R. (2003). Surgical treatment of malignant melanoma. *Surg Clin North Am*, *83*, 109-156.

[43] Serpell, J. W., Carne, P. W. & Bailey, M. (2003). Radical lymph node dissection for melanoma. *ANZ J Surg*, *73*, 294-299.

[44] Garbe, C., Hauschild, A., Volkenandt, M., Schadendorf, D., Stolz, W., Reinhold, U., Kortmann, R. D., Kettelhack, C., Frerich, B., Keilholz, U., Dummer, R., Sebastian, G., Tilgen, W., Schuler, G., Mackensen, A. & Kaufmann, R. (2008). Evidence-based and interdisciplinary consensus-based German guidelines: systemic medical treatment of melanoma in the adjuvant and palliative setting. *Melanoma Res*, *18*, 152-160.

[45] Karakousis, C. P., Hena, M. A., Emrich, L. J. & Driscoll, D. L. (1990). Axillary node dissection in malignant melanoma: results and complications. *Surgery*, *108*, 10-17.

[46] Karakousis, C. P. (1998). Therapeutic node dissections in malignant melanoma. *Ann Surg Oncol*, *5*, 473-482.

[47] Namm, J. P., Chang, A. E., Cimmino, V. M., Rees, R. S., Johnson, T. M. & Sabel, M. S. (2012). Is a level III dissection necessary for a positive sentinel lymph node in melanoma? *J Surg Oncol*, *105*, 225-228.

[48] Gershenwald, J. E., Berman, R. S., Porter, G., Mansfield, P. F., Lee, J. E. & Ross, M. I. (2000). Regional nodal basin control is not compromised by previous sentinel lymph node biopsy in patients with melanoma. *Ann Surg Oncol*, *7*, 226-231.

[49] Clary, B. M., Brady, M. S., Lewis, J. J. & Coit, D. G. (2001). Sentinel lymph node biopsy in the management of patients with primary cutaneous melanoma: review of a large single-institutional experience with an emphasis on recurrence. *Ann Surg*, *233*, 250-258.

[50] Leiter, U., Buettner, P. G., Bohnenberger, K., Eigentler, T., Meier, F., Moehrle, M., Breuninger, H. & Garbe, C. (2010). Sentinel lymph node dissection in primary melanoma reduces subsequent regional lymph node metastasis as well as distant metastasis after nodal involvement. *Ann Surg Oncol*, *17*, 129-137.

[51] Veenstra, H. J., van der Ploeg, I. M., Wouters, M. W., Kroon, B. B. & Nieweg, O. E. (2010). Reevaluation of the locoregional recurrence rate in melanoma patients with a positive sentinel node compared to patients with palpable nodal involvement. *Ann Surg Oncol*, *17*, 521-526.

[52] Kretschmer, L. & Preusser, K. P. (2001). Standardized axillary lymphadenectomy improves local control but not survival in patients with palpable lymph node metastases of cutaneous malignant melanoma. *Langenbecks Arch Surg*, *386*, 418-425.

[53] Balch, C. M. *Cutaneous melanoma*, 4th edn. St. Louis, Mo.: Quality Medical Pub. 2003.

[54] Uren, R. F., Howman-Giles, R., Thompson, J. F., McCarthy, W. H., Quinn, M. J., Roberts, J. M. & Shaw, H. M. (2000). Interval nodes: the forgotten sentinel nodes in patients with melanoma. *Arch Surg*, *135*, 1168-1172.

[55] Lawton, G., Rasque, H. & Ariyan, S. (2002). Preservation of muscle fascia to decrease lymphedema after complete axillary and ilioinguinofemoral lymphadenectomy for melanoma. *J Am Coll Surg*, *195*, 339-351.

[56] Wrightson, W. R., Wong, S. L., Edwards, M. J., Chao, C., Reintgen, D. S., Ross, M. I., Noyes, R. D., Viar, V., Cerrito, P. B. & McMasters, K. M. (2003). Complications associated with sentinel lymph node biopsy for melanoma. *Ann Surg Oncol*, *10*, 676-680.

[57] Kretschmer, L., Thoms, K. M., Peeters, S., Haenssle, H., Bertsch, H. P. & Emmert, S. (2008). Postoperative morbidity of lymph node excision for cutaneous melanoma-sentinel lymphonodectomy versus complete regional lymph node dissection. *Melanoma Res*, *18*, 16-21.

[58] de Vries, M., Vonkeman, W. G., van Ginkel, R. J. & Hoekstra, H. J. (2005). Morbidity after axillary sentinel lymph node biopsy in patients with cutaneous melanoma. *Eur J Surg Oncol*, *31*, 778-783.

[59] Davis, P. G., Serpell, J. W., Kelly, J. W. & Paul, E. (2011). Axillary lymph node dissection for malignant melanoma. *ANZ J Surg*, *81*, 462-466.

[60] Mann, G. B. & Coit, D. G. (1999). Does the extent of operation influence the prognosis in patients with melanoma metastatic to inguinal nodes? *Ann Surg Oncol*, *6*, 263-271.

[61] Hughes, T. M., A'Hern, R. P. & Thomas, J. M. (2000). Prognosis and surgical management of patients with palpable inguinal lymph node metastases from melanoma. *Br J Surg*, *87*, 892-901.

[62] Kretschmer, L., Neumann, C., Preusser, K. P. & Marsch, W. C. (2001). Superficial inguinal and radical ilioinguinal lymph node dissection in patients with palpable melanoma metastases to the groin--an analysis of survival and local recurrence. *Acta Oncol*, *40*, 72-78.

[63] Sterne, G. D., Murray, D. S. & Grimley, R. P. (1995). Ilioinguinal block dissection for malignant melanoma. *Br J Surg*, *82*, 1057-1059.

[64] Strobbe, L. J., Jonk, A., Hart, A. A., Nieweg, O. E. & Kroon, B. B. (1999). Positive iliac and obturator nodes in melanoma: survival and prognostic factors. *Ann Surg Oncol*, *6*, 255-262.

[65] Shen, P., Conforti, A. M., Essner, R., Cochran, A. J., Turner, R. R. & Morton, D. L. (2000). Is the node of Cloquet the sentinel node for the iliac/obturator node group? *Cancer J*, *6*, 93-97.

[66] Allan, C. P., Hayes, A. J. & Thomas, J. M. (2008). Ilioinguinal lymph node dissection for palpable metastatic melanoma to the groin. *ANZ J Surg*, *78*, 982-986.

[67] Strobbe, L. J., Jonk, A., Hart, A. A., Peterse, J. L., Wobbes, T., Nieweg, O. E. & Kroon, B. B. (2001). The value of Cloquet's node in predicting melanoma nodal metastases in the pelvic lymph node basin. *Ann Surg Oncol*, *8*, 209-214.

[68] Jansen, L., Nieweg, O. E., Peterse, J. L., Hoefnagel, C. A., Olmos, R. A. & Kroon, B. B. (2000). Reliability of sentinel lymph node biopsy for staging melanoma. *Br J Surg*, *87*, 484-489.

[69] Estourgie, S. H., Nieweg, O. E., Valdes Olmos, R. A., Hoefnagel, C. A. & Kroon, B. B. (2003). Review and evaluation of sentinel node procedures in 250 melanoma patients with a median follow-up of 6 years. *Ann Surg Oncol*, *10*, 681-688.

[70] Santinami, M., Carbone, A., Crippa, F., Maurichi, A., Pellitteri, C., Ruggeri, R., Zoras, O. & Patuzzo, R. (2009). Radical dissection after positive groin sentinel biopsy in melanoma patients: rate of further positive nodes. *Melanoma Res*, *19*, 112-118.

[71] Chu, C. K., Delman, K. A., Carlson, G. W., Hestley, A. C. & Murray, D. R. (2011). Inguinopelvic lymphadenectomy following positive inguinal sentinel lymph node biopsy in melanoma: true frequency of synchronous pelvic metastases. *Ann Surg Oncol*, *18*, 3309-3315.

[72] Spillane, A. J., Haydu, L., McMillan, W., Stretch, J. R. & Thompson, J. F. (2011). Quality assurance parameters and predictors of outcome for ilioinguinal and inguinal dissection in a contemporary melanoma patient population. *Ann Surg Oncol*, *18*, 2521-2528.

[73] van der Ploeg, I. M., Kroon, B. B., Valdes Olmos, R. A. & Nieweg, O. E. (2009). Evaluation of lymphatic drainage patterns to the groin and implications for the extent of groin dissection in melanoma patients. *Ann Surg Oncol*, *16*, 2994-2999.

[74] van der Ploeg, I. M., Valdes Olmos, R. A., Kroon, B. B. & Nieweg, O. E. (2008). Tumor-positive sentinel node biopsy of the groin in clinically node-negative melanoma patients: superficial or superficial and deep lymph node dissection? *Ann Surg Oncol*, *15*, 1485-1491.

[75] Pearlman, N. W., Robinson, W. A., Dreiling, L. K., McIntyre, R. C., Jr. & Gonzales, R. (1995). Modified ilioinguinal node dissection for metastatic melanoma. *Am J Surg*, *170*, 647-649; discussion 649-650.

[76] Chang, S. B., Askew, R. L., Xing, Y., Weaver, S., Gershenwald, J. E., Lee, J. E., Royal, R., Lucci, A., Ross, M. I. & Cormier, J. N. (2010). Prospective assessment of postoperative complications and associated costs following inguinal lymph node dissection (ILND) in melanoma patients. *Ann Surg Oncol*, *17*, 2764-2772.

[77] Karakousis, C. P. & Driscoll, D. L. (1994). Groin dissection in malignant melanoma. *Br J Surg*, *81*, 1771-1774.

[78] Ravi, R. (1993). Morbidity following groin dissection for penile carcinoma. *Br J Urol*, *72*, 941-945.

[79] Spiess, P. E., Hernandez, M. S. & Pettaway, C. A. (2009). Contemporary inguinal lymph node dissection: minimizing complications. *World J Urol*, *27*, 205-212.

[80] Hughes, T. M. & Thomas, J. M. (1999). Combined inguinal and pelvic lymph node dissection for stage III melanoma. *Br J Surg*, *86*, 1493-1498.

[81] Beitsch, P. & Balch, C. (1992). Operative morbidity and risk factor assessment in melanoma patients undergoing inguinal lymph node dissection. *Am J Surg*, *164*, 462-465; discussion 465-466.

[82] Sabel, M. S., Griffith, K. A., Arora, A., Shargorodsky, J., Blazer, D. G., 3rd, Rees, R., Wong, S. L., Cimmino, V. M. & Chang, A. E. (2007). Inguinal node dissection for melanoma in the era of sentinel lymph node biopsy. *Surgery*, *141*, 728-735.

[83] Spratt, J. (2000). Groin dissection. *J Surg Oncol*, *73*, 243-262.

[84] Delman, K. A., Kooby, D. A., Rizzo, M., Ogan, K. & Master, V. (2011). Initial experience with videoscopic inguinal lymphadenectomy. *Ann Surg Oncol*, *18*, 977-982.

[85] Ising, I. M., Bembenek, A., Gutzmer, R., Kockerling, F. & Moesta, K. T. (2012). Enhanced postoperative lymphatic staging of malignant melanoma by endoscopically assisted iliacoinguinal dissection. *Langenbecks Arch Surg*, *397*, 429-436.

[86] Micheletti, L., Levi, A. C. & Bogliatto, F. (1998). Anatomosurgical implications derived from an embryological study of the Scarpa's triangle with particular reference to groin lymphadenectomy. *Gynecol Oncol*, *70*, 358-364.

[87] Baas, P. C., Schraffordt Koops, H., Hoekstra, H. J., van Bruggen, J. J., van der Weele, L. T. & Oldhoff, J. (1992). Groin dissection in the treatment of lower-extremity melanoma. Short-term and long-term morbidity. *Arch Surg*, *127*, 281-286.

[88] Mortenson, M. M., Xing, Y., Weaver, S., Lee, J. E., Gershenwald, J. E., Lucci, A., Mansfield, P. F., Ross, M. I. & Cormier, J. N. (2008). Fibrin sealant does not decrease seroma output or time to drain removal following inguino-femoral lymph node dissection in melanoma patients: a randomized controlled trial (NCT00506311). *World J Surg Oncol*, *6*, 63.

[89] Neuss, H., Raue, W., Koplin, G., Schwenk, W., Reetz, C. & Mall, J. W. (2009). A prospective randomized trial: the influence of intraoperative application of fibrin glue after radical inguinal/iliacal lymph node dissection on postoperative morbidity. *Eur J Surg Oncol*, *35*, 884-889.

[90] Nakamura, Y., Fujisawa, Y., Maruyama, H., Furuta, J., Kawachi, Y. & Otsuka, F. (2011). Intraoperative mapping with isosulfan blue of lymphatic leakage during

inguinal lymph node dissection (ILND) for skin cancer for the prevention of postoperative lymphocele. *J Surg Oncol*, *104*, 657-660.

[91] Lee, R. J., Gibbs, J. F., Proulx, G. M., Kollmorgen, D. R., Jia, C. & Kraybill, W. G. (2000). Nodal basin recurrence following lymph node dissection for melanoma: implications for adjuvant radiotherapy. *Int J Radiat Oncol Biol Phys*, *46*, 467-474.

[92] Ballo, M. T., Ross, M. I., Cormier, J. N., Myers, J. N., Lee, J. E., Gershenwald, J. E., Hwu, P. & Zagars, G. K. (2006). Combined-modality therapy for patients with regional nodal metastases from melanoma. *Int J Radiat Oncol Biol Phys*, *64*, 106-113.

[93] Ballo, M. T., Strom, E. A., Zagars, G. K., Bedikian, A. Y., Prieto, V. G., Mansfield, P. F., Lee, J. E., Gershenwald, J. E. & Ross, M. I. (2002). Adjuvant irradiation for axillary metastases from malignant melanoma. *Int J Radiat Oncol Biol Phys*, *52*, 964-972.

[94] Ballo, M. T., Bonnen, M. D., Garden, A. S., Myers, J. N., Gershenwald, J. E., Zagars, G. K., Schechter, N. R., Morrison, W. H., Ross, M. I. & Kian Ang, K. (2003). Adjuvant irradiation for cervical lymph node metastases from melanoma. *Cancer*, *97*, 1789-1796.

[95] Ballo, M. T., Zagars, G. K., Gershenwald, J. E., Lee, J. E., Mansfield, P. F., Kim, K. B., Camacho, L. H., Hwu, P. & Ross, M. I. (2004). A critical assessment of adjuvant radiotherapy for inguinal lymph node metastases from melanoma. *Ann Surg Oncol*, *11*, 1079-1084.

[96] Burmeister, B. H., Mark Smithers, B., Burmeister, E., Baumann, K., Davis, S., Krawitz, H., Johnson, C. & Spry, N. (2006). A prospective phase II study of adjuvant postoperative radiation therapy following nodal surgery in malignant melanoma-Trans Tasman Radiation Oncology Group (TROG) Study 96.06. *Radiother Oncol*, *81*, 136-142.

[97] Agrawal, S., Kane, J. M., 3rd, Guadagnolo, B. A., Kraybill, W. G. & Ballo, M. T. (2009). The benefits of adjuvant radiation therapy after therapeutic lymphadenectomy for clinically advanced, high-risk, lymph node-metastatic melanoma. *Cancer*, *115*, 5836-5844.

[98] Guadagnolo, B. A. & Zagars, G. K. (2009). Adjuvant radiation therapy for high-risk nodal metastases from cutaneous melanoma. *Lancet Oncol*, *10*, 409-416.

In: Melanoma
Editor: Alexander C. Jones

ISBN: 978-1-62808-608-9

Chapter 6

CUTANEOUS MELANOMA: MOLECULAR MECHANISMS AND CURRENT THERAPEUTIC APPROACHES

Nathan L. Avaritt, Fade Mahmoud, Matthew Reynolds, Deepanwita Sengupta, Issam Makhoul, Sara Shalin and Alan J. Tackett

University of Arkansas for Medical Sciences, Little Rock, Arkansas, US

ABSTRACT

Cutaneous melanoma arises in the skin from melanocytes and is one of the most deadly forms of skin cancer. Worldwide incidence of cutaneous melanoma has been increasing dramatically, particularly among young adults [1]. Fortunately, the skin is easily examined and biopsied, leading to early diagnosis, effective surgical treatment and positive clinical outcomes in most cases. However, the most important prognostic indicator of a primary tumor is the depth of invasion into the skin, and once the primary tumor has invaded lower layers of the skin and/or spread to lymph nodes or distant sites, mortality rates increase exponentially. This mortality rate is primarily due to the lack of effective treatment, particularly for metastatic melanoma, although recent advances have generated more effective therapy. Research into the molecular mechanisms that initiate and drive melanoma has improved our understanding of melanoma biology and may lead to new treatment options in the future.

Competing Interests: The authors declare that they have no competing interests

INTRODUCTION

Melanocytes: Origin and Biological Function

Melanocytes arise from the neural crest, a subset of migratory cells that form during embryonic development of many vertebrates. Neural crest cells generate a large number of other cell types including peripheral and enteric neurons, Schwann, bone and smooth muscle cells. Recent research holds that melanocytes derive from Schwann cell precursors associated with various nerves throughout the body and then migrate to the skin, as well as other locations [2]. Mature melanocytes are located in the basal layer of the epidermis and interact with surrounding keratinocytes through long plasma membrane extensions known as dendrites. Melanocytes produce melanin, a dark pigment derived from the amino acid tyrosine, through a process known as melanogenesis. Once formed, melanin is transported along melanocytic dendrites to surrounding keratinocytes in vesicles called melanosomes [3]. Within keratinocytes, melanin particles form an umbrella-like structure along the apical surface of nuclei, protecting nucleic acids contained therein from damage caused by ultra-violet radiation (UVR) [4-6].

Melanogenesis occurs at variable rates: basal activity is responsible for normal skin pigmentation levels. The difference in skin pigmentation among light or dark skin individuals is due to the resting rate of melanogenesis, not because of differences in number of melanocytes. In response to UVR-induced DNA damage, epidermal keratinocytes secrete factors that promote melanogenesis, increasing the rate of melanogenesis in neighboring melanocytes. Darkening of the skin, or tanning, occurs following UVR exposure and is the result of increased melanogenesis. The tanning phenomenon protects the skin from sunlight and contributes to thermoregulation. Unfortunately, many young people, particularly young women, utilize indoor tanning beds that artificially induce the tanning response, a behavior that increases their risk for developing melanoma, despite public health campaigns designed to limit these activities [7]. A recent study has shown that the incidence of melanoma increased 8-fold among young women and 4-fold among young men (mean age at diagnosis 29.9) from 1970 to 2009 and postulated that the higher increase in young women was likely due to tanning bed usage [8].

Nevi: Benign Melanocytic Tumors

The common mole, or melanocytic nevus, is a benign tumor composed of melanocytes. These lesions can be acquired or may be present at birth (congenital nevi). Melanocytic nevi are characterized clinically by circumscription and well-defined borders. They may be colored pink, tan or brown. They can be flat (macular) or raised (papular), and this corresponds histologically with the location of nevomelanocytes in the different levels of the skin. Many adults have several dozen nevi, typically found on the trunk or sun-exposed areas such as the arms, hands and face. Melanocytic nevi arise from activation of oncogenes, including mutant *BRAF* and *NRAS*, but are considered senescent and only rarely transform into melanoma [9-12].

Awareness of melanoma has been enhanced in the general public by campaigns publicizing the ABCDE acronym: Asymmetry: common moles are symmetrical, melanomas are generally asymmetrical in shape; Border: benign moles have a distinct, regular border whereas melanomas usually have an irregular border; Color: normal moles are typically one color but melanomas have an uneven distribution of color or may be more than one color; Diameter: common moles can vary in size but are usually less than the diameter of a pencil eraser, melanomas are usually greater than 6 millimeters in diameter; Evolution: a mole that is changing in color, shape or size could signal a melanoma. Any lesion that fails to respect these rules for benignity should be evaluated by a dermatologist and might be biopsied for histologic examination.

Dysplastic nevi are generally acquired nevi that are clinically atypical. Though still benign, they violate one or more of the ABCDE rules. They are may have irregular and indistinct borders with variable coloration. They can be greater than 5 millimeters in diameter with a flat or slightly textured surface. When examined under a microscope, dysplastic nevi are characterized by having abnormal architecture and cytologic atypia. They are considered by most to be a marker of increased risk of melanoma, especially in patients with numerous dysplastic nevi [13]. According to the Clark model of melanoma progression, dysplastic nevi are precursor lesions that ultimately lead to melanoma formation [14]. In one study of 289 cases of cutaneous melanoma, approximately 50% of melanomas were associated with a preexisting nevus, more than half of which were dysplastic nevi [15]. However, even patients with dysplastic nevus syndrome (>50 clinically atypical nevi) who have a higher risk of melanoma, will not necessarily develop melanomas from existing nevi [16,17]. Because of their increased risk, patients with many dysplastic nevi are generally closely followed by dermatologists for new or changing pigmented lesions.

Melanoma: Incidence and Risk Factors

One of the most alarming characteristics of melanoma of the skin is the fact that incidences of this disease have been increasing each year, particularly in young adults [1,8]. According to the Surveillance Epidemiology and End Results (SEER) program, from 2006-2010 the age-adjusted incidence of cutaneous melanoma in the United States was 21.1 per 100,000 individuals with rates slightly higher in men than women [18]. Risk for developing melanoma is considerably higher in Caucasians than in Asians or African-Americans, reflecting the protective effect of higher baseline melanogenesis among ethnic groups. Current estimates for new cases of melanoma in the United States for 2012 are approximately 76,250 with another 9,180 estimated deaths (National Cancer Institute). An estimated 76,690 men and women will be diagnosed with cutaneous melanoma in 2013; in almost 10,000 of these individuals the disease is predicted to be fatal. The rate of increase is currently 2.6% per year with an increase in mortality of 1.5% per year. One explanation for the slower increase in mortality compared to the increase in incidence is that more people are being diagnosed at earlier stages of disease, during which surgical removal of the lesion results in a high cure rate [19,20].

The development of cutaneous melanoma is contingent on a complex interaction of both environmental and endogenous risk factors. Behaviors that result in significant exposure to sunlight (natural or artificial) constitute the most important environmental risk factor in the development of cutaneous melanoma [21,22,7]. Intermittent intense sun exposure, generally resulting in sunburns and the acquisition of nevi on the shoulders, back and face, appears to be a significant determinant of risk for the development of melanoma [21]. Broad-spectrum sunscreen protects the skin from UV radiation and, presumably, lowers the risk of developing cutaneous melanoma, although studies attempting to establish this hypothesis have been inconclusive [23,24]. In fact, while sunscreen has been shown to reduce the number of acquired nevi and amount of freckling following sun exposure [25], in another study its usage resulted in increased duration of sun exposure, thereby possibly inducing a false sense of protection in people and negating the sunscreen's protective effect [26]. These results indicate that while sunscreen can provide protection during intentional sunlight exposure, other preventive measures should be taken (e.g. clothing that covers much of one's skin, limited duration of exposure, etc.).

Endogenous risk factors for the development of melanoma include the following physical characteristics: pale skin; numerous freckles; susceptibility to sunburn; more than 50 acquired nevi; one or more nevi greater than five mm in diameter; five or more histologically-confirmed dysplastic nevi; giant (greater than 20 cm) congenital nevi; and Xeroderma pigmentosum [27-31]. In addition to these physical characteristics that increase risk for melanoma, other endogenous risk factors have been identified. A family history of melanoma is a strong determinant of risk for the development of cutaneous melanoma. Individuals with a relative, particularly an immediate family member like a father or sister, who has a history of melanoma, are almost twice as likely to develop the disease [32]. Germline mutations in the *CDKN2A* locus (which encodes the tumor suppressor protein p16) represent a commonly identified molecular aberration found in familial melanoma, although these mutations are by no means the majority [33,34]. Other genetic aberrations have been identified in sporadic or familial melanomas; these will be described in later sections. These findings show that it is important to consider intrinsic factors, as well as behavior, when calculating risk for melanoma development in any one individual.

Melanoma: Molecular Aberrations

Alterations of multiple molecular pathways appear to be involved in progression of benign melanocytes to malignant melanoma [35]. The commitment and maturation of melanocytes is under tight regulation by different developmental transcription factors including microphthalmia transcription factor (MITF), PAX3, SOX10, and SLUG [36]. Alterations in expression of these transcription factors have been shown to contribute to the melanoma phenotype in various ways. *MITF* is frequently amplified in malignant melanoma, where it functions as a survival-promoting oncogene [37, 38]. PAX3 and SOX10 promote migration, invasion, survival and proliferation in melanoma cells [39,40]. SLUG transcription factor also contributes to survival in melanoma cells; small interfering RNA (siRNA) knockdown of SLUG increased the effectiveness of cisplatin and fotemustine chemotherapeutics [41]. These findings indicate that transformation of melanocytes into malignant melanoma cells likely involves pathways that normally function to constrain growth within tight parameters. Cellular changes, such as amplification or loss of components of these pathways, likely play an important role in melanoma initiation.

One of the most distinct cytological differences between nevomelanocytes and melanoma cells is the presence of multiple chromosomal aberrations in malignant cells, such as losses or gains of chromosomes [42]. These abnormalities have not been identified in common nevi, although some nevi variants such as Spitz nevi do contain reproducible chromosomal aberrations [43]. Studies have identified chromosomes 6q, 8p, 9p and 10q as absent as well as increases in number of chromosomes 1q, 6p, 7, 8q, 17q and 20q in many melanomas [43,44]. Using comparative genomic hybridization techniques in 186 melanocytic tumors (132 melanomas and 54 benign nevi), researchers showed numerous chromosomal aberrations in malignant melanomas with no detectable abnormalities in common nevi cells [43]. Loss of genomic stability is a feature common to most cancers and establishes conditions necessary for malignant transformation as well as cancer progression [45]. The starkly contrasting patterns of chromosomal abnormalities between benign nevi and melanomas indicate that the appearance of genomic instability could be an important step in the conversion of benign melanocytes into melanoma cells. Consequently, techniques such as array comparative genomic hybridization are being employed in histologically ambiguous melanocytic proliferations to help guide diagnosis, with the assumption that a melanocytic tumor with multiple chromosomal gains or losses is more likely malignant (melanoma) than benign (nevus).

Melanocytic nevi often express oncogenic forms of BRAF or NRAS, which results in sustained activation of the RAS/RAF/MEK/ERK (MAPK) pathway. Activation of this pathway causes phosphorylation of numerous downstream proteins, which in turn induce changes in gene expression that promote cell growth and proliferation [46]. However, while mutant BRAF (or NRAS) may initially stimulate proliferation of melanocytes, and formation of melanocytic nevi, sustained RAS/RAF/MEK/ERK activation in these cells appears to ultimately lead to growth arrest and cellular senescence [12,47].

BRAF mutations (most commonly a point mutation at codon 600 leading to a valine to glutamic acid substitution) are also detected in a large subset of melanomas. However, the observation of oncogene-induced senescence in nevomelanocytes reveals that expression of one or two oncogenes alone is not sufficient to transform melanocytes into malignant cells. Instead, additional changes must take place before melanomagenesis occurs. Recently, activation of the PI3K pathway has been shown to overcome senescence in melanocytes, and contributes to melanomagenesis [48]. Signals propagated through the PI3K pathway, and its intermediary AKT, a serine/threonine kinase, promote cell proliferation and survival through regulation of gene expression [49,50]. Levels of AKT activity correlate with melanoma progression: increased AKT activation was found in 17% of common nevi, 43% of dysplastic nevi, 49% of primary melanomas and 77% of metastatic melanomas [51].

Other evidence has shown that circumvention of senescence in nevi can occur through inhibition of the p16-Rb pathway, an integral component of senescence in nevi [52-54]. The tumor suppressor gene *CDKN2A* encodes both p14 and p16, a cyclin-dependent kinase inhibitor that prevents phosphorylation of retinoblastoma protein (Rb) by cyclinD/CDK4/6. The hypophosphorylated form of Rb binds to transcription factors of the E2F family; hyperphosphorylation of Rb by cyclinD/CDK4/6 frees E2F transcription factors, which can then activate transcription of genes necessary for cell cycle progression from G1 to S phase [35] and can, ultimately, overcome senescence. Expression of p16 is often reduced or missing, either through deletion, mutation or transcriptional repression, in melanoma cells [55-58]. Taken together, these data indicate that multiple oncogenic "hits," along with concurrent loss of tumor suppressor mechanisms, must take place before melanocytes become malignant melanoma cells. Importantly, increased RAS/RAF/MEK/ERK signaling and activation of the PI3K pathway continues to contribute to the melanoma phenotype, promoting disease progression long after the melanoma was initially formed.

The RAS/RAF/MEK/ERK pathway, as mentioned above, is a phosphorelay system in which protein kinases phosphorylate and activate downstream protein targets that, in turn, regulate cell growth, proliferation, migration and invasion [59-61]. Constitutive activation of this pathway is commonly observed in melanoma [62], and is not limited to melanomas harboring *BRAF* or *NRAS* mutations [63,64]. Signaling from this pathway is implicated in rapid melanoma cell proliferation [65] and has been shown to interact with the PI3K/AKT and NF-$_{\kappa}$B pathways, resulting in the generation of strong survival signals [66]. Therapeutic targeting of the RAS/RAF/MEK/ERK signaling pathway in melanoma, through small molecule inhibitors of mutant BRAF, has become a reality. The antineoplastic effects of these drugs may be due to inhibition of downstream MAPK signaling, by preventing activation of MEK1/2 by BRAF, or may be the result of inhibition of non-MEK, RAF-binding protein kinases [67]. Inhibition of mutant BRAF has also been shown to effectively block melanoma lung metastasis, a common site of melanoma cell migration [68]. The efficacy of these drugs, and their impact on overall patient survival, is detailed in the treatment section below.

The PI3K/AKT pathway integrates signals from multiple receptors on the plasma membrane, which leads to the activation of phosphoinositide 3-kinase (PI3K). Active PI3K converts the phospholipid PIP_2 into PIP_3. PIP_3 then can activate AKT, which promotes resistance to apoptotic signaling by activating transcription of antiapoptotic protein Bcl-XL and inhibition of proapoptotic proteins BAD and caspase 9 [69]. The tumor suppressor gene PTEN inhibits AKT activity by converting PIP_3 into PIP_2, effectively limiting the strength of PI3K-mediated prosurvival signaling [70]. In advanced melanoma, PTEN expression is often decreased or absent due to deletion, mutation or transcriptional repression [71-73]. Consequently, loss of this negative regulator of AKT activity results in sustained, unchecked AKT signaling that promotes proliferation and confers resistance to apoptosis [49,74]. Both the RAS/RAF/MEK/ERK and PI3K/AKT pathways modulate melanoma progression and may provide key points of susceptibility that could be targeted in combination to destroy melanoma cells.

Melanoma: Treatment Approaches

Metastatic melanoma continues to be a challenging disease to treat, with an estimated 9,180 related deaths in the United States in 2012 (National Cancer Institute). Many factors have been proposed to influence the prognosis in patients with metastatic melanoma. Melanoma remains the most lethal skin malignancy in the Western world [75]. Thus, there is an imperative need to identify new targets for developing novel therapeutics for malignant melanoma.

Metastatic (Stage IV) melanoma is when tumor cells have spread beyond the primary tumor site and regional lymph node basins into other parts of the body. The most common sites of metastases are to subcutaneous soft tissue, lymph nodes, the lungs, liver, brain, and bone. Some patients present with metastatic melanoma of an unknown primary site. The main goals of therapy in these patients are to prevent progression, prolong survival and provide comfort (palliation). Complicating treatment is the fact that melanoma cells are notoriously resistant to chemotherapy [76]. Recent advances in immunotherapy and targeted therapy have been shown to potentially prolong survival and provide hope for patients with melanoma [77]. Immunotherapy involves treatment that activates or enhances the immune response, with the goal being recognition of tumors by the immune system, resulting in destruction of cancer cells. Biochemotherapy combines chemotherapeutic agents with interleukin-2 (IL-2) or interferon alpha (IFNa) to simultaneously activate an immune response as well as inhibiting growth of proliferative cells. Targeted therapies are based on molecular features unique to specific types of cancers, such as the $BRAF^{V600E}$ mutation in melanoma, which can be selectively inhibited in cancer cells and not normal cells.

IMMUNOTHERAPY

I. Interleukin-2 (IL-2)

Response to high-dose IL-2 regimens (600,000 to 720,000 IU/kg) generally ranges from 10% to 20% [78,79]. No improvement in overall survival (OS) has been demonstrated in randomized trials, however there is a subgroup of patients (4-6%) who may derive a long term remission and that is why the FDA approved HD IL-2 in 1998. High dose IL-2 can cause serious side effects, including low blood pressure, irregular heart rhythms, accumulation of fluid in the lungs, fever, and rarely death. For that reason it is important to select patients who are young and fit to withstand these side effects.

II. Ipilimumab

Ipilimumab is an antibody against the cytotoxic T-lymphocyte antigen (anti-CTLA-4). It is used in the treatment of advanced melanoma (i.e. stage III, unresectable, or stage IV) [80]. The Eastern Cooperative Oncology Group (ECOG) study (E1609) in the United States is currently open to see if postoperative adjuvant ipilimumab or high-dose interferon α-2b can improve disease-free and OS in patients with resected high-risk melanoma. Until the results of E1609 become available, there is not a current role for ipilimumab in the adjuvant setting. In a phase III, international, randomized, double-blind trial; 676 previously treated, unresectable stage III or IV melanoma patients were randomized to receive ipilimumab alone, ipilimumab with glycoprotein 100 (gp100) peptide vaccine, or gp100 vaccine plus placebo. The median OS was 10 months and 10.1 months among patients receiving ipilimumab alone or with the gp100 vaccine, respectively, versus 6.4 months for patients receiving the vaccine alone (hazard ratio (HR), 0.68; $P < .001$; HR, 0.66; $P <.003$). 10-15% of patients developed immune related adverse effects (AEs) like colitis and hypopituitarism. There were 14 deaths related to study drugs (2.1%); half of them due to immune related adverse events [81].

Another phase III trial randomly assigned 502 patients with metastatic melanoma to ipilimumab (10 mg/kg) plus dacarbazine (850 mg/m^2) or to placebo plus dacarbazine (850 mg/m^2), in the first line setting, at weeks 1, 4, 7, and 10 followed by dacarbazine alone every 3 weeks through week 22. Patients with stable disease or an objective response received ipilimumab or placebo every 12 weeks thereafter as maintenance therapy. The median OS was 11.2 months (95% confidence interval [CI], 9.4–13.6) versus 9.1 months (95% CI, 7.8–10.5). Grade 3 to 4, immune-related AEs were seen in 38.1% of patients treated with ipilimumab plus dacarbazine versus 4.4% in the placebo arm. No drug-related deaths occurred [82].

Ipilimumab (Yervoy®) is given at a dose of 3 mg/kg intravenously every 3 weeks for 4 doses. There is no need for dose adjustment in renal failure or hepatic failure. However, if liver enzymes or bilirubin levels rise during therapy, then treatment may need to be temporarily held (for AST or ALT elevations between 2.5 and 5 times the upper limit of normal or bilirubin elevations 1.5 to 3 times the upper limit of normal) or discontinued completely (for ALT or AST greater than 5 times or total bilirubin greater than 3 times the upper limit of normal). It is extremely important to pay attention to the immune-mediated adverse reactions that may be severe and fatal at times [83].

BIOCHEMOTHERAPY

I. IL-2 Regimens

Combining IL-2 with dacarbazine produced considerable toxicity with a response rate in the range of only 13 to 33% [84]. Subsequent studies combined IL-2 with cisplatin alone or in combination with other chemotherapy agents and/or IFNα [84]. The first concurrent biochemotherapy regimen was developed by Legha et al. [85]. The "Legha" regimen consists of cisplatin, vinblastine and dacarbazine chemotherapy combined with a continuous infusion of IL-2 (9 MU/m2 per day) for 4 days and 5 days of subcutaneous IFNα (5 MU/m2 per day) at 21 day intervals. This regimen resulted in an overall response rate of 64% and a complete response rate of 21%. The median overall survival was 12 months and a 2-year survival rate of 10%. Although the toxicity of this regimen is less than high dose IL-2 therapy, it is high enough dosing that patients should be admitted to the hospital during treatment. Almost all patients develop fever, chills, rigors, myalgias, fatigue, anorexia, nausea, vomiting, diarrhea and headache to varying degrees. Neutropenia, anemia and thrombocytopenia necessitate the need for transfusion and use of growth factors. IL-2-specific toxicity includes varying degrees of capillary leakage syndrome with hypotension, fluid retention and third-spacing, pulmonary congestion and reversible end-organ dysfunction that could be severe enough to require admission to an intensive care unit.

II. IFNα Regimens

Combining cytotoxic chemotherapy with IFNα has been evaluated in many randomized controlled trials. Perhaps the two largest trials to test the efficacy of biochemotherapy in metastatic melanoma are the ECOG 3690 and the Dermatologic Cooperative Oncology Group (DCOG) phase III trial. In the ECOG 3690 trial, 271 patients were randomly assigned to one of four treatment arms: dacarbazine alone, dacarbazine with tamoxifen, dacarbazine with IFNα, or dacarbazine with the combination of tamoxifen plus IFNα [86]. The overall response rate was 18%, median time to treatment failure was 2.6 months and median survival was 9.1 months with no statistically significant difference amongst all 4 arms. A phase III trial from the DCOG randomly assigned 282 patients to temozolomide plus IFNα or temozolomide alone [87]. The addition of IFNα was associated with a significant increase in response rate (24 versus 13%), although the difference in survival was not significant (9.7 versus 8.4 months with temozolomide alone).

Targeted Therapy

I. *BRAF*^{V600E} Inhibitors

The identification of driver oncogenes has provided important targets for drugs that can change the landscape of melanoma therapies. The *BRAF*^{V600E} mutation is found in half of all melanomas [9]. Both vemurafenib and dabrafenib, inhibitors of oncogenic BRAF, have showed dramatic antitumor activity in patients with advanced melanomas that are positive for the *BRAF*^{V600E} mutation [88,89]. Unfortunately this impressive response to BRAF inhibitors is short lived and virtually every patient treated with these medications will have disease progression, likely due to activation of alternative survival pathways [90].

Vemurafenib (Zelboraf; Plexxikon/Roche) is approved by the FDA for patients with unresectable or metastatic melanoma possessing the *BRAF*^{V600E} mutation. In a randomized, open-label, multicenter, phase III trial; oral vemurafenib improved median overall survival (13.6 months) and progression free survival (PFS) (5.3 months) in patients with unresectable, previously untreated, *BRAF*^{V600E} mutation-positive, stage IIIC or IV melanoma compared to dacarbazine (median OS 9.7 months and PFS 1.6 months). Common adverse reactions are cutaneous squamous cell carcinoma and/or keratoacanthoma which were reported in 18% of patients [91].

A randomized phase III trial of 675 patients with previously untreated, *BRAF*^{V600E}-positive, locally advanced or metastatic melanoma received either vemurafenib (960 mg orally twice daily) or dacarbazine (1000 mg/m^2 IV every 3 weeks). At interim analysis, both OS and PFS met the statistical criteria in favor of vemurafenib, so patients in the dacarbazine group were allowed to cross over to receive vemurafenib. Despite the cross over, the OS in the vemurafenib arm was clearly superior to that in the dacarbazine arm. The estimated median PFS was 5.3 months versus 1.6 months in the vemurafenib and dacarbazine arms, respectively. Similar to the previous study, adverse events were common including cutaneous squamous cell carcinoma, keratoacanthoma, or both, developed in 18% of patients and were treated by simple excision [90].

Vemurafenib is effective even in heavily pretreated patients with metastatic melanoma. In another study, 132 patients with a *BRAF*^{V600E} mutation, who received one or more prior therapies for advanced melanoma, received 960 mg vemurafenib orally twice per day. Median follow-up was 12.9 months. The overall response rate was detected in 53% (95% CI, 44–62) with 6% achieving complete response. The median duration of response was 6.7 months (95% CI, 5.6–8.6) [92].

Dabrafenib is another specific BRAF kinase inhibitor. A phase III trial of 250 patients with locally advanced or metastatic melanoma, who harbor the *BRAF*^{V600E} mutation, were randomly assigned in a 3:1 ratio to either dabrafenib (150 mg orally twice a day) or dacarbazine (1000 mg/m2 IV every three weeks) [89]. Dabrafenib significantly increased PFS compared with dacarbazine (median 5.1 versus 2.7 months, HR 0.30, 95% CI 0.18-0.51). Objective responses were seen in 50% of patients treated with dabrafenib and only 6% of patients treated with dacarbazine. OS favored dabrafenib (HR 0.61, 95% CI 0.25-1.48), but was not statistically significant, however, patients allowed to cross over to dabrafenib might have affected the OS data. Dabrafenib is well tolerated with the most frequent grade 2 or greater toxicities being skin-related.

MEK Inhibition

I. Trametinib

Trametinib is a very potent and specific MEK1/MEK2 inhibitor that blocks sustained RAS/RAF/MEK/ERK pathway activation. In the METRIC trial, a phase II study, 322 patients with advanced melanoma (87% had V600E mutation and 18% had V600K mutation) were randomly assigned in a 2:1 ratio to either trametinib (2 mg/day orally) or chemotherapy (dacarbazine or paclitaxel). One third of patients had received prior chemotherapy and 30% had received prior immunotherapy. Trametinib compared to chemotherapy showed a statistically improvement in progression-free survival (median 4.8 versus 1.5 months, HR 0.45, 95% CI 0.33-0.63) and OS (6 month survival rate 81 versus 67 percent, HR for death 0.54, 95% CI 0.32-0.92). The most common side effects were rash, diarrhea, and edema. A decreased cardiac ejection fraction was seen in 7 percent of patients treated with trametinib [93].

Trametinib has been combined with dabrafenib to maximize inhibition of the RAS/RAF/MEK/ERK kinase cascade. In the phase II study, 162 patients who harbor the V600 mutation were randomly assigned to one of three regimens: Dabrafenib (150 mg twice daily) as monotherapy, dabrafenib plus trametinib (150 mg twice daily and 1 mg once daily, respectively), or dabrafenib plus trametinib (150 mg twice daily and 2 mg once daily, respectively). The combined dabrafenib and trametinib significantly prolonged progression-free survival compared with dabrafenib alone (median 9.4 versus 5.8 months, HR 0.39, 95% CI 0.25-0.62), and significantly increased the proportion of patients alive and progression-free at one year (41 versus 9 percent) [94].

Chemotherapy

I. Dacarbazine (DTIC)

Dacarbazine was approved in 1970 based on overall response rates of 10-20%. It is a non-targeted chemotherapeutic agent that is a purine analog, thereby interfering with DNA synthesis. However, the response rate is short lived and no impact on OS has been demonstrated in clinical trials [95-97].

II. Temozolomide

Temozolomide is an orally-delivered alkylating agent that appears to have similar efficacy to DTIC in melanoma but is not an FDA approved agent. It has an overall response rate of 10-20%, crosses the blood brain barrier and hence can be considered for use in melanoma that has metastasized to the brain. Lymphopenia could develop and patients should receive prophylaxis against opportunistic infections. A randomized trial of DTIC versus temozolomide showed an OS of 6.4 months versus 7.7 months, respectively (95% CI, 0.92-1.52) [96].

After decades of disappointing clinical trials of novel malignant melanoma therapeutics, several agents are showing promise in extending overall survival in patients with advanced stage disease. Both targeted and immunological therapies, sometimes combined with chemotherapeutics, are extending life for individuals with malignant melanoma. A greater understanding of the biology of melanoma, the functional effects of these therapeutic agents and identification of biomarkers that allow clinicians to select specific therapeutic approaches for each patient, should result in even more positive outcomes for individuals with malignant melanoma.

Conclusion

After more than a decade without the introduction of new treatments for advanced malignant melanoma (1999-2010), three agents: trametinib, vemurafenib and ipilimumab, have shown significant improvements in controlling melanoma progression increasing overall survival. While recent advances in the treatment of malignant melanoma have moderately improved patient outcomes, more insights into the molecular framework governing melanoma biology is necessary in order to develop new, targeted therapies that could greatly change the poor prognosis for advanced cases of this disease. The identification of common patterns of *BRAF* and *NRAS* mutations in many cases of melanoma has led to new targeted therapies; this underscores the need to more fully characterize molecular features of melanomas so that additional molecularly-targeted drugs can be developed. Also, the success of ipilimumab supports research into the complex interactions between melanoma cells and the immune system to create agents that promote immune recognition, and destruction, of these cells. One area of increasing excitement is the role that epigenetic regulation of gene transcription may play in malignant melanoma biology. For example, expression of the histone methyltransferase EZH2, a member of the polycomb repressive complex 2 that silences gene transcription through methylation of lysine 27 of histone H3, increases incrementally from benign nevi to metastatic melanomas, suppressing the protective senescence phenotype and contributing to tumorigenicity [98,99]. Small molecule inhibitors of EZH2 are currently being tested in various cancer backgrounds, such as lymphoma, with promising results [100,101]. In the future, pharmacological inhibition of EZH2 activity, perhaps combined with immunotherapy, targeted therapy and chemotherapy, in malignant melanoma may result in a whole new therapeutic approach for this disease.

Authors' Contributions

NLA, MF and SS drafted the manuscript. MF and SS provided critical clinical perspective. AJT finalized the draft of the manuscript. All authors read and approved the final manuscript.

References

[1] Purdue, M. P., Freeman, L. E. B., Anderson, W. F., & Tucker, M. A. (2008). Recent trends in incidence of cutaneous melanoma among US Caucasian young adults. *Journal of Investigative Dermatology*, *128*(12), 2905-2908.

[2] Adameyko, I., Lallemend, F., Aquino, J. B., Pereira, J. A., Topilko, P., Müller, T., ... & Ernfors, P. (2009). Schwann cell precursors from nerve innervation are a cellular origin of melanocytes in skin. *Cell*, *139*(2), 366-379.

[3] Ando, H., Niki, Y., Ito, M., Akiyama, K., Matsui, M. S., Yarosh, D. B., & Ichihashi, M. (2011). Melanosomes are transferred from melanocytes to keratinocytes through the processes of packaging, release, uptake, and dispersion. *Journal of Investigative Dermatology*, *132*(4), 1222-1229.

[4] Morison, W. L. (1985). What is the function of melanin?. *Archives of dermatology*, *121*(9), 1160.

[5] Hearing, V. J. (2005). Biogenesis of pigment granules: a sensitive way to regulate melanocyte function. *Journal of dermatological science*, *37*(1), 3-14.

[6] Brenner, M., & Hearing, V. J. (2008). The Protective Role of Melanin Against UV Damage in Human Skin†. *Photochemistry and photobiology*, *84*(3), 539-549.

[7] Gallagher, R. P., Spinelli, J. J., & Lee, T. K. (2005). Tanning beds, sunlamps, and risk of cutaneous malignant melanoma. *Cancer Epidemiology Biomarkers & Prevention*, *14*(3), 562-566.

[8] Reed, K. B., Brewer, J. D., Lohse, C. M., Bringe, K. E., Pruitt, C. N., & Gibson, L. E. (2012, April). Increasing incidence of melanoma among young adults: an epidemiological study in Olmsted County, Minnesota. In *Mayo Clinic Proceedings* (Vol. 87, No. 4, pp. 328-334). Elsevier.

[9] Pollock, P. M., Harper, U. L., Hansen, K. S., Yudt, L. M., Stark, M., Robbins, C. M., ... & Meltzer, P. S. (2002). High frequency of BRAF mutations in nevi.*Nature genetics*, *33*(1), 19-20.

[10] Poynter, J. N., Elder, J. T., Fullen, D. R., Nair, R. P., Soengas, M. S., Johnson, T. M., ... & Gruber, S. B. (2006). BRAF and NRAS mutations in melanoma and melanocytic nevi. *Melanoma Research*, *16*(4), 267-273.

[11] Bauer, J., Curtin, J. A., Pinkel, D., & Bastian, B. C. (2006). Congenital melanocytic nevi frequently harbor NRAS mutations but no BRAF mutations.*Journal of Investigative Dermatology*, *127*(1), 179-182.

[12] Michaloglou, C., Vredeveld, L. C., Soengas, M. S., Denoyelle, C., Kuilman, T., van der Horst, C. M., ... & Peeper, D. S. (2005). BRAFE600-associated senescence-like cell cycle arrest of human naevi. *Nature*, *436*(7051), 720-724.

[13] Goldstein, A. M., & Tucker, M. A. (2013). Dysplastic Nevi and Melanoma.*Cancer Epidemiology Biomarkers & Prevention*, *22*(4), 528-532.

[14] Clark, W. H., Elder, D. E., Guerry, D., Epstein, M. N., Greene, M. H., & Van Horn, M. (1984). A study of tumor progression: the precursor lesions of superficial spreading and nodular melanoma. *Human pathology*, *15*(12), 1147-1165.

[15] Skender-Kalnenas, T. M., English, D. R., & Heenan, P. J. (1995). Benign melanocytic lesions: risk markers or precursors of cutaneous melanoma?.*Journal of the American Academy of Dermatology*, *33*(6), 1000-1007.

[16] Elder, D. E., Goldman, L. I., Goldman, S. C., Greene, M. H., & Clark, W. H. (1980). Dysplastic nevus syndrome: a phenotypic association of sporadic cutaneous melanoma. *Cancer*, *46*(8), 1787-1794.

[17] Kraemer, K., Greene, M., Tarone, R., Elder, D., Clark, W., & Guerry, D. (1983). Dysplastic naevi and cutaneous melanoma risk. *The Lancet*, *322*(8358), 1076-1077.

[18] Howlader N, Noone AM, Krapcho M, Garshell J, Neyman N, Altekruse SF, Kosary CL, Yu M, Ruhl J, Tatalovich Z, Cho H, Mariotto A, Lewis DR, Chen HS, Feuer EJ, Cronin KA (eds). (2013) SEER Cancer Statistics Review, 1975-2010, National Cancer Institute. Bethesda, MD, http://seer.cancer.gov/csr/1975_2010/, based on November 2012 SEER data submission.

[19] Hiatt, R. A., & Fireman, B. (1986). The possible effect of increased surveillance on the incidence of malignant melanoma. *Preventive medicine*, *15*(6), 652-660.

[20] Clark, W. H., Elder, D. E., Guerry, D., Braitman, L. E., Trock, B. J., Schultz, D., ... & Halpern, A. C. (1989). Model predicting survival in stage I melanoma based on tumor progression. *Journal of the National Cancer Institute*, *81*(24), 1893-1904.

[21] Elwood, J. M., & Jopson, J. (1997). Melanoma and sun exposure: an overview of published studies. *International Journal of Cancer*, *73*(2), 198-203.

[22] Veierød, M. B., Weiderpass, E., Thörn, M., Hansson, J., Lund, E., Armstrong, B., & Adami, H. O. (2003). A prospective study of pigmentation, sun exposure, and risk of cutaneous malignant melanoma in women. *Journal of the National Cancer Institute*, *95*(20), 1530-1538.

[23] Vainio, H., Miller, A. B., & Bianchini, F. (2000). An international evaluation of the cancer–preventive potential of sunscreens. *International Journal of Cancer*,*88*(5), 838-842.

[24] Huncharek, M., & Kupelnick, B. (2002). Use of topical sunscreens and the risk of malignant melanoma: a meta-analysis of 9067 patients from 11 case–control studies. *Journal Information*, *92*(7).

[25] Gallagher, R. P., Rivers, J. K., Lee, T. K., Bajdik, C. D., McLean, D. I., & Coldman, A. J. (2000). Broad-spectrum sunscreen use and the development of new nevi in white children. *JAMA: the journal of the American Medical Association*, *283*(22), 2955-2960.

[26] Autier, P., Dore, J. F., Negrier, S., Lienard, D., Panizzon, R., Lejeune, F. J., ... & Eggermont, A. M. (1999). Sunscreen use and duration of sun exposure: a double-blind, randomized trial. *Journal of the National Cancer Institute*, *91*(15), 1304-1309.

[27] Beitner, H., Ringborg, U., Wennersten, G., & Lagerlöf, B. (1981). Further evidence for increased light sensitivity in patients with malignant melanoma. *British Journal of Dermatology*, *104*(3), 289-294.

[28] D'Arcy, C., Holman, J., & Armstrong, B. K. (1984). Pigmentary traits, ethnic origin, benign nevi, and family history as risk factors for cutaneous malignant melanoma. *Journal of the National Cancer Institute*, *72*(2), 257-266.

[29] Whiteman, D. C., Parsons, P. G., & Green, A. C. (1998). p53 expression and risk factors for cutaneous melanoma: A case-control study. *International journal of cancer*, *77*(6), 843-848.

[30] Mikkilineni, R., & Weinstock, M. A. (2000). Is the self-counting of moles a valid method of assessing melanoma risk?. *Archives of dermatology*, *136*(12), 1550.

[31] Naldi, L., Lorenzo Imberti, G., Parazzini, F., Gallus, S., & La Vecchia, C. (2000). Pigmentary traits, modalities of sun reaction, history of sunburns, and melanocytic nevi as risk factors for cutaneous malignant melanoma in the Italian population. *Cancer*, *88*(12), 2703-2710.

[32] Cho, E., Rosner, B. A., Feskanich, D., & Colditz, G. A. (2005). Risk factors and individual probabilities of melanoma for whites. *Journal of clinical oncology*,*23*(12), 2669-2675.

[33] Harland, M., Taylor, C. F., Bass, S., Churchman, M., Randerson-Moor, J. A., Holland, E. A., Mann, G.J., Bishop, T, & Newton Bishop, J. A. (2005). Intronic sequence variants of the CDKN2A gene in melanoma pedigrees. *Genes, Chromosomes and Cancer*,*43*(2), 128-136.

[34] Titus-Ernstoff, L., Perry, A. E., Spencer, S. K., Gibson, J., Ding, J., Cole, B., & Ernstoff, M. S. (2006). Multiple primary melanoma: two-year results from a population-based study. *Archives of dermatology*, *142*(4), 433.

[35] Palmieri, G., Capone, M., Ascierto, M., Gentilcore, G., Stroncek, D., Casula, M., Sini, M., Palla, M., Mozzillo, N., & Ascierto, P. (2009). Main roads to melanoma. *Journal of translational medicine*, *7*(1), 86.

[36] White, R. M., & Zon, L. I. (2008). Melanocytes in development, regeneration, and cancer. *Cell stem cell*, *3*(3), 242-252.

[37] Garraway, L. A., Widlund, H. R., Rubin, M. A., Getz, G., Berger, A. J., Ramaswamy, S., ... & Sellers, W. R. (2005). Integrative genomic analyses identify MITF as a lineage survival oncogene amplified in malignant melanoma.*Nature*, *436*(7047), 117-122.

[38] Levy, C., Khaled, M., & Fisher, D. E. (2006). MITF: master regulator of melanocyte development and melanoma oncogene. *Trends in molecular medicine*, *12*(9), 406-414.

[39] Scholl, F. A., Kamarashev, J., Murmann, O. V., Geertsen, R., Dummer, R., & Schäfer, B. W. (2001). PAX3 is expressed in human melanomas and contributes to tumor cell survival. *Cancer research*, *61*(3), 823-826.

[40] Mascarenhas, J. B., Littlejohn, E. L., Wolsky, R. J., Young, K. P., Nelson, M., Salgia, R., & Lang, D. (2010). PAX3 and SOX10 activate MET receptor expression in melanoma. *Pigment cell & melanoma research*, *23*(2), 225-237.

[41] Vannini, I., Bonafe, M., Tesei, A., Rosetti, M., Fabbri, F., Storci, G., ... & Zoli, W. (2007). Short interfering RNA directed against the SLUG gene increases cell death induction in human melanoma cell lines exposed to cisplatin and fotemustine. *Analytical Cellular Pathology*, *29*(4), 279-287.

[42] Cowan, J. M., Halaban, R., & Francka, U. (1988). Cytogenetic analysis of melanocytes from premalignant nevi and melanomas. *Journal of the National Cancer Institute*, *80*(14), 1159-1164.

[43] Bastian, B. C., Olshen, A. B., LeBoit, P. E., & Pinkel, D. (2003). Classifying melanocytic tumors based on DNA copy number changes. *The American journal of pathology*, *163*(5), 1765-1770.

[44] Cowan, J. M., Halaban, R., & Francka, U. (1988). Cytogenetic analysis of melanocytes from premalignant nevi and melanomas. *Journal of the National Cancer Institute*, *80*(14), 1159-1164.

[45] Hanahan, D., & Weinberg, R. A. (2011). Hallmarks of cancer: the next generation. *Cell*, *144*(5), 646-674.

[46] Seger, R., & Krebs, E. G. (1995). The MAPK signaling cascade. *The FASEB journal*, *9*(9), 726-735.

[47] Mooi, W. J., & Peeper, D. S. (2006). Oncogene-induced cell senescence—halting on the road to cancer. *New England Journal of Medicine*, *355*(10), 1037-1046.

[48] Vredeveld, L. C., Possik, P. A., Smit, M. A., Meissl, K., Michaloglou, C., Horlings, H. M. ... & Peeper, D. S. (2012). Abrogation of BRAFV600E-induced senescence by PI3K pathway activation contributes to melanomagenesis.*Genes & Development*, *26*(10), 1055-1069.

[49] Dhawan, P., Singh, A. B., Ellis, D. L., & Richmond, A. (2002). Constitutive activation of Akt/protein kinase B in melanoma leads to up-regulation of nuclear factor-κB and tumor progression. *Cancer research*, *62*(24), 7335-7342.

[50] Cully, M., You, H., Levine, A. J., & Mak, T. W. (2006). Beyond PTEN mutations: the PI3K pathway as an integrator of multiple inputs during tumorigenesis. *Nature Reviews Cancer*, *6*(3), 184-192.

[51] Dai, D. L., Martinka, M., & Li, G. (2005). Prognostic significance of activated Akt expression in melanoma: a clinicopathologic study of 292 cases. *Journal of clinical oncology*, *23*(7), 1473-1482.

[52] Bartkova, J., Lukas, J., Guldberg, P., Alsner, J., Kirkin, A. F., Zeuthen, J., & Bartek, J. (1996). The p16-cyclin D/Cdk4-pRb pathway as a functional unit frequently altered in melanoma pathogenesis. *Cancer research*, *56*(23), 5475-5483.

[53] Straume, O., Sviland, L., & Akslen, L. A. (2000). Loss of nuclear p16 protein expression correlates with increased tumor cell proliferation (Ki-67) and poor prognosis in patients with vertical growth phase melanoma. *Clinical Cancer Research*, *6*(5), 1845-1853.

[54] Ross, A. L., Sanchez, M. I., & Grichnik, J. M. (2011). Nevus senescence.*ISRN dermatology*, *2011*.

[55] Cairns, P., Polascik, T. J., Eby, Y., Tokino, K., Califano, J., Merlo, A., ... & Sidransky, D. (1995). Frequency of homozygous deletion at p16/CDKN2 in primary human tumours. *Nature genetics*, *11*(2), 210-212.

[56] Pollock, P. M., Pearson, J. V., & Hayward, N. K. (1996). Compilation of somatic mutations of the CDKN2 gene in human cancers: Non-random distribution of base substitutions. *Genes, Chromosomes and Cancer*, *15*(2), 77-88.

[57] Platz, A., Ringborg, U., Lagerlöf, B., Lundqvist, E., Sevigny, P., & Inganäs, M. (1996). Mutational analysis of the CDKN2 gene in metastases from patients with cutaneous malignant melanoma. *British journal of cancer*, *73*(3), 344.

[58] Gonzalez-Zulueta, M., Bender, C. M., Yang, A. S., Nguyen, T., Beart, R. W., Van Tornout, J. M., & Jones, P. A. (1995). Methylation of the 5′ CpG island of the

p16/CDKN2 tumor suppressor gene in normal and transformed human tissues correlates with gene silencing. *Cancer research*, *55*(20), 4531-4535.

[59] Johnson, G. L., & Lapadat, R. (2002). Mitogen-activated protein kinase pathways mediated by ERK, JNK, and p38 protein kinases. *Science*,*298*(5600), 1911-1912.

[60] Giehl, K. (2005). Oncogenic Ras in tumour progression and metastasis.*Biological chemistry*, *386*(3), 193-205.

[61] Campbell, P. M., & Der, C. J. (2004, April). Oncogenic Ras and its role in tumor cell invasion and metastasis. In *Seminars in cancer biology* (Vol. 14, No. 2, pp. 105-114). Academic Press.

[62] Fecher, L. A., Amaravadi, R. K., & Flaherty, K. T. (2008). The MAPK pathway in melanoma. *Current opinion in oncology*, *20*(2), 183-189.

[63] Dong, J., Phelps, R. G., Qiao, R., Yao, S., Benard, O., Ronai, Z., & Aaronson, S. A. (2003). BRAF oncogenic mutations correlate with progression rather than initiation of human melanoma. *Cancer Research*, *63*(14), 3883-3885.

[64] Greene, V. R., Johnson, M. M., Grimm, E. A., & Ellerhorst, J. A. (2009). Frequencies of NRAS and BRAF mutations increase from the radial to the vertical growth phase in cutaneous melanoma. *Journal of Investigative Dermatology*, *129*(6), 1483-1488.

[65] Davies, H., Bignell, G. R., Cox, C., Stephens, P., Edkins, S., Clegg, S., ... & Davis, N. (2002). Mutations of the BRAF gene in human cancer. *Nature*,*417*(6892), 949-954.

[66] Malumbres, M., & Pellicer, A. (1998). RAS pathways to cell cycle control and cell transformation. *Front Biosci*, *3*, d887-912.

[67] O'Neill, E., Rushworth, L., Baccarini, M., & Kolch, W. (2004). Role of the kinase MST2 in suppression of apoptosis by the proto-oncogene product Raf-1.*Science Signaling*, *306*(5705), 2267.

[68] Sharma, A., Tran, M. A., Liang, S., Sharma, A. K., Amin, S., Smith, C. D., ... & Robertson, G. P. (2006). Targeting mitogen-activated protein kinase/extracellular signal–regulated kinase kinase in the mutant (V600E) B-Raf signaling cascade effectively inhibits melanoma lung metastases. *Cancer research*, *66*(16), 8200-8209.

[69] Cantley, L. C. (2002). The phosphoinositide 3-kinase pathway. *Science Signaling*, *296*(5573), 1655.

[70] Maehama, T., Taylor, G. S., & Dixon, J. E. (2001). PTEN and myotubularin: novel phosphoinositide phosphatases. *Annual review of biochemistry*, *70*(1), 247-279.

[71] Tsao, H., Goel, V., Wu, H., Yang, G., & Haluska, F. G. (2004). Genetic interaction between NRAS and BRAF mutations and PTEN/MMAC1 inactivation in melanoma. *Journal of Investigative Dermatology*, *122*(2), 337-341.

[72] Wu, H., Goel, V., & Haluska, F. G. (2003). PTEN signaling pathways in melanoma. *Oncogene*, *22*(20), 3113-3122.

[73] Mirmohammadsadegh, A., Marini, A., Nambiar, S., Hassan, M., Tannapfel, A., Ruzicka, T., & Hengge, U. R. (2006). Epigenetic silencing of the PTEN gene in melanoma. *Cancer research*, *66*(13), 6546-6552.

[74] Davies, M. A., Stemke-Hale, K., Lin, E., Tellez, C., Deng, W., Gopal, Y. N., ... & Gershenwald, J. E. (2009). Integrated molecular and clinical analysis of AKT activation in metastatic melanoma. *Clinical Cancer Research*, *15*(24), 7538-7546.

[75] Jemal, A., Siegel, R., Ward, E., Hao, Y., Xu, J., Murray, T., & Thun, M. J. (2008). Cancer statistics, 2008. *CA: a cancer journal for clinicians*, *58*(2), 71-96.

[76] Soengas, M. S., & Lowe, S. W. (2003). Apoptosis and melanoma chemoresistance. *Oncogene*, *22*(20), 3138-3151.

[77] Leong, S. P., Mihm Jr, M. C., Murphy, G. F., Hoon, D. S., Kashani-Sabet, M., Agarwala, S. S., ... & Kirkwood, J. M. (2012). Progression of cutaneous melanoma: implications for treatment. *Clinical & experimental metastasis*,*29*(7), 775-796.

[78] Atkins, M. B., Lotze, M. T., Dutcher, J. P., Fisher, R. I., Weiss, G., Margolin, K., ... & Rosenberg, S. A. (1999). High-dose recombinant interleukin 2 therapy for patients with metastatic melanoma: analysis of 270 patients treated between 1985 and 1993. *Journal of Clinical Oncology*, *17*(7), 2105-2105.

[79] Atkins, M. B., Kunkel, L., Sznol, M., & Rosenberg, S. A. (2000). High-dose recombinant interleukin-2 therapy in patients with metastatic melanoma: long-term survival update. *The cancer journal from Scientific American*, *6*, S11.

[80] Wolchok, J. D., Neyns, B., Linette, G., Negrier, S., Lutzky, J., Thomas, L., ... & Lebbé, C. (2010). Ipilimumab monotherapy in patients with pretreated advanced melanoma: a randomised, double-blind, multicentre, phase 2, dose-ranging study. *The lancet oncology*, *11*(2), 155-164.

[81] Hodi, F. S., O'Day, S. J., McDermott, D. F., Weber, R. W., Sosman, J. A., Haanen, J. B., ... & Urba, W. J. (2010). Improved survival with ipilimumab in patients with metastatic melanoma. *New England Journal of Medicine*, *363*(8), 711-723.

[82] Robert, C., Thomas, L., Bondarenko, I., O'Day, S., Weber, J., Garbe, C., ... & Wolchok, J. D. (2011). Ipilimumab plus dacarbazine for previously untreated metastatic melanoma. *New England Journal of Medicine*, *364*(26), 2517-2526.

[83] Weber, J. S., Kähler, K. C., & Hauschild, A. (2012). Management of immune-related adverse events and kinetics of response with ipilimumab. *Journal of Clinical Oncology*, *30*(21), 2691-2697.

[84] O Day, S. J., Kim, C. J., & Reintgen, D. S. (2002). Metastatic melanoma: chemotherapy to biochemotherapy. *Cancer Control*, *9*(1), 31-38.

[85] Legha, S. S., Ring, S., Eton, O., Bedikian, A., Buzaid, A. C., Plager, C., & Papadopoulos, N. (1998). Development of a biochemotherapy regimen with concurrent administration of cisplatin, vinblastine, dacarbazine, interferon alfa, and interleukin-2 for patients with metastatic melanoma. *Journal of Clinical Oncology*, *16*(5), 1752-1759.

[86] Falkson, C. I., Ibrahim, J., Kirkwood, J. M., Coates, A. S., Atkins, M. B., & Blum, R. H. (1998). Phase III trial of dacarbazine versus dacarbazine with interferon alpha-2b versus dacarbazine with tamoxifen versus dacarbazine with interferon alpha-2b and tamoxifen in patients with metastatic malignant melanoma: an Eastern Cooperative Oncology Group study. *Journal of clinical oncology*, *16*(5), 1743-1751.

[87] Kaufmann, R., Spieth, K., Leiter, U., Mauch, C., von den Driesch, P., Vogt, T., ... &

[88] Dummer, R. (2005). Temozolomide in combination with interferon-alfa versus temozolomide alone in patients with advanced metastatic melanoma: a randomized, phase III, multicenter study from the Dermatologic Cooperative Oncology Group. *Journal of clinical oncology*, *23*(35), 9001-9007.

[89] Bollag, G., Tsai, J., Zhang, J., Zhang, C., Ibrahim, P., Nolop, K., & Hirth, P. (2012). Vemurafenib: the first drug approved for BRAF-mutant cancer. *Nature Reviews Drug Discovery*, *11*(11), 873-886.

[90] Hauschild, A., Grob, J. J., Demidov, L. V., Jouary, T., Gutzmer, R., Millward, M., ... & Chapman, P. B. (2012). Dabrafenib in *BRAF*-mutated metastatic melanoma: a multicentre, open-label, phase 3 randomised controlled trial. *The Lancet*.

[91] Chapman, P. B., Hauschild, A., Robert, C., Haanen, J. B., Ascierto, P., Larkin, J., ... & McArthur, G. A. (2011). Improved survival with vemurafenib in melanoma with BRAF V600E mutation. *New England Journal of Medicine*, *364*(26), 2507-2516.

[92] Keating, G. M. (2012). Vemurafenib. *Biodrugs*, *26*(5), 325-334.

[93] Sosman, J. A., Kim, K. B., Schuchter, L., Gonzalez, R., Pavlick, A. C., Weber, J. S., ... & Ribas, A. (2012). Survival in BRAF V600–mutant advanced melanoma treated with vemurafenib. *New England Journal of Medicine*, *366*(8), 707-714.

[94] Kim, K. B., Kefford, R., Pavlick, A. C., Infante, J. R., Ribas, A., Sosman, J. A., ... & Lewis, K. D. (2013). Phase II study of the MEK1/MEK2 inhibitor trametinib in patients with metastatic BRAF-mutant cutaneous melanoma previously treated with or without a BRAF inhibitor. *Journal of Clinical Oncology*, *31*(4), 482-489.

[95] Flaherty, K. T., Robert, C., Hersey, P., Nathan, P., Garbe, C., Milhem, M., ... & Schadendorf, D. (2012). Improved survival with MEK inhibition in BRAF-mutated melanoma. *New England Journal of Medicine*, *367*(2), 107-114.

[96] Chapman, P. B., Einhorn, L. H., Meyers, M. L., Saxman, S., Destro, A. N., Panageas, K. S., ... & Kirkwood, J. M. (1999). Phase III multicenter randomized trial of the Dartmouth regimen versus dacarbazine in patients with metastatic melanoma. *Journal of Clinical Oncology*, *17*(9), 2745-2745.

[97] Middleton, M. R., Grob, J. J., Aaronson, N., Fierlbeck, G., Tilgen, W., Seiter, S., ... & Thatcher, N. (2000). Randomized phase III study of temozolomide versus dacarbazine in the treatment of patients with advanced metastatic malignant melanoma. *Journal of Clinical Oncology*, *18*(1), 158-158.

[98] Avril, M. F., Aamdal, S., Grob, J. J., Hauschild, A., Mohr, P., Bonerandi, J. J., ... & Menu, Y. (2004). Fotemustine compared with dacarbazine in patients with disseminated malignant melanoma: a phase III study. *Journal of Clinical Oncology*, *22*(6), 1118-1125.

[99] McHugh, J. B., Fullen, D. R., Ma, L., Kleer, C. G., & Su, L. D. (2007). Expression of polycomb group protein EZH2 in nevi and melanoma. *Journal of cutaneous pathology*, *34*(8), 597-600.

[100] Fan, T., Jiang, S., Chung, N., Alikhan, A., Ni, C., Lee, C. C. R., & Hornyak, T. J. (2011). EZH2-dependent suppression of a cellular senescence phenotype in melanoma cells by inhibition of p21/CDKN1A expression. *Molecular Cancer Research*, *9*(4), 418-429.

[101] McCabe, M. T., Ott, H. M., Ganji, G., Korenchuk, S., Thompson, C., Van Aller, G. S., ... & Creasy, C. L. (2012). EZH2 inhibition as a therapeutic strategy for lymphoma with EZH2-activating mutations. *Nature*.

[102] Qi, W., Chan, H., Teng, L., Li, L., Chuai, S., Zhang, R., ... & Li, E. (2012). Selective inhibition of Ezh2 by a small molecule inhibitor blocks tumor cells proliferation. *Proceedings of the National Academy of Sciences*, *109*(52), 21360-21365.

In: Melanoma
Editor: Alexander C. Jones

ISBN: 978-1-62808-608-9

Chapter 7

EPIDEMIOLOGY OF MELANOMA IN YOUNG INDIVIDUALS: A SYSTEMATIC REVIEW

Adeel S. Zubair and Jerry D. Brewer*
Division of Dermatologic Surgery, Department of Dermatology
Mayo Clinic/Mayo Clinic College of Medicine, Rochester, MN, US

ABSTRACT

Skin cancer is the most common type of cancer affecting patients today. Cutaneous melanoma is one of the more serious forms of skin cancer, which originates from melanocytes usually in the dermal-epidermal junction. [1, 2] The rates of cutaneous melanoma have been steadily increasing; 1/500 in 1935, 1/600 in 1960, and 1/75 in 2000 with a projected steady increase in incidence in the future; current estimates suggest that the rates are 1/50. [2] Particularly, melanoma rates continue to grow, especially in younger individuals. [2]

There are a variety of different epidemiological studies which have shown that younger individuals are at an ever increasing risk for developing melanoma. Childhood and adolescence are considered to be "critical periods of vulnerability" when individuals are vulnerable to the effects ultraviolet radiation. [3] 25% of sun exposure occurs before the age of 18 and sun exposure during those years is often more intense than those in later years due to the behavior of the younger individuals. [3] In addition to being at a much higher risk for sunlight exposure young individuals are also less likely to practice proper sun-protection. [4] Studies have shown that there is an increased risk of melanoma after receiving a sunburn during the adolescent and childhood periods. This is hypothesized to occur because exposure may lead to alteration in the DNA of melanocytes which increases the risk of malignant degeneration as the individual ages. [3, 5, 6]

Many younger individuals also spend time tanning in indoor tanning machines which exposes them to increased levels of UV radiation which can lead to DNA damage and skin cancer in the long term. Many studies have shown strong associations between UV exposure via tanning beds and risk of melanoma. [3, 7, 8]

---

* Corresponding Author: Dr. Jerry D Brewer, MD. Associate Professor of Dermatology, Chair, Division of Dermatologic Surgery, Department of Dermatology, Mayo Clinic, 200 First Street SW, Rochester, MN 55905. E-mail address: brewer.jerry@mayo.edu. Phone: (507) 284-3579. Fax: (507) 284-2072.

In young individuals, social pressures have contributed to increased desire to achieve greater skin pigmentation, often through use of tanning beds. [9-11] Tanning bed use leads to a great deal of negative health effects, including melanoma. [8] In young adults, cutaneous melanomas from 1975-2000 were the most common cancers in the 25-29 year old population of females and was 12% of cancers in 20-40 year old females. [3, 7] In the past few years there has been a sharp uptick in the number of patients with cutaneous malignancies; from 1970 to 2009, the incidence of melanoma has skyrocketed in males aged 18 to 39 (4-fold increase) and females in the same age range (8-fold increase). [12]

Younger individuals may be at a greater risk for developing melanoma due to tanning bed use and greater exposure to the ultraviolet radiation. [9] Education programs targeted at highlighting risky behaviors and leading to increased protection from UV radiation and other toxic exposures can limit the incidence of melanoma as the individual progresses from childhood to adulthood.

Melanoma: What Is It?

Skin cancer is one of the most common types of malignancy in the United States with over 1,000,000 cases of skin cancer diagnosed yearly. [13] Melanoma accounts for 4% of dermatologic cancers but is responsible for 80% of the deaths from skin cancer. [14] Patients who develop metastatic melanoma have a poor prognosis with only 14% surviving five years. [14]

The model for progression of melanoma is the Clark Model which describes the stepwise transformation of melanocytes to melanoma. [15] The process for this is melanocytes begin to replicate and proliferate in the process of forming nevi which then leads to the subsequent development of dysplasia, hyperplasia, invasion, and metastasis. [16, 17]

The first change in melanocytes is the formation of benign nevi; these cells have disrupted growth regulation. These cells have atypical activation of mitogen-activated protein kinase (MAPK) which leads to growth in these cells. [18] Many of these benign nevi develop mutations in BRAF and p53 which lead to progression of cancer. [19]

The next step in the path to tumorigenesis is the development of dysplastic nevi which have molecular irregularities. These irregularities include problems with DNA repair and susceptibility to cell death, associated with the previously mentioned BRAF and p53 mutations. [18]

Mortality and morbidity in melanoma come through local invasion and metastatic spread which occur when melanocytes continue to pick up mutations. [18, 20] Tumor cells begin to dissociate from the primary lesion and invade lymaphtics and blood vessels to establish tumors at differing sites.

Genetic Background of Melanoma

There have been many genetic factors which are thought to increase an individual's chances towards developing melanoma. Recent studies have shown that 10% of melanoma patients have a family history of melanoma as well, and thus have a twofold increased risk of developing melanoma. [21] Additionally, many factors which convey an increased risk of melanoma such as familial atypical mole/melanoma (FAMM) syndrome and a light skin complexion, among others, are heritable risk factors passed on from parents to children. [21] Epidemiological studies have elucidated the fact that there is a positive correlation between light skin color and risk for melanoma. One gene associated with this is melanocortin-1 receptor (MC1R), a gene for the transmembrane receptor which leads to the induction of transcription for pigment synthetic genes. [22] These genes result in the production of eumelanin which is the major player in the tempering of UV radiation in individuals with darkly pigmented skin. [21, 22] Having a predisposition to the genetic factors which can lead to melanoma can manifest through early onset of the disease or multiple primary melanomas in the patient as well as multiple cases of melanoma in the family history.

There are a few different loci in the human genome which confer a greater risk to patients in terms of developing melanoma. One such locus is RB1. Patients with inactivated copies of RB1 in the germline have a significantly high risk of developing melanoma; it is estimated that they have a 4-fold to 80-fold increase in the chance to develop melanoma. [21]

Another important locus which has been linked with greater risk of developing melanoma is CDKN2A, a gene located on the chromosome 9p21 region. CDKN2A codes for p16, a protein which is a potent tumor suppressor that inhibits CDK4; a mutation in CDKN2A, as present in many melanoma families, leads to G1-S transition and resumption of the cell cycle. [22, 23] The role of CDKN2A in leading to melanomas has been shown in murine models. In mice who were CDKN2A-- and contained alleles which activated the oncogene NRAS where shown to form cutaneous melanoma like tumors. [22-24] Additionally, when these mice were exposed to UV radiation they quickly formed cutaneous melanomas.

The risks for patients to develop cutaneous melanoma who have a CDKN2A mutation are increased significantly. [21-24] According to one study, the penetrance of developing melanoma in these familial cases is 30% by age 50 and 67% by age 80. [25] Mutations in this gene can lead to an increased risk of developing melanoma, especially when exposed to UV radiation.

PROGNOSTIC FACTORS FOR MELANOMA

As the incidence of melanoma continues to increase in the general population it becomes more critical to have accurate histopathologic diagnosis of melanocytic lesions, particularly in initial biopsies, because histopathologic parameters are critical components of both staging and diagnosis of melanoma. [26-28] There are a variety of different parameters that are used; these parameters are useful in staging the tumor and determining the prognosis of the patient but also in analyzing the potential for future treatment options or determining metastatic lesions. [27, 29]

Breslow Thickness

The Brewslow thickness is one of the most important prognostic factors for melanoma clinical behavior and it also has been shown to have the least interobserver variability. [27, 29, 30] The Brewslow thickness is a measurement taken from the top of the epidermal granular layer down to the deepest melanocyte of the invasive component of melanoma. [27]

Mitotic Figures

Mitotic figures are an important part of staging and are used in defining T1 categories. [27, 31, 32] This involves counting mitotic figures and should only be done in invasive dermal components of melanoma. [31] This is done by reporting the mitotic count per square millimeter. A high mitotic rate is associated with worse survival.

Vertical and Radial Growth Phase

Radial and vertical growth phase can be an important prognostic indicator for melanoma. All in situ melanomas only have radial (Nontumorigenic) growth phases. [27, 32-34] Vertical (tumorigenic) growth phases, on the other hand, have dermal nests which are bigger than any nests located in the junctional component of the lesion. [27, 32-34] Vertical growth is strongly correlated with metastatic potential of melanoma and can be related to the tumor volume.

Ulceration

Ulceration is regarded as an independent prognostic factor for melanoma-associated survival and the rates of patients with ulcerated melanoma are lower than those of patients with nonulcerated melanoma. [27]

It is worth noting that there have been several biomarkers which have been identified as a means to aid in prognostication of primary melanoma. Methods employed in trying to aid in prognostication include polymerase chain reaction (PCR), gene expression arrays, immunohistochemistry, and comparative genomic hybridization (CGH). [35] However, no biomarkers for prognosis in melanoma have been translated to clinical practice. An introduction of biomarkers into the clinical setting would allow for more accurate diagnoses and a better chance of catching melanoma in earlier stages.

Incidence in Young Individuals

It is well established that melanoma is a major cause of mortality and morbidity in the U.S. that the rates of cancers are going up in the population as a whole. [13, 14] The predominance of melanoma incidence in the U.S. is in the age group above 55 years of age. In the U.S. and the U.K., the incidence of melanoma from 1973 to 2002 in the male population aged between 55 and 64 years old went up from 12.4 cases/100,000 to 56.1 cases/100,000 whereas in the age group over 65 years of age the incidence went from 18.8 to 104.4/100,000, a sharp increase. [13, 14, 36]

However, there are few studies which examine the incidence in young individuals. One such epidemiological study done in Olmsted County, Minnesota showed that the incidence of cutaneous melanoma is increasing among young adults and that the incidence has increased 6-fold from 1970 to 2009. [12] It is known that the lifetime risk for melanoma is higher in males rather than in females. [13, 14, 36] However, the opposite is true in young adults; the female-male incidence ratio among young adults aged 20-24 is reported to be as high as 1.8. Over the time period of 1970 to 2009, the incidence for women increased 8-fold while the incidence for men increased 4-fold. [12] In addition melanoma is the third most common cancer of men in their 20s.

CAUSES FOR THE INCREASING INCIDENCE

There are a host of factors which could be leading to an increase in the incidence of melanoma in young individuals. These factors include environmental factors such as decrease in the earth's ozone layer to behavioral changes such as increased exposure to artificial UVR for tanning, changes in clothing preference to those that expose more skin, and spending more time in sunny locations. [2] Additionally, increases in development and prescription of photo-sensitive drugs as well as use of cosmetic agents have also led to increased incidence of melanoma.

Ozone Depletion

Ozone depletion has been linked with higher UVB radiation reaching the ground, which in turn is thought to be a factor for the increasing incidence of melanoma. [37] Governments across the world have banned production of ozone delpleting substances such as hydrobromoflourocarbons, cholorofluorocarbons (CFCs), and other substances such as halons. Ozone delpleting substances such as these were used in a variety of everyday appilances such as refrigiators, aerosol products, air conditioning systems, and even automobiles. [2] The damage to the ozone is allowing more UV radiation to hit the earth, resulting in more DNA damage in those exposed to it. [37]

Photosensitive Drugs

Photo-sensitive drugs can also be a cause for increased incidence of melanoma. Drug-induced photosensitivity can occur in a plethora of different mechanisms. The photo-sensitivity that results can be classified as either photosensitization reactions or as phototoxic. Photosensitization reactions to drugs can lead to indirect DNA damage through the formation of ROS species and can occur due to topical drugs. [38] Phototoxic reactions cause cellular damage by resulting in deeper penetration of UVA light; this can be seen in initial exposure to medication. [39] Medications which are associated with photosensitivity include oral contraceptives, retinoids, tetracyclines, and phenothiazines. [40] Many of those drugs are used by younger individuals to prevent pregnancy (oral contraceptives) or to treat acne (tetracyclines) and as such can lead to higher photoreactivity. [2]

Cosmetic Agents

Chemical agents, such as those used in cosmetics, have been shown to play an increased role developing cancer. The ingredients of these cosmetic products are absorbed through the skin, particularly when they are applied for long periods of time, such as facial makeup. [41] Substances such as diethanolamine (DEA) or 2-bromo-2-nitropropane-1,3-diol can end up leading to the formation of nitrosamines which are considered to be carcinogenic. [42] DEA is found in shampoos, creams, and skin lotions, among other applications and is widely used.

Other cosmetic products, such as hair dyes and temporary tattoos, contain products such as para-phenylenediamine (PPD) which have been shown to transform human skin and are considered carcinogenic. [43] The absorption spectra of hair dye compounds also absorb UVA and UVB which could result in UV-induced DNA damage indirectly. [42] These products are often targeted at younger individuals and those individuals are more likely to use these cosmetic agents. [2]

Sex Hormones

Many different hormones target both normal and malignant melanocytes; these hormones include testosterone and estrogen, among others which stimulate the pigment cells. [44] There has been research done on the link between sex hormones and the biological behavior of melanoma which have elucidated different survival prognoses for men and women as well as the scarcity in incidence of melanoma in children who have not undergone puberty. [2, 44, 45]

Ultraviolet Radiation

Ultraviolet radiation, resulting from exposure to the sun, is the wavelength (100nm-350nm) directly implicated with development of the disease.1, 2 Between the UV radiation wavelengths of 100 to 280nm is called UVA and the wavelengths between 280 and 350nm is UVB (Table 1). [1, 7, 46] The international Agency for Research on Cancer (IARC) and the National Toxicology programs have classified UVA and UVB wavelengths as human carcinogens, stating that “there is sufficient evidence in humans for the carcinogenicity of solar radiation. Solar radiation causes cutaneous malignant melanoma and non-melanocytic skin cancer.” [47]

Table 1. UV radiation range

Wavelength Range (nm)	Type of UV Radation
100-280	UVA
280-350	UVB

The earth’s atmosphere filters UVB using ozone (O3) so that the UV light which hits the surface is 5% UVB and 95% UVA. UVR has many effects on skin including erythema, sunburn, inflammation, pigmentation, and cancer. [34, 37-39, 48-50]

UV radiation leads to DNA damage in the skin which can lead to carcinogenesis; in particular, UVB is especially dangerous as DNA absorbs strongly in this wavelength which leads to cyclobutane pyrimidine dimers. [51, 52] These cyclobutane dimers are considered to be unique to UVB irradiation; these dimers lead to steric hindrance which leads to problem in replication and transcription of DNA. [34, 48-50] This damage is repaired through the tumor suppressor p53. [19, 24] However, p53 can also be affected by the damage, leading to dysregulation of repair. This is how UV-mediated damage of the DNA leads to carcinogenic potential in those individuals with repeated high exposure to UV radiation. [19, 24]

UVA penetrates skin deeper than UVB and can cause oxidative damage to DNA that has the potential to be mutagenic. UVA is not absorbed by DNA but rather by chromophores in the skin. [52] Upon excitation, these chromophores generate reactive intermediates which include oxygen free radicals. [53-55] These oxygen free radicals can cause DNA breaks and although UVA is not as efficient as UVB it still results in oncogenesis [55]

Studies in animals have also suggested that UVR exposure is a critical step in the pathogenesis of melanoma. It has been shown in opossums, fish, and other animals that melanoma can be induced by UV radiation. [56-58]

Aside from this, there is strong epidemiologic evidence that UVR is linked with melanoma. In studies does examining links of melanoma with latitude, higher incidence rates of skin cancer were found in locations closer to the equator where sunlight exposure was the greatest. [48, 59, 60]

Lighter skin color is also linked with higher rates of melanoma. Superficial epidermal melanin lowers the transmission of UVR resulting in the protection of basal layer melanocytes from UVR damage that can lead to malignancy. [48, 59, 60] Melanin is seen as a natural sunscreen that regulates UVR penetration into the skin, resulting in lower levels of DNA damage. People with lighter skin have lesser amount of melanin and are at greater risk for developing melanoma without adequate photo-protection. [19, 21, 50, 61]

History of sun exposure is also important in terms of etiology of melanoma skin cancer. Increased amounts of sun exposure, especially in areas of elevated UVR radiation, result in higher levels of skin cancer. [19, 21, 50, 61] Development of cancer often occurs in areas that receive the most sun exposure (hands, neck, face) and others were protective measures such as sun-screen do not cover (backs of the ear). [20, 62, 63]

Exposures as an adolescent to young adult are termed to be "critical periods of vulnerability," periods when people are at higher risks to the effects of toxic exposure. Studies have shown that approximately 25% of lifetime sun exposure occurs before 18 years of age. [3, 4, 10] This sun exposure can result in the alteration of melanocyte DNA which can lead to increased risk of development of malignant nevi (moles). Children with light skin tend to develop more nevi in comparison to children who are darker. Peak melanocytic activity occurs early in life as shown by the acquisition of nevi and freckling during childhood and adolescence. [3, 10, 44] Freckles appear in children after high levels of sun exposure and are considered to be clones of mutated melanocytes; the presence of freckling is associated with an increased risk of melanoma. [3, 64] Children who have been exposed to high sunlight in childhood have more initiated melanocytes than those who have less sunlight exposure – this is thought to be due to increased UVR exposure. [3, 10, 44, 65]

TANNING BED USE AND MELANOMA

Since the 1970's, more and more individuals have started using tanning beds as a means of obtaining tanner skin. Over the course of the past 40 years there have been significant changes in the practice of indoor tanning. [52] Sunlamps which were used in the 1970s primarily emitted UVB and artificial tanning most commonly occurred at home. A shift took place in the 1980s when people started tanning at salons and the machines there began to use UVA radiation instead of UVB. [7, 9] Most modern sunlamps emit in the UVA range and the amount of radiation received in one exposure from a powerful unit is 10-15 times the strength of midday sunlight.

Tanning beds or artificial sunlamps work by exposing individuals to UVR which leads to a biphasic response: immediate pigment darkening (IPD) and delayed tanning. Immediate pigment darkening does not lead to synthesis of new melanin but rather the oxidation of previous melanin. [52] IPD also leads to redistribution of melanosomes throughout the cell. [66, 67] This process is considered to be minimally photoprotective but results in more pigmented looking skin. Delayed tanning leads to melanogenesis as well as increased melanocytic proliferation and activity. [68, 69] Additionally, the stratum corneum and epidermis get thicker. These changes become apparent three days after exposure to UVR and they serve to form a nuclear cap of melanin that defends against damage to the cell's genetic content. [66-69]

Research has shown that tanning bed use is dangerous, especially when conducted in the adolescent to young adult years. A meta-analysis done showed that individuals who began to use tanning devices such as sunlamps before the age of 30 had up to a 75% increase in the risk for melanoma. [3, 67, 70] Surveys conducted in the US have shown that 60% of all tanning bed users were under the age of 45, illustrating that the prevalence of tanning bed use is partly responsible for the rising incidence of melanoma. [47, 71] A study of 73,494 female nurses conducted showed that use of artificial tanning resulted in more moles and higher incidence of melanoma (Table 2). [72]

Many studies on the demographics of tanning bed users have shown that indoor tanning is most prevalent in younger populations. Additionally, more indoor tanning facilities were used more frequently by females in comparison. A 1996 study conducted by the American Academy of Dermatology found that the frequency of tanning bed use had increased among women despite programs which were aimed at increasing public exposure to the dangers of UVR. [11] Other studies have shown young women have a greater tendency to use indoor tanning machines. [9] This increased use of tanning beds among young females in comparison to males can be seen as one of the factors for the 8-fold increase in melanoma incidence in females. [12]

There are a variety of factors which could be the impetus behind the higher incidence of younger individuals, especially females, using the indoor tanning machines. One such factor is media influence. Many TV shows, including reality TV, show tan individuals creating the desire in many individuals' minds that they want to look like that. [73] One study showed that female college students who viewed images of tan models in magazines which targeted young women had an increasing desire to "get a tan." Other studies on female college students have shown that attitudes towards media portrayal of tanning are associated with a greater incidence of indoor tanning among them. [74] Men did not have an increased incidence of tanning after watching reality TV shows or other portrayals in the media. [73]

Tanning is also considered to be an appearance management behavior; women are more concerned with their appearance and may engage in more tanning activities. Many women get tan to remediate what they perceive to be a flawed appearance. [73] Men also participate in indoor tanning but to a more limited numbers.

Table 2. Incidence of tanning bed use as well as melanoma development in young individuals {Zhang, 2012 #17}

	1-2 Times/year	3-5 times/year	>6 times/year
	During High School/College		
Mean age	33.0	32.5	31.8
Family History of Melanoma (%)	5.8	7.2	6.5
Outdoor sun exposure >5 hrs, (%)	65.2	72.2	75.8
No. of moles on legs >3, (%)	34.3	34.8	35.6
Melanoma, No.	17	8	12
	Between Age 25-35		
Mean age	33.5	33.0	32.5
Family History of Melanoma (%)	5.7	4.9	5.7
Outdoor sun exposure >5 hrs, (%)	54.0	56.9	65.8
No. of moles on legs >3, (%)	33.9	32.9	34.2
Melanoma, No.	25	14	32

PREVENTION

With the increasing incidence and cost of melanoma, it becomes crucial to take steps to prevent the disease or delay its onset. There are many steps which can be taken towards prevention, changes that can make an immediate impact.

A first step towards prevention could be reducing the prevalence of tanning bed use in young individuals. This could be accomplished in a variety of different ways including raising costs for artificial tanning, making machines less accessible, or limiting the amount of tanning available per person. [71, 75, 76] A more aggressive measure would be to ban tanning beds completely, making artificial exposure to UVR much less prevalent.

Other steps which could be taken during childhood would be to limit children's exposure to midday-sun and encouraging use of sunscreen when going outside, such as the SunSmart program implemented in Australia. [77] Sunscreens block out UVR affecting the epidermis which prevents against sunburn. [50, 71, 78] By applying sunscreen in conditions when children and adolescents are exposed to sunlight on a regular basis it would become possible to lower incidence of melanoma and avoid DNA damage in the "critical years." [3] The SunSmart program targets primary and secondary school children through strong intervention techniques. This program includes staff intervention requiring children put on sunscreen before going out to play in the sun as well as other methods targeting safe and limited sun exposure. [77]

Some final steps which could be taken to combat rising incidence of melanoma could be smaller things such as increasing window tinting in cars and homes as well using sunglasses to help prevent uveal melanoma. [34, 79] More and more time is being spent in cars during childhood and in adolescence. Car windows allow a great deal of UVA exposure which could be limited by tinting windows

Conclusion

The most common type of cancer affecting patients today is skin cancer; cutaneous melanoma is a serious type of skin cancer originating from melanocytes. Incidence rates of skin cancer and melanoma have been steadily increasing over the past 75 years, with rates increasing from 1/500 in 1935 to 1/50 more recently. [2] Younger individuals are at increasing risk for melanoma due to changes in the ozone layer, cosmetic agents, genetic predispositions, increased hormones, behavioral modifications, and increased exposure to UV light through artificial means such as tanning beds.

Tanning bed use leads to increased exposure to UV radiation with the primary type being UVA. UVA leads to oxidative damage which can be mutagenic. As individuals expose themselves repeatedly to UVA light, these mutagenic changes add up and can lead to the development of melanoma.

Targeting this younger group of individuals with preventive measures such as stricter regulations of tanning beds and other photo-preventive measures can lower the incidence of melanoma. Most importantly, there is a need for a change in mindset and behavior to result in significant differences in the rates of melanoma. Skin cancer and melanoma are diseases that effect a large segment of our population but with advances in medicine and strategic planning, it may be possible to lower incidence and morbidity.

References

[1] Chang, A. E., Karnell, L. H. and Menck, H. R., The National Cancer Data Base report on cutaneous and noncutaneous melanoma: a summary of 84,836 cases from the past decade. The American College of Surgeons Commission on Cancer and the American Cancer Society, Cancer, 1998, 83(8):1664-1678.

[2] Volkovova, K., Bilanicova, D., Bartonova, A., Letasiova, S. and Dusinska, M., Associations between environmental factors and incidence of cutaneous melanoma. Review, Environ Health, 2012, 11 Suppl 1:S12.

[3] Balk, S. J., Ultraviolet radiation: a hazard to children and adolescents, Pediatrics, 2011, 127(3):e791-817.

[4] Cripps, D. J. and Hegedus, S., Protection factor of sunscreens to monochromatic radiation, Arch Dermatol, 1974, 109(2):202-204.

[5] Davies, H., Bignell, G. R., Cox, C., Stephens, P., Edkins, S., Clegg, S., Teague, J., et al., Mutations of the BRAF gene in human cancer, Nature, 2002, 417(6892):949-954.

[6] Dennis, L. K., Vanbeek, M. J., Beane Freeman, L. E., Smith, B. J., Dawson, D. V. and Coughlin, J. A., Sunburns and risk of cutaneous melanoma: does age matter? A comprehensive meta-analysis, Ann Epidemiol, 2008, 18(8):614-627.

[7] Gallagher, R. P., Spinelli, J. J. and Lee, T. K., Tanning beds, sunlamps, and risk of cutaneous malignant melanoma, Cancer Epidemiol Biomarkers Prev, 2005, 14(3):562-566.

[8] Ting, W., Schultz, K., Cac, N. N., Peterson, M. and Walling, H. W., Tanning bed exposure increases the risk of malignant melanoma, Int J Dermatol, 2007, 46(12):1253-1257.

[9] Choi, K., Lazovich, D., Southwell, B., Forster, J., Rolnick, S. J. and Jackson, J., Prevalence and characteristics of indoor tanning use among men and women in the United States, Arch Dermatol, 2010, 146(12):1356-1361.

[10] Cokkinides, V., Weinstock, M., Glanz, K., Albano, J., Ward, E. and Thun, M., Trends in sunburns, sun protection practices, and attitudes toward sun exposure protection and tanning among US adolescents, 1998-2004, Pediatrics, 2006, 118(3):853-864.

[11] Robinson, J. K., Rigel, D. S. and Amonette, R. A., Trends in sun exposure knowledge, attitudes, and behaviors: 1986 to 1996, J Am Acad Dermatol, 1997, 37(2 Pt 1):179-186.

[12] Reed, K. B., Brewer, J. D., Lohse, C. M., Bringe, K. E., Pruitt, C. N. and Gibson, L. E., Increasing incidence of melanoma among young adults: an epidemiological study in Olmsted County, Minnesota, Mayo Clin Proc, 2012, 87(4):328-334.

[13] American Cancer Society: Cancer facts and figures, 2009.

[14] National Cancer Institute: Surveillance Epidemiology and End Results: Cancer Statistics Review., 2012.

[15] Frishberg DP, B. C., Balzer BL, Protocol for the examination of specimens from patients with melanoma of the skin, College of American Pathologists, 2011.

[16] Farber, M. J., Heilman, E. R. and Friedman, R. J., Dysplastic nevi, Dermatol Clin, 2012, 30(3):389-404.

[17] Ferris, L. K. and Harris, R. J., New diagnostic aids for melanoma, Dermatol Clin, 2012, 30(3):535-545.

[18] Miller, A. J. and Mihm, M. C., Melanoma, New England Journal of Medicine, 2006, 355(1):51-65.

[19] Box, N. F. and Terzian, T., The role of p53 in pigmentation, tanning and melanoma, Pigment Cell Melanoma Res, 2008, 21(5):525-533.

[20] Russak, J. E. and Rigel, D. S., Risk factors for the development of primary cutaneous melanoma, Dermatol Clin, 2012, 30(3):363-368.

[21] Tsao, H., Chin, L., Garraway, L. A. and Fisher, D. E., Melanoma: from mutations to medicine, Genes Dev, 2012, 26(11):1131-1155.

[22] Demenais, F., Mohamdi, H., Chaudru, V., Goldstein, A. M., Newton Bishop, J. A., Bishop, D. T., Kanetsky, P. A., et al., Association of MC1R variants and host phenotypes with melanoma risk in CDKN2A mutation carriers: a GenoMEL study, J Natl Cancer Inst, 2010, 102(20):1568-1583.

[23] Wu, H., Goel, V. and Haluska, F. G., PTEN signaling pathways in melanoma, Oncogene, 2003, 22(20):3113-3122.

[24] Chudnovsky, Y., Adams, A. E., Robbins, P. B., Lin, Q. and Khavari, P. A., Use of human tissue to assess the oncogenic activity of melanoma-associated mutations, Nat Genet, 2005, 37(7):745-749.

[25] Bishop, D. T., Demenais, F., Goldstein, A. M., Bergman, W., Bishop, J. N., Paillerets, B. B.-d., Chompret, A., et al., Geographical Variation in the Penetrance of CDKN2A Mutations for Melanoma, Journal of the National Cancer Institute, 2002, 94(12):894-903.

[26] Hawryluk, E. B., Sober, A. J., Piris, A., Nazarian, R. M., Hoang, M. P., Tsao, H., Mihm, M. C., Jr., et al., Histologically challenging melanocytic tumors referred to a tertiary care pigmented lesion clinic, J Am Acad Dermatol, 2012, 67(4):727-735.

[27] Ivan, D. and Prieto, V. G., An update on reporting histopathologic prognostic factors in melanoma, Arch Pathol Lab Med, 2011, 135(7):825-829.

[28] Leiter, U., Buettner, P. G., Eigentler, T. K. and Garbe, C., Prognostic factors of thin cutaneous melanoma: an analysis of the central malignant melanoma registry of the german dermatological society, J Clin Oncol, 2004, 22(18):3660-3667.

[29] Scolyer, R. A., Thompson, J. F., Stretch, J. R., Sharma, R. and McCarthy, S. W., Pathology of melanocytic lesions: new, controversial, and clinically important issues, J Surg Oncol, 2004, 86(4):200-211.

[30] Sartore, L., Papanikolaou, G. E., Biancari, F. and Mazzoleni, F., Prognostic factors of cutaneous melanoma in relation to metastasis at the sentinel lymph node: a case-controlled study, Int J Surg, 2008, 6(3):205-209.

[31] Kesmodel, S. B., Karakousis, G. C., Botbyl, J. D., Canter, R. J., Lewis, R. T., Wahl, P. M., Terhune, K. P., et al., Mitotic rate as a predictor of sentinel lymph node positivity in patients with thin melanomas, Ann Surg Oncol, 2005, 12(6):449-458.

[32] Ruiter, D. J., Spatz, A., van den Oord, J. J. and Cook, M. G., Pathologic staging of melanoma, Semin Oncol, 2002, 29(4):370-381.

[33] Long, G. V., Menzies, A. M., Nagrial, A. M., Haydu, L. E., Hamilton, A. L., Mann, G. J., Hughes, T. M., et al., Prognostic and clinicopathologic associations of oncogenic BRAF in metastatic melanoma, J Clin Oncol, 2011, 29(10):1239-1246.

[34] Svetlosakova, Z., Krasnik, V., Gergisakova, H., Babal, P. and Kusenda, P., [Selected prognostic factors of malignant uveal melanoma], Cesk Slov Oftalmol, 2012, 68(1):38-42.

[35] Wisco, O. J. and Sober, A. J., Prognostic factors for melanoma, Dermatol Clin, 2012, 30(3):469-485.

[36] Alexander, R. L., Skin cancer: causes and groups at risk, Nurs Times, 2012, 108(30-31):23-25.

[37] Pandey, R., Mehrotra, S., Ray, R. S., Joshi, P. C. and Hans, R. K., Evaluation of UV-radiation induced singlet oxygen generation potential of selected drugs, Drug Chem Toxicol, 2002, 25(2):215-225.

[38] O'Donovan, P., Perrett, C. M., Zhang, X., Montaner, B., Xu, Y. Z., Harwood, C. A., McGregor, J. M., et al., Azathioprine and UVA light generate mutagenic oxidative DNA damage, Science, 2005, 309(5742):1871-1874.

[39] Xia, Q., Yin, J. J., Cherng, S. H., Wamer, W. G., Boudreau, M., Howard, P. C. and Fu, P. P., UVA photoirradiation of retinyl palmitate--formation of singlet oxygen and superoxide, and their role in induction of lipid peroxidation, Toxicol Lett, 2006, 163(1):30-43.

[40] Lee A, T. J., Adverse Drug Reactions: Pharmaceutical Press, 2006.

[41] Nohynek, G. J., Duche, D., Garrigues, A., Meunier, P. A., Toutain, H. and Leclaire, J., Under the skin: Biotransformation of para-aminophenol and para-phenylenediamine in reconstructed human epidermis and human hepatocytes, Toxicol Lett, 2005, 158(3):196-212.

[42] Nohynek, G. J., Fautz, R., Benech-Kieffer, F. and Toutain, H., Toxicity and human health risk of hair dyes, Food Chem Toxicol, 2004, 42(4):517-543.

[43] Rojanapo, W., Kupradinun, P., Tepsuwan, A., Chutimataewin, S. and Tanyakaset, M., Carcinogenicity of an oxidation product of p-phenylenediamine, Carcinogenesis, 1986, 7(12):1997-2002.

[44] Lasithiotakis, K., Leiter, U., Meier, F., Eigentler, T., Metzler, G., Moehrle, M., Breuninger, H., et al., Age and gender are significant independent predictors of survival in primary cutaneous melanoma, Cancer, 2008, 112(8):1795-1804.

[45] Zell, J. A., Cinar, P., Mobasher, M., Ziogas, A., Meyskens, F. L., Jr. and Anton-Culver, H., Survival for patients with invasive cutaneous melanoma among ethnic groups: the effects of socioeconomic status and treatment, J Clin Oncol, 2008, 26(1):66-75.

[46] Lim, J. H., Park, S. H., Kim, M. R., Yoo, B. S., Yang, J. C., Cheong, I. W., Kim, J. H., et al., Cyclohexanediol bis-ethylhexanoate inhibits melanogenesis of murine b16 melanoma and uv-induced pigmentation in human skin, *Biol Pharm Bull,* 2012.

[47] Boniol, M., Autier, P., Boyle, P. and Gandini, S., Cutaneous melanoma attributable to sunbed use: systematic review and meta-analysis, BMJ, 2012, 345:e4757.

[48] Besaratinia, A. and Pfeifer, G. P., Sunlight ultraviolet irradiation and BRAF V600 mutagenesis in human melanoma, Hum Mutat, 2008, 29(8):983-991.

[49] Farhat, E. K., Top-accessed article: UV light tanning as a type of substance-related disorder, Arch Dermatol, 2012, 148(10):1182.

[50] Kanavy, H. E. and Gerstenblith, M. R., Ultraviolet radiation and melanoma, Semin Cutan Med Surg, 2011, 30(4):222-228.

[51] Dore, J. F. and Chignol, M. C., Tanning salons and skin cancer, Photochem Photobiol Sci, 2012, 11(1):30-37.

[52] Ibrahim, S. F. and Brown, M. D., Tanning and cutaneous malignancy, Dermatol Surg, 2008, 34(4):460-474.

[53] Barker, C. A. and Lee, N. Y., Radiation therapy for cutaneous melanoma, Dermatol Clin, 2012, 30(3):525-533.

[54] Nielsen, K., Masback, A., Olsson, H. and Ingvar, C., A prospective, population-based study of 40,000 women regarding host factors, UV exposure and sunbed use in relation to risk and anatomic site of cutaneous melanoma, Int J Cancer, 2012, 131(3):706-715.

[55] Villanueva, J., Vultur, A., Lee, J. T., Somasundaram, R., Fukunaga-Kalabis, M., Cipolla, A. K., Wubbenhorst, B., et al., Acquired resistance to BRAF inhibitors mediated by a RAF kinase switch in melanoma can be overcome by cotargeting MEK and IGF-1R/PI3K, Cancer Cell, 2010, 18(6):683-695.

[56] Gevertz, A. K., Tucker, A. J., Bowling, A. M., Williamson, C. E. and Oris, J. T., Differential tolerance of native and nonnative fish exposed to ultraviolet radiation and fluoranthene in Lake Tahoe (California/Nevada), USA, Environ Toxicol Chem, 2012, 31(5):1129-1135.

[57] Maksimovich, A. A. and Gniubkina, V. P., [Response of the retina of Pacific salmon fry to magnetic field and ultraviolet radiation], Morfologiia, 2012, 142(5):34-38.

[58] Robinson, E. S., Hubbard, G. B., Colon, G. and Vandeberg, J. L., Low-dose ultraviolet exposure early in development can lead to widespread melanoma in the opossum model, Int J Exp Pathol, 1998, 79(4):235-244.

[59] Coelho, S. G. and Hearing, V. J., UVA tanning is involved in the increased incidence of skin cancers in fair-skinned young women, Pigment Cell Melanoma Res, 2010, 23(1):57-63.

[60] Weinstock, M. A. and Fisher, D. E., Indoor ultraviolet tanning: what the data do and do not show regarding risk of melanoma and keratinocyte malignancies, J Natl Compr Canc Netw, 2010, 8(8):867-872; quiz 873.

[61] Allen, B. C., Mohammed, T. L., Tan, C. D., Miller, D. V., Williamson, E. E. and Kirsch, J. S., Metastatic melanoma to the heart, Curr Probl Diagn Radiol, 2012, 41(5):159-164.

[62] Schulman, J. M. and Fisher, D. E., Indoor ultraviolet tanning and skin cancer: health risks and opportunities, Curr Opin Oncol, 2009, 21(2):144-149.

[63] Wehner, M. R., Shive, M. L., Chren, M. M., Han, J., Qureshi, A. A. and Linos, E., Indoor tanning and non-melanoma skin cancer: systematic review and meta-analysis, BMJ, 2012, 345:e5909.

[64] Surber, C., [Children, adolescents, young adults and sun protection], MMW Fortschr Med, 2012, 154(8):43-46.

[65] Situm, M., Buljan, M., Bulic, S. O. and Simic, D., The mechanisms of UV radiation in the development of malignant melanoma, Coll Antropol, 2007, 31 Suppl 1:13-16.

[66] Routaboul, C., Denis, A. and Bohbot, M., Proposal for a new UVA protection factor: use of an in vitro model of immediate pigment darkening, Eur J Dermatol, 2002, 12(5):439-444.

[67] Sklar, L. R., Almutawa, F., Lim, H. W. and Hamzavi, I., Effects of ultraviolet radiation, visible light, and infrared radiation on erythema and pigmentation: a review, Photochem Photobiol Sci, 2013, 12(1):54-64.

[68] Hwang, Y. J., Park, H. J., Hahn, H. J., Kim, J. Y., Ko, J. H., Lee, Y. W., Choe, Y. B., et al., Immediate pigment darkening and persistent pigment darkening as means of measuring the ultraviolet A protection factor in vivo: a comparative study, Br J Dermatol, 2011, 164(6):1356-1361.

[69] Moan, J., Nielsen, K. P. and Juzeniene, A., Immediate pigment darkening: its evolutionary roles may include protection against folate photosensitization, FASEB J, 2012, 26(3):971-975.

[70] Lazovich, D., Vogel, R. I., Berwick, M., Weinstock, M. A., Anderson, K. E. and Warshaw, E. M., Indoor tanning and risk of melanoma: a case-control study in a highly exposed population, Cancer Epidemiol Biomarkers Prev, 2010, 19(6):1557-1568.

[71] Buller, D. B., Cokkinides, V., Hall, H. I., Hartman, A. M., Saraiya, M., Miller, E., Paddock, L., et al., Prevalence of sunburn, sun protection, and indoor tanning behaviors among Americans: review from national surveys and case studies of 3 states, J Am Acad Dermatol, 2011, 65(5 Suppl 1):S114-123.

[72] Zhang, M., Qureshi, A. A., Geller, A. C., Frazier, L., Hunter, D. J. and Han, J., Use of tanning beds and incidence of skin cancer, J Clin Oncol, 2012, 30(14):1588-1593.

[73] Fogel, J. and Krausz, F., Watching reality television beauty shows is associated with tanning lamp use and outdoor tanning among college students, J Am Acad Dermatol, 2012.

[74] Gillen, M. M. and Markey, C. N., The role of body image and depression in tanning behaviors and attitudes, Behav Med, 2012, 38(3):74-82.

[75] Lim, H. W., James, W. D., Rigel, D. S., Maloney, M. E., Spencer, J. M. and Bhushan, R., Adverse effects of ultraviolet radiation from the use of indoor tanning equipment: time to ban the tan, J Am Acad Dermatol, 2011, 64(4):e51-60.

[76] Lostritto, K., Ferrucci, L. M., Cartmel, B., Leffell, D. J., Molinaro, A. M., Bale, A. E. and Mayne, S. T., Lifetime history of indoor tanning in young people: a retrospective assessment of initiation, persistence, and correlates, BMC Public Health, 2012, 12:118.

[77] Makin, J. K., Warne, C. D., Dobbinson, S. J., Wakefield, M. A. and Hill, D. J., Population and age-group trends in weekend sun protection and sunburn over two decades of the SunSmart programme in Melbourne, Australia, Br J Dermatol, 2013, 168(1):154-161.

[78] Mulliken, J. S., Russak, J. E. and Rigel, D. S., The effect of sunscreen on melanoma risk, Dermatol Clin, 2012, 30(3):369-376.

[79] Topcu-Yilmaz, P., Kiratli, H., Saglam, A., Soylemezoglu, F. and Hascelik, G., Correlation of clinicopathological parameters with HGF, c-Met, EGFR, and IGF-1R expression in uveal melanoma, Melanoma Res, 2010, 20(2):126-132.

In: Melanoma
Editor: Alexander C. Jones

ISBN: 978-1-62808-608-9

Chapter 8

CARDIAC INVOLVEMENT IN MALIGNANT MELANOMA

Antonella Fontana*

Department of Cardiology, St. Gerardo Hospital and
University of Milan-Bicocca, Monza, Italy

ABSTRACT

Skin is a complex tissue, whose outer layer, epidermis, protects against ultraviolet radiation and several pathogens. Thus, epidermal cells have a high risk of acquiring gene mutations leading to cancer. Malignant melanoma is a tumor derived from genetically altered epidermal melanocytes; it is highly aggressive, often associated with rapid progression. Familial melanomas represent about 10% of all melanoma cases. The study of familiar cases led to the identification of several melanoma susceptibility genes in chromosomes 1, 6, 7, 9, and 10. Some of the molecular pathways altered in malignant melanoma regard tyrosine kinase receptors pathways, cell cycle regulation pathways, epigenetic gene expression regulation, apoptosis pathways, common apoptosis effectors, and protein chaperoning and degradation.

The presence of lymph-node metastases decreases the 5-year survival rate by approximately 40%. However, 25% of patients free of lymphatic metastasis have disease recurrence and die.

Malignant melanoma has a high rate of cardiac metastases. It is rarely detected ante mortem, and can involve almost any cardiac structure. Heart involvement is usually silent, or the patient complains of nonspecific symptoms. Right or left heart failure, cardiac tamponade and atrioventricular block can also occur. Echocardiography is a first-line imaging technique for heart evaluation. Disease staging is performed by means of tomographic scanning of chest, abdomen, and brain, magnetic resonance imaging of and whole-body 18 Fluorodeoxyglucose. Prognosis is poor, as therapeutic options are usually limited to palliative treatments. However, patients with metastases in the form of single intra-cardiac masses can undergo excision, at least for symptoms relief.

---

* Corresponding author: Address: via Borsa 12, 20900 Monza, Italy, Research and Professional Experience: Cardiology Resident Trainee at St Gerardo Hospital, Monza.

Introduction

Skin derives from both mesoderm and ectoderm and is organized in a multi-layered manner, in which the outer one is represented by the epidermis, a squamous epithelium constantly renewed by stem cells transforming into keratinocytes.

Other types of cells compose the epidermis: the melanocytes, the Langerhans cells and the Merkel cells. The epidermis protects the body from ultraviolet radiation, chemicals, viruses and other pathogens, acting as barrier to separate internal organs from the external environment. For this reason, epidermal cells can easily acquire gene mutations, expressions of DNA instability caused by ultraviolet light or failures in DNA repair. Moreover, also the generation of reactive oxygen species ends up to the development of cancer.

Several predisposing factors linked to melanoma development have been discovered, and are mainly physical characteristics such as red hair and blue eyes, the presence of multiple pigmented lesions and a strong family history of melanoma.

Malignant melanoma is the worse type of skin cancer, with high mortality rates varying by country, gender (women tend to survive longer than men), and ethnic origin. Malignant melanoma has a very poor prognosis, the median survival rate being only 7 to 9 months. Outcome depends on the depth into the skin reached by the melanoma, and it has not improved despite the recent implementations in therapeutic strategies. Malignant melanoma is a tumor of the melanocytes, which may affect also other tissues apart from skin, as is the case of uveal or meningeal melanomas.

Malignant melanoma is the consequence of a multi-step process derived from the dysregulation of two different types of genes. Dysregulation may consist of down-regulation of tumor suppressor genes or up-regulation and enhancement of oncogenes, are altered proto-oncogenes essential to cell growth and proliferation in normal conditions. After the onset of genetic instability and the beginning of enhanced and inappropriate cellular proliferation, other two relevant molecular phases characterize the development of melanoma: the acquisition of invasive metastatic capacity and promotion of tumor angiogenesis.

Genetic lesions involved in the genesis of melanoma were discovered analyzing the inherited form of familial melanoma, which represent about 10% of all melanoma cases. The first gene responsible for melanoma to be identified was *CDKN2A*.

Among other commonly mutated oncogenes in malignant melanoma there are genes of the *ras* family; p53; p16 and cyclin-dependent kinase 4. Also BRAF is another oncogene commonly mutated in malignant melanoma.

Activating BRAF mutations are the most prevalent somatic genetic mutations in human malignant melanoma. BRAF produces a protein that regulates physiologic skin cells growth, allowing cells proliferation only when necessary. However, a specific mutated version of BRAF called V600E confers to the protein constitutive activation, preventing its switching off and thus determining continued cells proliferation. The main mutation consists of a single phosphomimetic substitution in the kinase activation domain V600E. It has been supposed that BRAFV600E mutation may be induced by ultraviolet damage, since this BRAF mutation is highly prevalent in cutaneous melanoma, a tumors which is also known to be epidemiologically linked to ultraviolet light exposure. However, this supposition may not be true, as the typical mutation at amino acid 600 (V600E) is the T→A transversion that converts valine to glutamic acid, and it is not a classically ultraviolet-induced damage.

Moreover, BRAF mutations are common in melanomas arising in skin with intermittent sun exposure, such as trunk and arms, and are less frequent in more extensively sun exposed areas.

It has also been supposed that constitutional activation of BRAFV600E in a context of otherwise normal genes may not be determinant for melanoma development. In fact, although BRAF mutations appear early in melanoma genesis, they are insufficient for melanocyte transformation, suggesting that BRAFV600E may be a weaker melanoma oncogene than the RAS family genes.

Staging of primary cutaneous malignant melanoma is made through evaluation of thickness, ulceration, cutaneous layers penetration, mitotic rate, lymph nodes involvement and metastasis spread, although the biological meaning of tumor thickness and ulceration is uncertain. Lymph-nodes involvement decreases the five-year survival rate by approximately 40%, and the presence of distant metastasis may suggest end-stage disease, especially in case of heart involvement.

Several prognostic serum biomarkers for malignant melanoma were identified, among which Lactate dehydrogenase and S100B, which might serve as a prognostic factor in late-stage malignant melanoma as they are directly correlated to survival and progression of the disease.

Heart Involvement in Malignant Melanoma

Frequency of Cardiac Metastasis and Dissemination Pathways

Metastatic involvement of the heart is almost twenty times more frequent than primary heart tumors. In an autopsy series, metastases to the heart were found in up to 12% of all autopsies in cancer patients, with malignant melanoma accounting for 4.4% of all cardiac metastases.

The incidence of metastatic heart involvement has recently increased, both for improvements of diagnostic techniques and for prolonged survival secondary to better treatment strategies.

Potentially, all tumors can metastasize to the heart, but among the tumors with known propensity for cardiac tissue infiltration, malignant melanoma plays a central role. Malignant melanoma is biologically aggressive, and neoplastic melanocytes have great affinity for heart tissues: thus cardiac metastases from malignant melanomas are common, with the highest metastatic rates compared to all other sites. Only lung and breast cancers and lymphomas are superior to malignant melanoma for cardiac metastatic potential.

Since the incidence of melanoma is in continuous and rapid increase compared to other malignancy, its high metastatic potential should be kept in mind, with almost one third of patients with malignant melanoma developing metastases. Although the most common sites of metastatic involvement from malignant melanoma are lungs, liver, brain, and bones, cardiac involvement is not so rare: postmortem heart involvement was reported in up to 70% of cases in malignant melanoma autopsy series.

On the contrary, ante mortem diagnosis of cardiac metastases is reported only in about 1-2% of patients, since heart metastases are rarely responsible for clinical manifestations, with less than 10% of patients presenting symptoms of cardiac involvement.

Moreover, cardiac metastases (as well as metastases in other tissues), may appear years after initial diagnosis of the primary tumor.

The heart may be affected in a multifocal way, following hematological dissemination, although lymphatic dissemination has also been reported. The epicardium, the myocardium and the pericardium may be simultaneously or separately affected, but cardiac involvement may also present as isolated intra-cavitary lesions. The myocardium is most often affected (98%), suggesting the possible predominance of hematogenous spread. However, contemporary involvement of both the pericardium and the epicardium is also frequent.

Endocardial lesions are usually intra-cavitary, and may develop anywhere in the heart: they can invade the wall of any of the cardiac chambers, with the right heart frequently involved. The right atrium in particular usually presents sessile metastasis arising from its free wall. Extensive invasion of the right atrial wall may also occur, whereas massive involvement of the myocardium is known as 'charcoal heart'. The left ventricular free wall and the ventricular septum are other common sites of cardiac metastasis from malignant melanoma, whereas valvular involvement is rare.

The majority of heart metastases are multiple small metastases throughout the heart, although some reports of solitary intra-cardiac pedunculated masses in the right atrium attached to the interatrial septum in the area of the *fossa ovalis* exists.

Hematogenous metastases to the heart are often associated with hematogenous dissemination to other organs, and once the heart is affected, the disease is generally extensively disseminated. However, several cases of solitary cardiac involvement in the absence of any other extra cardiac metastasis have been reported.

Clinical Presentation of Cardiac Metastasis

Symptoms of cardiac involvement are infrequent and non-specific, and they rarely represent the initial clinical manifestation of the primary tumor. Moreover, the patient is usually asymptomatic until the advanced stage of the disease, when cardiac involvement is massive, affecting the normal activity of the heart.

Thus, melanoma metastases to the heart are clinically silent in the majority of the cases, with patients completely asymptomatic due to the small size of cardiac infiltration, which does not affect cardiac function. Symptoms or signs of cardiac dysfunction, if present, are rarely isolated or the initial presenting symptoms.

Symptoms may be constitutional or depend strictly on the location of the metastasis, consisting of generic signs of cardiovascular alteration, according to the site and amount of the involved portion of the heart. Constitutional symptoms include fatigue and weakness, asthenia or exercise intolerance, generally attributed to other causes. More specific symptoms of cardiac origin are represented by dyspnea, and edema, with right or left congestive heart failure, acute pericarditis, cardiac tamponade, arrhythmias, superior vena cava obstruction syndrome with raised jugular venous pressure, right and/or left ventricular outflow and inflow obstruction, transient ischemic attacks and pulmonary or systemic embolisms, or even syncope.

However, patients with cardiac metastases from malignant melanoma may present symptoms only caused by diffused metastatic involvement of other organs, without any cardiac dysfunction. As well, common symptoms of possible cardiac origin can also depend on other specific tissue metastasis. That is the case of dyspnea, which can depend on heart failure or tamponade or be caused by pulmonary metastases, and of chest pain, possible expression of myocardial ischemia or of bony metastases.

Several possible specific tumor-related symptoms have been reported, the majority of which are rhythm disturbances: brady-arrhythmias and tachy-arrhythmias, sick sinus syndrome, tachycardia-bradycardia syndrome, atrial tachycardia, atrioventricular block, atrial fibrillation, left and right bundle branches block and ventricular arrhythmias. These occur usually in case of extensive invasion of the right atrium and of other parts of the heart, such as the conduction system, by nodular lesions, with a specific cause-effect relationship suggested by the association between the onset of rhythm disturbances and the time of widespread metastatic dissemination. Pulmonary or systemic embolization in case of grossly pedunculated intra-cavitary metastases can also occur.

Not frequently valve dysfunction may be the consequence of cardiac involvement in malignant melanoma.

In general, cardiac metastasis is correlated with wide metastatic spread from the primary tumor, and thus it carries a worse prognosis, representing a premorbid event. However, death may be caused more often by cerebral hemorrhage rather than cardiac involvement.

Diagnosis of Heart Involvement

Electrocardiographic findings are in general nonspecific, and they usually occur late, unrelated to disease extent. Moreover, several possible etiologies of electrocardiographic alterations should be excluded before attributing those alterations to a possible cardiac metastatic invasion by malignancies.

It should be kept in mind during follow-up visits of patients with known malignancies (especially those with high frequency of cardiac metastasis) that the involvement of the conduction system may produce any of the possible rhythm disturbances previously enounced, ranging from small prolongations in the PR interval successively leading to complete atrioventricular block, to fatal ventricular tachycardia, and any other rhythm disturbance. On the other hand, in case of pericardial effusion, small amplitude QRS complexes can be identified.

Diagnostic Imaging

Imaging techniques have the unique possibility of directly show the heart and its surrounding structures, representing a first-line diagnostic tool in case of cardiac metastasis.

Echocardiography is the very first diagnostic technique to be used for imaging the heart. It is a non-invasive and low-cost technique of heart visualization, with high sensitivity for the detection of intra-cardiac masses. It should be performed in any patient with known tumors, in order to assess possible cardiac dysfunction related to chemotherapy, or in case of new-onset cardiac symptoms to exclude metastatic cardiac involvement, or during patient follow-up.

Echocardiography is rapidly available, and allows the definition of the size, mobility, and site of attachment of cardiac metastases, if present.

Trans-thoracic approach is often sufficient to orient diagnosis, especially in cases of gross morphologic alterations of the normal cardiac anatomy. However, thickening of the myocardium cannot be considered as a specific sign of cardiac metastatic involvement, especially in case of isolated cardiac disease.

Trans-esophageal echocardiography can thus be used for better evaluation of specific cardiac sites and valves structure and function, or in cases of difficult patients such as obese or pneumopatic patients, in whom small details can be missed during a difficult trans-thoracic evaluation. Trans-esophageal echocardiography carries out a better image quality which improves the ability to diagnose the nature of intra-cardiac involvement. In some cases of particularly typical morphology and appearance of cardiac metastases, it has been suggested that trans-esophageal visualization may obviate the need for biopsy.

At present, three-dimensional technology represents a useful advantage over standard two-dimensional imaging in the context of ultrasonography. This is true in particular for cardiac metastases from malignant melanoma. In fact, since the frequency of right heart involvement is high and the shape of the right ventricle is complex, three-dimensional trans-thoracic and three-dimensional trans-esophageal echocardiographic techniques have an incremental value in the assessment of right ventricular masses. Three-dimensional trans-thoracic echocardiography can correctly identify the real dimensions of intra-cardiac masses, as well as their intimate structural characteristics and relationship to ventricular walls, differencing also fine trabeculations.

Findings from three-dimensional echocardiography were validated against computed tomography, angiograms and surgery/pathology findings, in a study which revealed that three-dimensional trans-thoracic echocardiography allows for the better identification of the attachments of the masses, their volumes, and inner characteristics. Moreover, three-dimensional trans-thoracic echocardiography improves the diagnostic properties of standard two-dimensional echocardiography as it allows the measurement of the real dimensions of cardiac tumors, which are intimately connected to prognosis. Another advantage of three-dimensional trans-thoracic echocardiography is that it is less dependent on the operator experience for the acquisition of good sections of the heart.

Three-dimensional trans-thoracic echocardiography allows the acquisition of pyramidal volumes of information that can then be visualized from different angles and cropped on any desired plane to focus on any region of interest contained in the volume acquired.

Three-dimensional trans-thoracic echocardiography is not inferior to computed tomography, and it can add important information over standard two-dimensional imaging. In fact three-dimensional trans-thoracic echocardiography is now almost comparable to cardiac magnetic resonance imaging for the characterization of cardiac anatomy and abnormalities, and only lacks the possibility of imaging the vascularization of the masses.

However, the diagnostic work-up of an intra-cardiac mass should not be limited to echocardiography alone. In fact, although echocardiography may orient diagnosis, confirmation of the nature of an intra-cardiac mass should be obtained with cardiac magnetic resonance imaging, which is by now the gold standard imaging technique for the definition of the nature of intra-cardiac masses and their relationship to adjacent structures, particularly to study the possible extension to other structures of the mediastinum.

Conventionally, in case of metastatic widespread of tumors, disease staging is usually performed by means of several diagnostic imaging modalities, starting from ultrasonography, followed by tomographic scanning of chest and abdomen, magnetic resonance imaging of brain, and bone scanning. However, these examinations have limited sensitivity and specificity for the detection of melanoma metastases, particularly in asymptomatic patients. Cardiac magnetic resonance imaging is added in case of heart involvement.

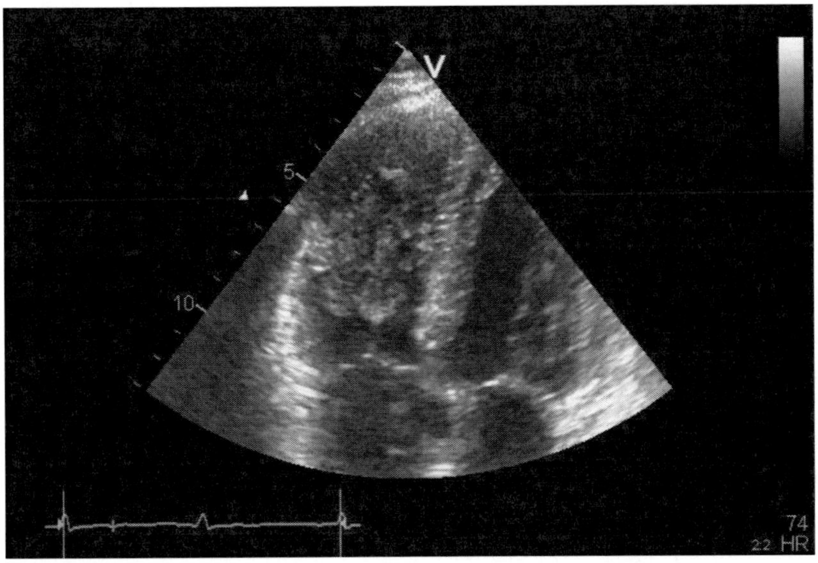

Figure 1. Two dimensional echocardiographic section from the echocardiographic apical four chamber view modified for right ventricular visualization revealing the presence of an intra-ventricular mass occupying almost the whole right ventricular cavity.

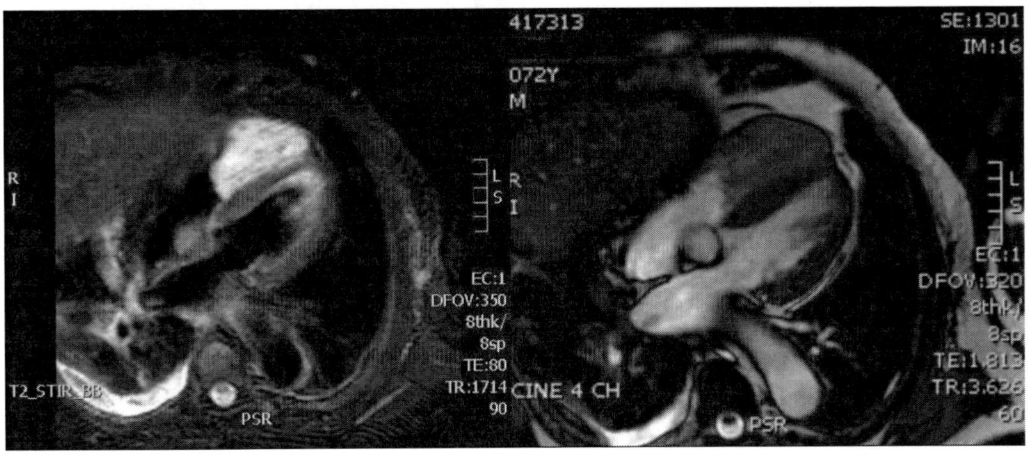

Figure 2. Cardiac Magnetic Resonance Imaging view of the right ventricle demonstrating the presence of a mass inside the whole right ventricular cavity and infiltrating the right ventricular walls, whereas extra cardiac structures do not seem to be involved by the infiltration. Due to its characteristics, according to patient's history, this mass was highly suspected for being an intra-cardiac metastasis from malignant melanoma.

Computed tomography and cardiac magnetic resonance imaging are important because they offer also additional information about the whole chest. The role of computed tomography, however, could be limited by motion artifacts leading to poor image quality. Resolution can be substantially improved by gating the computed tomography acquisition to the cardiac cycle. Gated cardiac magnetic resonance imaging enables to image each cardiac segment with equal clarity, and multiplanar reconstruction allows the accurate definition of size, location, borders, and surface characteristics of cardiac masses. Magnetic resonance imaging has been shown to be superior to two-dimensional echocardiography (both trans-thoracic and trans-esophageal) in defining the site of mural attachment and the extension of tumor into adjacent mediastinal structures. Malignant melanoma produces a characteristic hyper intense signal on T1-weighted images due to paramagnetic scavenging by melanin, which contrasts with the low signal produced by other tumors.

Currently positron-emission tomography (PET) scanning is clinically indicated to differentiate between cardiac tumor and other space-occupying lesions such as intra-cardiac thrombus, the most encountered lesion. However, in this sense echocardiography is sufficient to discriminate between them.

The higher accuracy of combined PET/computed tomography scan has recently been demonstrated in a study comparing contrast-enhanced computed tomography and non-enhanced low dose computed tomography. 18f-fluorodeoxyglucose (18F-FDG) PET was also evaluated in the diagnostic process of metastatic malignant melanoma, and its superiority over the other diagnostic techniques for the detection of distant metastases has been demonstrated, with sensitivity, specificity, and accuracy of 18 F-FDG PET for detecting recurrent melanoma ranging from 70% to 100%.

However, smaller lesions (less than 1 cm in diameter) are usually missed by 18 F-FDG PET, and can be detected by computed tomography or magnetic resonance imaging. For this reason, all these diagnostic techniques should be regarded as complementary and not replace one another in patients with suspected melanoma disease.

The final diagnosis of confirmation should be obtained through histology, with successful trans-esophageal echocardiography guided trans-venous biopsy reported as a possible way of obtaining a histology specimen, especially in cases of right atrial metastasis. Other attempts can be made accordingly to metastasis location and mainly comprehend left thoracotomy, or sub-xifoid intervention, whereas the creation of a pericardial window is used to relieve symptoms.

Therapeutic Options Available and Prognosis

Malignant melanoma behaves in an atypical way as compared to other malignancies. In fact, it can be highly aggressive with immediate widespread of distant metastasis, or it can also remain silent for several years and give metastases after a long disease free interval (some cases of prolonged disease free intervals, as long as 27 years, have been reported).

Prognosis for patients with malignant melanoma metastatic to the heart is poor. Since cardiac involvement occurs usually in the advanced stages of the disease, in general as a late step in the metastatic dissemination of malignant melanoma, therapeutic options are usually limited to palliative treatments, because patients typically have also extra cardiac disease, which affects their quality of life and survival as well as cardiac involvement.

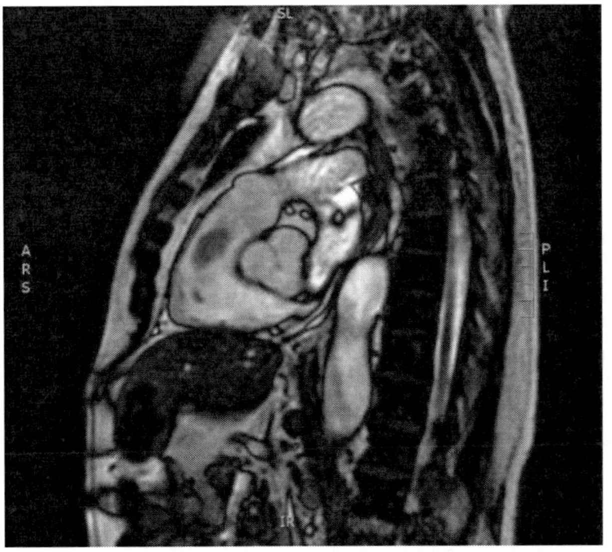

Figure 3. Cardiac Magnetic Resonance Imaging view of the right ventricular outflow tract showing the extension of the mass suspected to be a metastasis from malignant melanoma, into the right ventricular infundibulum. The image depicts the strict relationship of the intra-ventricular mass with the right ventricular outflow tract and the pulmonary valve.

It has been suggested that, if cardiac function is severely compromised by the tumor mass, operative intervention should be considered even if total resection is not possible. In fact, conservative surgery can be performed with minimal morbidity in an attempt to relieve symptoms and prevent imminent cardiac failure (and death). Several cases of single cardiac metastasis undergoing surgical excision have been reported. These options though not curative, at least relieve symptoms. On the other hand, other types of significant intervention are difficult, and outcome is always poor.

The anatomic location of the heart metastasis and the extent of invasion determine the feasibility of surgical intervention. The complete resection of an intra-cardiac melanoma metastasis prevents potential morbidities associated with progressive intra-cardiac growth. In general, conservative surgery improves the quality of a patient's life.

Also, chemotherapy itself can be only a palliative support in many cases, as its benefits are limited. It usually comprehends cisplatin and tamoxifen. Moreover, patients presenting metastatic dissemination of malignant melanoma while already on systemic chemotherapy are unlikely to respond to second-line treatment.

Conclusion

The occurrence of cardiac metastasis from malignant melanoma dramatically decreases prognosis, even in case of negative sentinel lymph-node surveillance biopsy. Specific treatment lacks, and even in case of early diagnosis patients' survival rate is limited.

To diagnose cardiac metastasis, several diagnostic imaging techniques can be used, with echocardiography as the first-line, non-invasive approach for heart evaluation. Moreover, the recent improvements in technology allow for correct evaluation of any cardiac mass with three-dimensional echocardiography, reducing the need for more invasive strategies. However, at least cardiac magnetic resonance imaging should be performed in case of heart involvement from neoplastic disease, since this technique represents by now the gold standard technique for heart evaluation. Moreover, as in case of other malignancies, complete disease staging should also be performed by means of chest, abdomen and brain evaluation with computed tomography. Therapeutic options are usually limited to palliative treatments, although patients with single intra-cardiac metastasis can undergo excision for symptoms relief.

References

[1] Radinsky, R. Modulation of tumor cell gene expression and phenotype by the organ specific metastatic environment. *Cancer Metastasis Rev*, 1995; 14, 323–38.

[2] Fidler, IJ; Kripke, ML. Metastasis results from preexisting variant cells within a malignant tumor. *Science*, 1977, 197, 893–5.

[3] Hussein, MR. Ultraviolet radiation and skin cancer, molecular mechanisms. *J Cutan Pathol*, 2005; 32, 191-205.

[4] de Snoo, FA; Hayward, NK. Cutaneous melanoma susceptibility and progression genes. *Cancer Lett*, 2005; 230, 153-86.

[5] Chin, L. The genetics of malignant melanoma, lessons from mouse and man. *Nat Rev Cancer*. 2003; 8,559-70.

[6] Daya-Grosjean, L; Sarasin, A. The role of UV induced lesions in skin carcinogenesis, an overview of oncogene and tumor suppressor gene modifications in xeroderma pigmentosum skin tumors. *Murat Res*, 2005; 571, 43-56.

[7] Boukamp, P. Non melanoma skin cancer, what drives tumor development and progression? *Carcinogenesis*, 2005; 10, 1657-67.

[8] Tsai, FY; Tsao, H. The genetics of skin cancer. *Am J Med Genet C Semin Med Genet*, 2004; 131 C1, 82-92.

[9] Lomas, J; Martin-Duque, P; Pons, M; Quintanilla, M. The genetics of malignant melanoma. *Front Biosci*, 2008, 13, 5071-93.

[10] Pons, M; Mancheño-Corvo, P; Martín-Duque, P; Quintanilla, M. Molecular biology of malignant melanoma. *Adv Exp Med Biol*, 2008, 624, 252-64.

[11] Fecher, LA; Cummings, SD; Keefe, MJ; Alani, RM. Toward a molecular classification of melanoma. *J Clin Oncol*, 2007, 25 (12), 1606-20.

[12] Gray-Schopfer, V; Wellbrock, C; Marais, R. Melanoma biology and new targeted therapy. *Nature*, 2007, 445, 851-7.

[13] Hayward, NK. Genetics of melanoma predisposition. *Oncogene*, 2003, 22, 3053-62.

[14] Merlino, G; Noonan, FP. Modeling gene-environment interactions in malignant melanoma. *Trends Mol Med*, 2003, 9, 102-8.

[15] Kabbarah, O; Chin, L. Revealing the genomic heterogeneity of melanoma. *Cancer Cell*, 2005; 8 (6), 439-41.

[16] Winnepenninckx, V; Lazar, V; Michiels, S; Dessen, P; Stas, M; Alonso, SR; Avril, MF; Ortiz Romero, PL; Robert, T; Balacescu, O; Eggermont, AM; Lenoir, G; Sarasin, A; Tursz, T; van den Oord, JJ; Spatz, A. Melanoma Group of the European Organization

for Research and Treatment of Cancer. Gene expression profiling of primary cutaneous melanoma and clinical outcome. *J Natl Cancer Inst*, 2006; 98 (7), 472-82.

[17] Rigel, DS. Epidemiology and prognostic factors in malignant melanoma. *Ann Plast Surg*, 1992; 28 (1), 7–8.

[18] Crombie, IK. Racial differences in melanoma incidence. *Br J Cancer*, 1979; 40, 185–193.

[19] Fuchs, J; Packer, L. Ultraviolet irradiation and the skin antioxidant system. *Photodermatol Photoimmunol Photomed*, 1990; 7 (2), 90–92.

[20] van Elsas, A; Zerp, SF; van der Flier, S; Krüse, KM; Aarnoudse, C; Hayward, NK; Ruiter, DJ; Schrier, PI. Relevance of ultraviolet-induced N-ras oncogene point mutations in development of primary human cutaneous melanoma. *Am J Pathol*, 1996; 149 (3), 883-893.

[21] Bale, SJ; Dracopoli, NC; Tucker, MA; Clark, WH Jr; Fraser, MC; Stanger, BZ; Green, P; Donis-Keller, H; Housman, DE; Greene, MH. Mapping the gene for hereditary cutaneous malignant melanoma-dysplastic nevus to chromosome 1p. *N Engl J Med*, 1989; 320, 1367-1372.

[22] Platz, A; Ringborg, U; Brahme, EM; Lagerlof, B. Melanoma metastases from patients with hereditary cutaneous malignant melanoma contain a high frequency of N-*ras* activating mutations. *Melanoma Res*, 1994; 4,169-177.

[23] Volkenandt, M; Schlegel, U; Nanus, DM; Albino, AP. Mutational analysis of the human p53 gene in malignant melanoma. *Pigment Cell Res*, 1991; 4, 35-40.

[24] Stretch, JR; Gatter, KC; Ralfkiaer, E; Lane, DP; Harris, AL. Expression of mutant p53 in melanoma. *Cancer Res*, 1991; 51, 5976-79.

[25] Bishop, JAN. Molecular pathology of melanoma. *Cancer Metastasis Rev*, 1997; 16, 141-154.

[26] Maelandsmo, GM; Flørenes, VA; Hovig, E; Oyjord, T; Engebraaten, O; Holm, R; Børresen, AL; Fodstad, O. Involvement of the pRb/p16/cdk4/cyclin D1 pathway in the tumorigenesis of sporadic malignant melanomas. *Br J Cancer*, 1996; 73, 909-916.

[27] Holzmann, B; Bröcker, EB; Lehmann, JM; Ruiter, DJ; Sorg, C; Riethmüller, G; Johnson, JP. Tumor progression in human malignant melanoma, five stages defined by either antigenic phenotypes. *Int J Cancer*, 1987; 39, 466-471.

[28] Davies, H; Bignell, GR; Cox, C; Stephens, P; Edkins, S; Clegg, S; Teague, J; Woffendin, H; Garnett, MJ; Bottomley, W; Davis, N; Dicks, E; Ewing, R; Floyd, Y; Gray, K; Hall, S; Hawes, R; Hughes, J; Kosmidou, V; Menzies, A; Mould, C; Parker, A; Stevens, C; Watt, S; Hooper, S; Wilson, R; Jayatilake, H; Gusterson, BA; Cooper, C; Shipley, J; Hargrave, D; Pritchard-Jones, K; Maitland, N; Chenevix-Trench, G; Riggins, GJ; Bigner, DD; Palmieri, G; Cossu, A; Flanagan, A; Nicholson, A; Ho, JW; Leung, SY; Yuen, ST; Weber, BL; Seigler, HF; Darrow, TL; Paterson, H; Marais, R; Marshall, CJ; Wooster, R; Stratton, MR; Futreal, PA. Mutations of the BRAF gene in human cancer. *Nature*, 2002; 417 (6892), 949-954.

[29] Finck, SJ; Giuliano, AE; Morton, DL. LDH and melanoma. *Cancer*, 1983; 51, 840–843.

[30] Campora, E; Repetto, L; Giuntini, P; Bertelli, G; Amoroso, D; Sertoli, MR; Rosso, R. LDH in the follow-up of stage I malignant melanoma. *Eur J Cancer Clin Oncol*, 1988; 24, 277–278.

[31] Deichmann, M; Benner, A; Bock, M; et al. S100-Beta, melanoma-inhibiting activity, and lactate dehydrogenase discriminate progressive from non-progressive American Joint Committee on Cancer stage IV melanoma. *J Clin Oncol*, 1999; 17, 1891–1896.

[32] Stahlecker, J; Gauger, A; Bosserhoff, A; Büttner, R; Ring, J; Hein, R. MIA as a reliable tumor marker in the serum of patients with malignant melanoma. *Anticancer Res*, 2000; 20, 5041-5044.

[33] Krahn, G; Kaskel, P; Sander, S; Waizenhöfer, PJ; Wortmann, S; Leiter, U; Peter, RU. S100 beta is a more reliable tumor marker in peripheral blood for patients with newly occurred melanoma metastases compared with MIA, albumin and lactate-dehydrogenase. *Anticancer Res*, 2001; 21, 1311–1316.

[34] Albino, AP. Genes involved in melanoma susceptibility and progression. *Curr Opin Oncol*, 1995; 7, 162–169.

[35] Tornaletti, S; Pfeiffer, GP. Slow repair of pyrimidine dimers at P53 mutation hot spots in skin cancer. *Science*, 1994; 263, 1436–1438.

[36] Gibbs, P; Cebon, JS; Calafiore, P; Robinson, WA. Cardiac metastases from malignant melanoma. *Cancer*, 1999; 85, 78–84.

[37] Houmsse, M; Raman, SV; Leier, CV; Orsinelli, DA. Metastatic melanoma of the left ventricle, cardiac imaging in the diagnosis and surgical approach. *Int J Cardiovasc Imaging*, 2004; 20 (6), 523–6.

[38] Tesolin, M; Lapierre, C; Oligny, L; Bigras, JL; Champagne, M. Cardiac metastases from melanoma. *Radiographics*, 2005; 25 (1), 249-53.

[39] Klatt, EC; Heitz, DR. Cardiac metastases. *Cancer*, 1990; 65 (6), 1456-9.

[40] Poggi, R; Pantaleo, MA; Benedetti, G; Biasco, G. Cardiac metastasis of melanoma. *Melanoma Res*, 2005; 15 (4), 315-6.

[41] Thurber, DL; Eduards, JE; Achor, RW. Secondary malignant tumors of the pericardium. *Circulation*, 1962; 26, 228-41.

[42] Glancy, DL; Roberts, WC. The heart in malignant melanoma, a study of 70 autopsy cases. *Am J Cardiol*, 1968; 21(4), 555-71.

[43] Waller, BF; Gottdiener, JS; Virmani, R; Roberts, WC. The "charcoal heart", melanoma to the core. *Chest*, 1980; 77 (5), 671–76.

[44] Malouf, JF; Thompson, RC; Maples, WJ; Wolfe, JT. Diagnosis of right atrial metastatic melanoma by transesophageal echocardiographic-guided transvenous biopsy. *Mayo Clin Proc*, 1996; 71 (12), 1167–70.

[45] Matturri, L; Nappo, A; Varesi, C; Rossi, L. Cardiac metastasis of malignant melanoma. *Pathologica*, 1993; 85, 97–102.

[46] Sheldon, R; Isaac, D. Metastatic melanoma to the heart presenting with ventricular tachycardia. *Chest*, 1991; 99 (5), 1296–98.

[47] Ozyuncu, N; Sahin, M; Altin, T; Karaoguz, R; Guldal, M; Akyurek, O. Cardiac metastasis of malignant melanoma, a rare cause of complete atrioventricular block. *Europace*, 2006; 8, 545-8.

[48] MacGee, W. Metastatic and invasive tumors involving the heart in a geriatric population, a necropsy study. *Virchows Arch A Pathol Anat Histopathol*, 1991; 419 (3), 183–9.

[49] Schneider, B; Zienkiewicz, T; Langenstein, B; Vierbuchen, M; Meinertz, T. Metastatic malignant melanoma initially seen as congestive heart failure, diagnosis by transesophageal echocardiography. *Am Heart J*, 1994; 128, 414–6.

[50] Hanfling, SM. Metastatic cancer to the heart, review of the literature and report of 127 cases. *Circulation*, 1960; 22, 474–83.

[51] Harvey, WP. Clinical aspects of cardiac tumors. *Am J Cardiol*, 1968; 21, 328–43.

[52] Vetto, JT; Heelan, RT; Burt, M. Malignant melanoma metastatic to the right atrium, an asymptomatic solitary metastasis diagnosed incidentally by magnetic resonance imaging. *J Thor Cardiovasc Surg*, 1992; 104, 843–4.

[53] Canver, CC; Lajos, TZ; Bernstein, Z; Dubois, DP; Mentzer, RM. Intracavitary melanoma of the left atrium. *Ann Thor Surg*, 1990; 49, 312–3.

[54] Emmot, WW; Vacek, JL; Agee, K; Moran, J; Dunn, MI. Metastatic malignant melanoma presenting clinically as obstruction of the right ventricular inflow and outflow tracts, characterization by magnetic resonance imaging. *Chest*, 1987; 92, 362–4.

[55] Merer, DM; Dutcher, JP; Mercando, AA; Brodman, R; Sutherland, MJ; Bhandari, A; Zimmerman, D; Mitchell, MS; Wiernik, PH. Case report, clinical findings and successful resection of melanoma metastatic to the right atrium. *Cancer Invest*, 1994; 12 (4), 409–13.

[56] Chen, R; Gaos, C; Frazier, O. Complete resection of a right atrial intracavitary metastatic melanoma. *Ann Thor Surg*, 1996; 61, 1255–7.

[57] Bortolotti, U; Tursi, V; Milano, A; Mazzucco, A; Galluci, V. Intracardiac metastatic melanoma, report of a case mimicking a right atrial myxoma with a review of the literature. *Tex Heart Inst J*, 1990; 17, 136–8.

[58] Thomas, JH; Panoussopoulos, DG; Jewell, WR; Pierce, GE. Tricuspid stenosis secondary to metastatic melanoma. *Cancer*, 1977; 39, 1732–7.

[59] Lam, KY; Dickens, P; Chan, AC. Tumors of the heart, a 20-year experience with a review of 12,485 consecutive autopsies. *Arch Pathol Lab Med*, 1993; 117, 1027-31.

[60] Reddy, VK; Faulkner, M; Bandarupalli, N; Nanda, NC; Singh, P; Dutta, R; Singh, A; Pothineni, KR; Dod, HS; Bhardwaj, R; Warden, BE; Beto, RJ; Jain, AC. Incremental value of live/real time three-dimensional transthoracic echocardiography in the assessment of right ventricular masses. *Echocardiography*, 2009; 26, 598-609.

[61] Asch, FM; Bieganski, SP; Panza, JA; Weissman, NJ. Real time 3-dimensional echocardiography evaluation of intracardiac masses. *Echocardiography*, 2006; 23, 218–224.

[62] Freedberg, RS; Kronzon, I; Rumancik, WM; Rumancik, WM; Liebeskind, D. The contribution of magnetic resonance imaging to the evaluation of intracardiac tumours diagnosed by echocardiography. *Circulation*, 1988; 77, 96–103.

[63] Gulati, G; Sharma, S; Kothari, SS; Juneja, R; Saxena, A; Talwar, KK. Comparison of echo and MRI in the imaging evaluation of intracardiac masses. *Cardiovasc Intervent Radiol*, 2004; 27, 459–469.

[64] Espinola-Zabaleta, N; Hernandez Morales, G; Vargas-Barron, J; Espinola-Zavaleta, N; Morales, GH; Vargas-Barrón, J; Keirns, C; Fraustro, AA. Three-dimensional transesophageal echocardiography in tumors of the heart. *J Am Soc Echocardiogr*, 2002; 15, 972–979.

[65] Pfluger, T; Melzer, HI; Schneider, V; La Fougere, C; Coppenrath, E; Berking, C; Bartenstein, P; Weiss, M. PET/CT in malignant melanoma, contrastenhanced CT versus plain low-dose CT. *Eur J Nucl Med Mol Imaging*, 2011; 38, 822–831.

[66] Kumar, R; Alavi, A. Clinical applications of fluorodeoxyglucose-positron emission tomography in the management of malignant melanoma. *Curr Opin Oncol*, 2005; 17, 154-9.

[67] Schöder, H; Larson, SM; Yeung, HW. PET/CT in oncology, Integration into clinical management of lymphoma, melanoma, and gastrointestinal malignancies. *J Nucl Med*, 2004; 45 (1S), 72-81.

[68] Mijnhout, GS; Hoekstra, OS; Van Tulder, MW; Teule, GJ; Deville, WL. Systematic review of the diagnostic accuracy of 18F-FDG PET in melanoma patients. *Cancer*, 2001; 91, 1530-42.

[69] Rubin, DC; Ziskind, AA; Hawke, MW; Plotnick, GD. Transesophageal echocardiographically guided percutaneous biopsy of a right atrial mass. *Am Heart J*, 1994; 127, 935–6.

[70] Hanley, PC; Shub, C; Seward, JB; Lester, EW. Intracavitary cardiac melanoma diagnosed by endomyocardial left ventricular biopsy. *Chest*, 1983; 84, 195–8.

[71] Chello, M; Marchese, AR; Panza, A; Mastroroberto, P; Dillello, F. Primary malignant melanoma of the esophagus with a left atrial metastasis. *Thorax*, 1993; 48, 185–6.

[72] Gosalakkal, JA; Sugrue, D. Malignant melanoma of the right atrium, antemortem diagnosis by transvenous biopsy. *Br Heart J*, 1989; 62, 159–60.

[73] Gindea, AJ; Steele, P; Runanich, WM; Culubret, M; Feiner, H; Sanger, JJ; Kronzon, I. Biventricular cavity obliteration by metastastic melanoma, role of magnetic resonance imaging in the diagnosis. *Am Heart J*, 1987; 114, 1249–53.

[74] Ellis, CJ; Dennison, EM; Simpson, IA. Imaging of cardiac metastatic melanoma, transesophageal echocardiography or magnetic resonance imaging. *Int J Cardiol*, 1993; 41, 176–9.

[75] Belhocine, TZ; Scott, AM; Even-Sapir, E; Urbain, JL; Essner, R. Role of nuclear medicine in the management of cutaneous malignant melanoma. *J Nucl Med*, 2006; 47, 957-67.

[76] Lynch, M; Clements, SD; Shanewise, JS; Chen, CC; Martin, RP. Right sided cardiac tumours detected by transesophageal echocardiography and its usefulness in differentiating the benign from the malignant ones. *Am J Cardiol*, 1997; 790, 781–4.

[77] Obeid, AI; Mudamgha, AA; Smulyan, H. Diagnosis of right atrial mass lesions by transesophageal and transthoracic echocardiography. *Chest*, 1993; 103, 1447–51.

[78] Reeder, GS; Khandheria, BK; Seward, JB; Tajik, AJ. Transesophageal echocardiography and cardiac masses. *Mayo Clin Proc*, 1991; 66, 1101–9.

[79] Mugge, A; Daniel, WG; Haverich, A; Lichtlen, PR. Diagnosis of non-infective cardiac mass lesions by two dimensional echocardiography, comparison of the transthoracic and transesophageal approaches. *Circulation*, 1991; 83, 70–8.

[80] Gross, BH; Glazer, GM; Francis, IR. CT of intracardiac and intrapericardial masses. *AJR Am J Roentgenol*, 1983; 140, 903–6.

[81] Godwin, JD; Axel, L; Adams, JR; Schiller, NB; Simpsom, PC; Gertz, EW. Computed tomography, a new method for diagnosing tumor of the heart. *Circulation*, 1981; 63, 448–51.

[82] Bleiweis, MS; Georgiou, D; Brundage, BH. Detection of intracardiac masses by ultrafast computed tomography. *Am J Card Imaging*, 1994; 8, 63– 8.

[83] Fujita, N; Caputo, GR; Higgins, CB. Diagnosis and characterization of intracardiac masses by magnetic resonance imaging. *Am J Card Imaging*, 1994; 8, 69–80.

[84] Freedberg, RS; Kronzon, I; Rumancik, WM; Liebskind, D. The contribution of magnetic resonance imaging to the evaluation of intracardiac tumors diagnosed by echocardiography. *Circulation*, 1988; 77, 96 –103.

[85] Winkler, M; Higgins, CB. Suspected intracardiac masses, evaluation with MR imaging. *Radiology*, 1987; 165, 117–22.

[86] Premkumar, A; Marincola, F; Taubenberger, J; Chow, C; Venzon, D; Schwartzentruber, D. Metastatic melanoma, correlation of MRI characteristics and histopathology. *J Magn Reson Imaging*, 1997; 6, 190–4.

[87] Enochs, WS; Petherick, P; Bogdanova, A; Mohr, U; Weiisler, R. Paramagnetic metal scavenging by melanin, MR imaging. *Radiology*, 1997; 204, 417–23.

[88] Mindell, SM; Chernick, AW; Sugarman, MH; Zirkin, MZ; Bloom, RE. Right ventricular metastatic melanoma 27 years after resection of the primary tumour. *Cancer*, 1989; 63, 1237–9.

[89] Eigentler, TK; Caroli, UM; Radny, P; Garbe, C. Palliative therapy of disseminated malignant melanoma, a systematic review of 41 randomised clinical trials. *Lancet Oncol*, 2003; 4, 748-59.

[90] Lee, KS. Resection of cardiac metastasis of malignant melanoma. *Korean Circ J*, 2000; 30, 1170-4.

In: Melanoma
Editor: Alexander C. Jones
ISBN: 978-1-62808-608-9

Chapter 9

POOR KARNOFSKY PERFORMANCE STATUS AND HIGH SERUM LACTATE DEHYDROGENASE LEVEL (KPS / LDH INDEX) IDENTIFIES PATIENTS WITH BRAIN METASTASES FROM MALIGNANT MELANOMA WHO DO NOT BENEFIT FROM PALLIATIVE WHOLE BRAIN RADIOTHERAPY

Richard Partl,[1,*] Erika Richtig,[2] Alexander Avian,[3] Andrea Berghold[3] and Karin S. Kapp[1]

[1]Department of Therapeutic Radiology and Oncology, Medical University of Graz, Graz, Austria
[2]Department of Dermatology, Medical University of Graz, Graz, Austria
[3]Institute for Medical Informatics, Statistics and Documentation, Medical University of Graz, Graz, Austria

ABSTRACT

Malignant melanoma has a high propensity for intracranial seeding. By the time brain metastases are diagnosed, the majority of patients also suffer from uncontrolled extracranial disease.

For this prognostically unfavorable group, and especially for patients with multiple or progressive intracranial metastases, there are no existing scores that are able to reliably predict whether the patients can benefit from palliative whole brain radiotherapy (WBRT) or best supportive care.

In a previous analysis, Karnofsky Performance Status (KPS) and lactate dehydrogenase level (LDH) independently predicted overall survival. The present study was undertaken to test these parameters in a larger patient cohort.

* Phone: ++43-316-385-80775, Fax: ++43-316-385-13426, E-mail: richard.partl@medunigraz.at

We present a retrospective analysis of 107 patients with initial multiple intracranial lesions or with progression of brain metastases after resection and/or radiosurgery, who were treated with palliative WBRT between 1988 and 2012. Uni- and multivariate analyses were used to analyze the impact of the following patient-, tumor- and treatment-related parameters on overall survival: age, sex, KPS, neurologic symptoms, serum LDH, number of intracranial metastases, prior neurosurgical resection or stereotactic radiosurgery as well as the number and site of extracranial metastases prior to WBRT.

In accordance with our previous findings, low KPS (defined as <70) and high serum LDH (defined as >240 U/L) were identified as the only independent prognostic factors for overall survival with a hazard ratio of 4.8 [95% CI 2.8–8.1] and 2.5 [95% CI 1.6–4.1] The combination of these two parameters (KPS/LDH Index) classified the patients into 4 distinct survival groups.

The median overall survival was 175 days for patients with high KPS and low LDH; 111 days for patients with high KPS and high LDH; 47 days for patients with low KPS and low LDH; and 34 days for patients with low KPS and high LDH. 76 patients presented with neurological symptoms at the time of WBRT. At the end of therapy no improvement, or even a deterioration of neurological symptoms had been recorded in 64.2% of these patients.

Our updated analysis confirmed that the KPS/LDH Index was highly predictive in identifying patients with a more favorable or a very unfavorable prognosis. Patients of the latter group did not benefit from WBRT in terms of improved survival. Disappointing results were also obtained in terms of improving quality of life in patients with neurological symptoms.

Keywords: Malignant melanoma, brain metastasis, whole brain radiotherapy, prognostic factors, KPS/LDH Index, survival, lactate dehydrogenase, Karnofsky Performance Status

INTRODUCTION

Brain metastases are by far the most common intracranial tumors. The risk of developing clinically manifest brain metastases for patients with malignant melanoma has been estimated to be between 6 and 43%. [1, 2, 3]. However, the fact that up to 74% of malignant melanoma patients were found to have brain metastases at autopsy implies that the risk is probably even higher than those estimates [4, 5]. These data show that malignant melanoma has a very strong tendency to metastasize to the brain and [6] thus ranks as the third most common cause of brain metastases after carcinomas of the lung and breast.

Sampson et al. [7] analyzed potential risk factors for development of brain metastases in a demographic study of 6953 patients with histologically confirmed malignant melanoma. Male sex, an extended, thick or ulcerated primary tumor, location of the primary tumor on the mucous membranes, the trunk or the head and neck area, and the histological subtypes acral lentiginous and nodular melanoma were all associated with an elevated probability of intracranial metastases. Patients who, at the time of initial diagnosis, already had metastases in lymph nodes or in internal organs (especially in the lung or in more than one internal organ), were also found to have an increased risk of brain metastases.

The brain metastases of malignant melanoma also differ from those resulting from other primary cancers in the length of time after first diagnosis of the cancer when they appear. The median time from first diagnosis to discovery of brain metastases is 0.2–2 months for lung carcinoma and 22 months for colorectal carcinoma, but 36 months (range 3–83 months) for malignant melanoma. Brain metastases not only become evident at a later time than with other cancers, but also at a later stage in the overall disease progression after extracranial metastases are manifest [8].

The most common clinical symptoms are headache (50%), unilateral paralysis (50%), personality changes (30%) and seizures (15-20%). The most sensitive diagnostic method is magnetic resonance tomography with and without contrast agents. Histological investigation should be considered if the presence of a cerebral lesion is not plausible on the basis of the patient's history (e.g. thin melanomas) and their condition allows a targeted biopsy or resection to be done.

The onset of metastases in the brain represents a significant worsening of the patient's prognosis. If the tumor growth is advanced, none of the outcomes reachable with currently available therapeutic approaches can really be described as satisfactory [9, 10, 11]; one result of this is that these patients are often excluded from clinical trials on melanoma [12]. The individual therapeutic strategy should always take account of the number and size of the intracranial lesions, the patient's general condition and the extracranial tumor load.

The current therapeutic options include surgical resection, stereotactic radiosurgery, stereotactic radiotherapy, whole brain radiotherapy (WBRT) and use of systemic drugs that can pass the blood-brain barrier.

In all studies, the therapy chosen has turned out to be an important prognostic factor. Resection and stereotactic irradiation are associated with better overall survival than WBRT or "best supportive care" (Table 1). Whether this effect is a result of the therapies themselves or of the selection of patients with better Karnofsky Performance Status (KPS) is not clear, due to the lack of prospective randomized studies. In order to avoid this selection bias, a number of prognostic scoring systems have been developed, with the aim of predicting the median survival of patients with brain metastases. Among the best-established scores are the Recursive Partitioning Analysis (RPA) and the Graded Prognostic Assessment Score (GPA), both of which are applicable to patients with brain metastases independent of origin. Differences between both scores are that GPA takes the number of brain metastases into account and evaluates systemic tumor control more consistently [13, 14].

Table 1. Treatment and Prognosis

	(median OS)
No treatment	1 month
BSC	1–2 months
WBRT	3–6 months
Resection or SRS	10–20 months
Resection or SRS with WBRT	10–20 months

Abbreviations: BSC: best supportive care; WBRT: whole brain radiotherapy; SRS: stereotactic radiosurgery

In the course of the further development of the GPA to create the diagnosis-specific DS-GPA, the KPS and the number of brain metastases have emerged as significant and independent predictors of overall survival [15]. Many melanoma patients who are diagnosed with advanced intracranial metastasis already have a history with the disease lasting from several to many years and also have an extracranial tumor load that is no longer controllable. In this situation, the decision whether to recommend palliative WBRT is medically and ethically difficult. In many health systems, this decision must also be made in a context of increasing pressure on costs. Since the existing scoring systems are weak when it comes to differentiating among patients with the most unfavorable overall diagnoses, we carried out the present retrospective analysis on a larger patient group in a single center. The particular aim was to search for patient-related and tumor-related factors that could be used to better identify the subgroup of patients who will not benefit from WBRT.

Methods and Materials

We analyzed the data on 107 patients with intra- and extracranial metastases of malignant melanoma who had been treated in our Department of Therapeutic Radiology and Oncology in the period 1988–2012. The classification of these patients' primary tumors is shown in Table 2.

Table 2. Primary Tumor Characteristics

	No. of patients (%)
Localization	
Trunk	47 (43.9)
Lower extremity	19 (17.8)
Upper extremity	14 (13.1)
Head & neck, acral	16 (14.9)
Mucosa, unknown primary	11 (10.2)
Histological subtype	
Superficial spreading melanoma (SSM)	45 (42.1)
Nodulary melanoma	34 (31.8)
Unknown primary	9 (8.4)
Acral lentiginious melanoma (ALM)	10 (9.3)
Lentigo maligna melanoma (LMM)	4 (3.7)
Non-cutaneous melanoma	5 (4.6)
Breslow thickness	
≤2 mm	32 (29.9)
2–4 mm	21 (19.6)
>4 mm	54 (50.5)

Table 3. Patient- and tumor-related parameters of 107 patients, including results of univariate survival analysis

Parameter	No.	p-value
Sex		
Male	66 (61.7 %)	0.345
Female	41 (38.3 %)	
Median age (years)	64 (range 20-87)	0.536
KPS		
≥70	59 (55.1 %)	<0.001
<70	40 (37.4 %)	
Unknown	8 (7.5 %)	
Neurological symptoms		
Yes	76 (71.0)	0.046
No	23 (21.5)	
Unknown	8 (7.5)	
LDH		
≤240 U/l	37 (34.6)	<0.001
>240 U/l	56 (52.3)	
Unknown	14 (13.1)	
No. of intracranial metastases		
≤3	46 (43.0)	0.006
>3	61 (57.0)	
Intracranial therapy prior to WBRT		
Resection or/and stereotactic radiosurgery	40 (37.4)	0.056
No prior intracranial treatment	64 (59.8)	
Unknown	3 (2.8)	
No. of extracranial metastatic locations		
≤2	62 (57.9)	0.181
>2	44 (41.1)	
Unknown	1 (0.9)	
Local recurrence and lymph node metastases		
Yes	69 (64.5)	0.175
No	32 (29.9)	
Unknown	6 (5.6)	

Abbreviations: KPS: Karnofsky Performance Status; LDH: serum lactate dehydrogenase; WBRT: hole brain radiotherapy.

The following patient-related and tumor-related parameters were extracted from the files: sex, age, KPS ≥70 vs. <70, neurological symptoms (yes/no), serum lactate dehydrogenase level (LDH ≤ 240 U/l or >240 U/l; normal range 120 – 240), number of intracranial metastases (1-3 or >3), prior resection or stereotactic radiosurgery (SRS), number of extracranial metastatic locations (≤2 or >2 different organs or structures involved), local recurrence and regional lymph node metastases (yes/no) at the time of WBRT (Table 3). With initial diagnoses of 1–3 brain metastases, 21.5% (23/107) of the patients were treated by resection and 15.9% (17/107) by SRS. A further 7 patients received SRS in response to a progression observed after resection.

WBRT was administered in cases of progression after surgical and/or SRS treatment of metastases (n= 47) or with an initial diagnosis of multiple brain metastases (n= 60). The radiation was given using photons via opposing fields with a daily dose of 3 Gy 5 times per week up to a planned total dose of 30 Gy.

Statistical Analysis

Data are presented as mean and standard deviation or median and range for continuous data, and absolute and relative frequency for categorical data, respectively. Overall survival was calculated from the beginning of palliative WBRT until death. Univariate analysis was performed to assess the impact of all variables on survival using the Kaplan-Meier method and the log-rank test for comparison. A stepwise multivariate Cox regression analysis was then performed, including all variables with a P-value of ≤0.1. P-values of <0.05 were considered statistically significant. For data analysis, PASW 18 (PASW Statistics; SPSS Inc, Chicago, IL) was used.

Results

The median age of the 107 patients (66 male, 41 female) at the time of WBRT was 64 years (range 20–87). 101 patients received the planned total dose of 30 Gy, and in 6 patients treatment was discontinued after a median total dose of 18 Gy (range 9 – 27) due to deteriorating health.

All but 6 of the patients had uncontrolled extracranial metastases at the time of WBRT. The distribution of metastases was as follows: lungs, 59 patients (55.1%); liver, 33 patients (30.8%); cutis and/or subcutis, 41 patients (38.3%); lymph nodes, 61 patients (57.0%); abdominal wall, peritoneum or retroperitoneal space, 20 patients (18.7%); and bones, 16 patients (14.7%). 26 patients (23.4%) had metastases in less common locations such as the eye, pericardium, thymus, muscle, spleen or kidney. 62 patients (57.9%) had one or two extracranial metastases and 44 patients (41.1%) had more than two extracranial metastases. Patients with liver metastases had a higher probability of also having metastases in other locations, and had a worse prognosis, than patients without liver metastases.

76 patients (71%) had neurological symptoms at the time of WBRT. The most frequent of these was headache, followed by various forms of paresis, vertigo and nausea.

Information on the clinical course of the illness subsequent to WBRT was found for 99 patients. After WBRT, 34 patients (35.8%) experienced an improvement of neurological symptoms, while for 61 patients (64.2%) no change or a worsening of intracranial-related symptoms was recorded.

The median survival of all patients was 86 days (range 1–1792). 59 patients had a KPS of ≥70 prior to WBRT. LDH values were present for 93 of 107 patients (87%), and 56 of them (52.3%) had an LDH value >240 U/l.

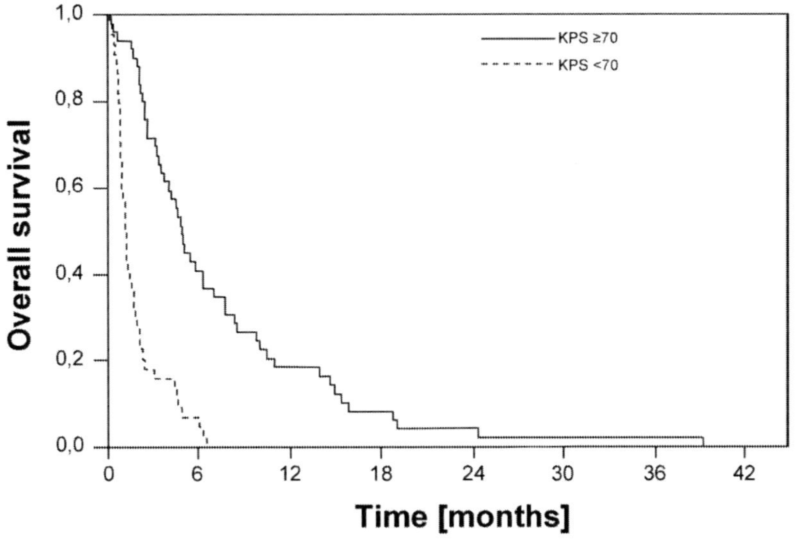

Figure 1. Kaplan-Meier analysis for overall survival form start of whole-brain radiation therapy; P<0.001. KPS= Karnofsky Performance Status.

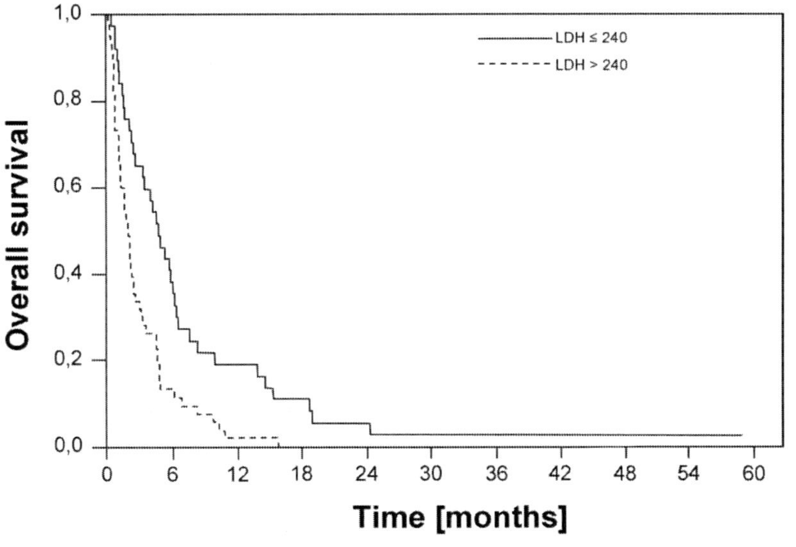

Figure 2. Kaplan-Meier analysis for overall survival form start of whole-brain radiation therapy; P<0.001. LDH= lactate dehydrogenase level.

Table 4. Result of multivariate survival analysis

Parameter	HR	95% CI	p-value
KPS			
≥70	Ref.		
<70	4.8	2.8–8.1	<0.001
LDH			
≤240	Ref.		
>240	2.5	1.5–4.1	<0.001

Abbreviations: HR: hazard ratio; CI: confidence interval; KPS: Karnofsky Performance Status; LDH: serum lactate dehydrogenase.

The univariate analysis revealed that patients with a KPS ≥70 had a median survival of 147 days (range 6–1195), compared with 34 days (range 1–197) for patients with a KPS <70 (p<0.001). Kaplan-Meier plot is shown in Figure 1. Patients with LDH ≤240 U/l had a median survival of 144 days (range 12–1792), compared with 59 days (range 1–483) for patients with LDH >240 U/l (p<0.001) (Figure 2). Patients had a median survival of 62 days (range 1–1792) if they had neurological symptoms at the time of WBRT, but 150 days (range 6–743) if they were free of neurological symptoms (p=0.046). Patients with 1–3 intracranial metastases had a median survival of 147 days (range 1–1792), compared to 65 days (range 6–578) for patients with more than 3 metastases (p=0.006). Patients who had had a resection and/or SRS before WBRT had a median survival of 147 days (range 7–1792), compared to 72 days (range 1–1195) for patients who had not had these interventions (p=0.056). The remaining parameters – sex, age, number of extracranial metastatic locations, local recurrence und regional lymph node metastases at the time of WBRT – showed no statistically significant effect on survival. The results of the Cox regression analysis are presented in Table 4. Patients with a KPS <70 had a significantly worse prognosis than patients with a KPS ≥70, with a 4.8-fold higher risk of dying sooner. Patients with LDH values >240 had a 2.5-fold higher mortality risk. Based on these results, we classified patients into four subgroups based on the possible permutations of KPS (<70 or ≥70) and LDH (≤ 240 or >240) and evaluated the prognostic significance of the resulting KPS/LDH score. The group with the best prognosis were the patients with KPS ≥70 and LDH ≤240 who had a median survival of 175 days (range 46–743). The second-best survival of 111 days (range 6–483) was found in the group with KPS ≥70 and LDH >240. The third-best group had KPS <70, LDH ≤240 and a survival of 47 days (range 12–197). Finally, the group with the worst prognosis had KPS <70, LDH >240 and a median survival of just 34 days (range 1–139). The survival probabilities are shown in Figure 3. Comparable results were obtained for patients who had undergone prior resection/SRS and patients who received upfront WBRT for multiple brain metastases. Those with a KPS ≥70 and a LDH ≤240 had the longest survival (234 days with prior resection/SRS, 144 days without). Patients with a KPS <70 and LDH >240 had the shortest survival (23 days with prior resection/SRS, 34 days without). Of the 6 patients who discontinued WBRT, 2 had a KPS ≥70 / LDH >240, 3 had a KPS <70 / LDH ≤240, and 1 patient had a KPS <70 / LDH >240, respectively.

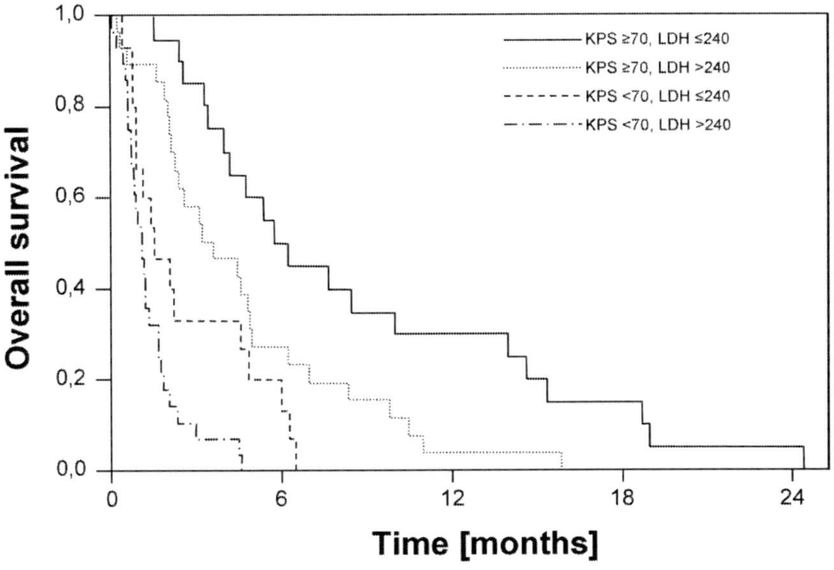

Figure 3. Kaplan-Meier analysis for overall survival of the KPS/LDH Index from start of whole-brain radiation therapy; P<0.001. KPS= Karnofsky Performance Status; LDH= lactate dehydrogenase level.

Discussion

Brain metastases are a common complication of cancer that occurs with many kinds of primary tumors. They are 10 times more common than primary brain tumors and they are an unfavorable prognostic factor for morbidity and mortality. In the case of malignant melanoma as the primary tumor, as many as 43% of all patients develop clinically manifest brain metastases. [16,12].

For physicians treating cancer patients, knowledge of prognostic factors is essential in order to make an assessment of the patient's prospects on the basis of the available evidence, and to explain the probable risks and benefits of systemic and local therapy options.

A multivariate analysis with 1137 melanoma patients revealed that the type of therapy chosen had the strongest impact on survival [17]. Patients who were treated with resection, with or without adjuvant WBRT, survived significantly longer than patients who had been given WBRT alone. In the patients who were treated by resection, no effect of adjuvant WBRT on survival was found. However, WBRT was found to be significantly better than best supportive care (BSC). Stratification according to the treatment revealed median survival times of 2.1 months with BSC, 3.4 months after WBRT, 8.7 months after resection and 8.9 months after resection with adjuvant WBRT.

The three-stage RPA classification was developed using the data from 3 prospective randomized RTOG studies [13]. Class 1 includes patients with a KPS ≥70, age <65 years, primary tumor control and without extracranial metastases. In this group with the most favorable prognosis, the median survival was 7.1 months. In contrast, class 3, which includes all patients with KPS <70 (regardless of age, primary tumor control status and extracranial metastasis) had the least favorable prognosis, with a median survival of 2.3 months.

The four-armed GPA developed by Sperduto et al. [14] is based on data from 1960 patients from 5 randomized RTOG studies. The advantage of this score over the previously used RPA classification is that it takes into account the number of brain metastases and avoids the imprecise evaluation of systemic tumor control. The GPA applies a three-point classification (giving the scores 0, 0.5 or 1) to the parameters age (≥ 60; 50– 59; <50 Jahre), KPS (<70; 70–80; >80), number of brain metastases (>3; 2–3; 1) and extracranial metastases (present; not applicable; none). The overall score is the sum of the individual parameter scores. The least favorable score in this study corresponded to a survival of 2.6 months.

Two years after publication of the GPA, the diagnosis-specific version DS-GPA was presented [15]. This is based on data from 5067 patients, 483 of them with malignant melanoma. As a result of this study it emerged that only KPS and the number of brain metastases influenced overall survival (p<0.0001). Like the GPA, this method also used a four-armed scoring scheme; the median survival of the patients in the least favorable arm was 3.38 months.

According to Lagerwaard et al. [18] the prognosis for patients with brain metastases (independent of the primary diagnosis) is influenced not only by the therapy chosen (BSC, WBRT, resection in combination with WBRT) and the KPS, but also by the response to steroid treatment, systemic tumor activity, and serum LDH. The independent prognostic influence of LDH was confirmed by Staudt et al. [19] for 265 patients with malignant melanoma.

LDH is a cytoplasmic enzyme which catalyzes the interconversion of lactate and pyruvate. Since it is present in all tissues, an elevated LDH value is a general marker for raised cell turnover or cell death. This makes it a suitable indicator of overall tumor load. The highest LDH activity is found in the heart, the brain, skeletal muscles, the liver and the kidney. Lower activities are present in erythrocytes, thrombocytes, and leukocytes, as well as in the spleen, the lung and the adrenal glands.

A study with 51 patients by Nieder et al. [20] investigated whether current prognostic scores reliably guide treatment decisions and concluded that GPA und DS-GPA reliably identify patients with favorable prognosis, who are known to benefit from more aggressive local treatment, but that they do not reliably predict survival in patients with unfavorable prognosis. The authors postulated that the combination of KPS and LDH would predict the cases with the shortest survival more reliably than GPA or DS-GPA (although LDH values were only available for 31 patients and the statistical significance could not be shown). A subsequent study retrospectively evaluated data from 100 patients with a variety of primary tumors, for whom LDH values from the time of WBRT were available [21]. The upper limit of normal serum LDH was set at ≥205 U/l. Patients with normal LDH had a significantly longer survival (median 4 months) than patients with elevated LDH (median 3.1 months). The authors were able to show that if they applied an LDH cutoff value of 1.5 times the normal value (i.e., LDH <307 U/l), the difference between the survival of patients in the "normal" and "elevated" LDH categories was maximized. Stratification by tumor histology revealed that this difference was especially clear for patients with malignant melanoma (median overall survival 1.1 compared with 5.5 months). However, only 10% of the patients in this study had malignant melanoma.

Eigentler et al. [22] also confirmed the prognostic influence of serum LDH measured before the beginning of treatment for melanoma patients, in a retrospective multi-center study of 672 patients done for the German Cancer Society. From the multivariate analysis, the number of brain metastases (single or multiple) and the serum LDH (normal or elevated; without specification of the cutoff value) emerged as the only statistically significant prognostic factors for the whole cohort. Patients with a single brain metastasis had a median survival of 7 months, falling to 4 months for patients with multiple metastases. A normal-range LDH at the beginning of therapy corresponded to a median overall survival of 6 months but with elevated LDH a survival of 3 months was observed. In the subgroup analysis of patients with a single brain metastasis, the therapy chosen (SRS or resection versus WBRT and/or chemotherapy) was the only statistically significant parameter.

While the study by Eigentler et al. also included patients with very favorable prognoses, a recent study by our research group was the first to focus exclusively on patients with unfavorable prognoses. This analysis identified KPS and LDH as independent prognostic factors for survival and found that a score combining KPS and LDH (KPS/LDH Index) was able to identify patients with an especially short overall survival [23].

The disease progression that we observed in our group was on average markedly more aggressive than that seen in the comprehensive studies of Sampson et al. [7] and Five et al. [17] with large numbers of patients.

In those studies, the median time from the first diagnosis of the primary tumor to the first diagnosis of a brain metastasis was 3.7 years, but in our group it was only 2 years (range 0–29). Possible explanations for this discrepancy include earlier diagnosis of the primary tumor in their study population or a higher prevalence of advanced primaries or tumor types with a strong tendency towards formation of brain metastases or simply a bias due to the much smaller size of our cohort.

The present evaluation of 107 patients with initially multiple and/or progressive brain metastases and extracranial metastases, confirms the conclusions of our previous study: the four-armed KPS/LDH Index shows statistically significant differences in median survival.

To test the prognostic ability of the DS-GPA, we applied it retrospectively to our patient group. It revealed no statistically significant difference in median overall survival between the least favorable prognosis class DS-GPA 0 and the next more favorable class DS-GPA 1 (data not shown). In contrast, our KPS/LDH Index found a statistically significant difference in survival of the groups KPS <70, LDH >240 and KPS <70, LDH ≤ 240.

CONCLUSION

The results of our follow-up study confirm that the KPS/LDH index can identify patients with particularly short survival better than the existing prognostic scores. For patients in our least favorable prognosis group with a median survival of 34 days, the appropriateness of WBRT is questionable for medical and ethical reasons and in terms of the proper use of resources.

Especially relevant is the fact that this treatment does not promise a satisfactory relief of already manifest neurological symptoms. These patients are unlikely to benefit from WBRT and should be considered for BSC instead.

We intend to follow up this study with a larger retrospective study at national level. If this confirms the usefulness of the KPS/LDH Index for this purpose, it should be tested in a prospective study on a larger patient group.

References

[1] Amer MH, Al-Sarraf M, Vaitkevicius VK. Clinical presentation, natural history and prognostic fators in advanced malignant melanoma. *Surg. Gynecol. Obstet.* 1979;149:687-692.

[2] Atkinson L. Melanoma of the central nervous system. *Aust. N. Z. J. Surg.* 1978;48:14-16.

[3] Mc Neer G, Das Gupta T. Problem of recurrence in the management of melanoma. *CA Cancer J. Clin.* 1965;15:270-274.

[4] Beresford HR. Melanoma of the nervous system: treatment with corticosteroids and radiation. *Neurology* 1969;19:59-65.

[5] de la Monte SM, Moore GW, Hutchins GM. Patterned distribution of metastases from malignant melanoma in humans. *Cancer Res.* 1983;43:3427-3433.

[6] Chason JL, Walker FB, Landers JW. Metastatic carcinoma in the central nervous system and dorsal root ganglia. A retrospective autopsy study. *Cancer* 1963; 57: 781-787.

[7] Sampson J, Carter J, Friedman A, et al. Demographics, prognosis, and therapy in 702 patients with brain metastases from malignant melanoma. *J. Neurosurg.* 1998;88:11-20.

[8] Weller M. Therapeutische Ansätze bei Hirnmetastasen. *Im Focus Onkologie*, 2005. 57-60.

[9] Catell E, Kelly C, Middleton MR. Brain metastases in melanoma: a European perspective. *Sem. Oncol.* 2002;29:513-517.

[10] Douglas JG, Margolin K. The treatment of brain metastases from malignant melanoma. *Sem. Oncol.* 2002;29:518-524.

[11] Barth A, Wanek LA, Morton DL. Progostic factors in 1,521 melanoma patients with distant metastases. *J. Am. Coll. Surg.* 1995;181(3):193-201.

[12] Budman DR, Camacho E, Wittes RE. The current cause of death in patients with malignant melanoma. *Eur. J. Cancer,* 1978; 14(4):327-330.

[13] Gaspar L, Scott C, Rotman M, et al. Recursive partitioning analysis (RPA) of prognostic factors in three Radiation Therapy Oncology Group (RTOG) brain metastases trials. *Int. J. Radiat. Oncol. Biol. Phys.* 1997;37(4):745-751.

[14] Sperduto PW, Berkley B, Gaspar LE, et al. A new prognostic index and comparison to three other indices for patients with brain metastases: An analysis of 1,960 patients in the RTOG database. *Int. J. Radiat. Oncol. Biol. Phys.* 2008;70:510-514.

[15] Sperduto PW, Chao ST, Sneed PK, et al. Diagnosis-specific prognostic factors, indexes, and treatment outcomes for patients with newly diagnosed brain metastases: A multi-institutional analysis of 4,259 patients. *Int. J. Radiat. Oncol. Biol. Phys.* 2010;77: 655-661.

[16] Barnholtz-Sloan JS, Sloan AE, Davis FG, et al. Incidence proportions of brain metastases in patients diagnosed (1973-2001) in the Metropolitan Detroit Cancer Surveillance System. *J. Clin. Oncol.* 2004;22(14):2865-2872.

[17] Fife KM, Colman MH, Stevens GN, et al. Determinants of Outcome in Melanoma Patients With Cerebral Metastases. *J. Clin. Oncol.* 2004;22:1293-1300.

[18] Lagerwaard F, Levendag P, Nowak P, et al. Idendifikation of prognostic factors in patients with brain metastases: A review of 1292 patients. *Int. J. Radiat. Oncol. Biol. Phys.* 1999;43:795-803.

[19] Staudt M, Lasithiotakis K, Leiter U, et al. Determinats of survival in patients with brain metastases from cutaneous meanoma. *Br. J. Cancer,* 2010; 102:1213-1218.

[20] Nieder C, Marienhagen K, Geinitz H, et al. Can current prognostic scores reliably guide treatment decisions in patients with brain metastases form malignant melanoma?. *J. Can. Res. Ther.* 2011;7:47-51.

[21] Nieder C, Marienhagen K., Dalhaug A., et al. Towards Improved Prognostic Scores Predicting Survival in Patients with Brain Metastases: A pilot Study of Serum Lactate Dehydrogenase Levels. *Scientific world journal* 2012; Epub 2012 Apr 19.

[22] 22 Eigentler TK, Figl A, Krex D, et al. Number of Metastases, Serum Lactat Dehydrogenase Level, and Type of Treatment are Prognostic Factors in Patients with Brain Metastases of Malignant Melanoma. *Cancer* 2011;117:1697-1703.

[23] 23 Partl R, Richtig E, Avian A, et al. Karnofsky Performance Status and Lactate Dehydrogenase Predict the Benefit of Palliative Whole-Brain Irradiation in Patients With Advanced Intra- and Extracranial Metastases From Malignant Melanoma. *Int. J. Radiat. Oncol. Biol. Phys.* 2013; 85(3):662-666.

SHORT COMMUNICATIONS

In: Melanoma
Editor: Alexander C. Jones

ISBN: 978-1-62808-608-9

Chapter 10

INTERFERON-BETA THERAPY FOR MELANOMA: A REVIEW OF THE LITERATURE

Yuta Kurashige * ***and Tetsuo Nagatani***
Department of Dermatology,
Hachioji Medical Center of Tokyo Medical University, Tokyo, Japan

ABSTRACT

Interferon (IFN)-β is a naturally occurring secretary glycoprotein. At present two subtypes of IFN-β, "natural" IFN-β (nIFN-β) and "recombinant" IFN-β (rIFN-β), are being used clinically. According to *in vitro* studies examining the anti-tumor activity of IFN-β, both nIFN-β and rIFN-β inhibited the proliferation of, and showed apoptotic effects on, melanoma cells. Moreover, some *in vivo* studies have demonstrated that the local administration of nIFN-β and rIFN-β leads to anti-tumor activity on human melanoma xenograft models. Despite such experimental outcomes, the results of phase II clinical trials involving metastatic melanoma patients indicated that systemic administration of neither nIFN-β nor rIFN-β was significantly effective. In contrast, clinical trials in Japan involving intratumoral injections of nIFN-β resulted in an efficacy rate of 50% against cutaneous metastatic melanomas. Due to this finding, nIFN-β is now approved in Japan and is frequently used, especially as a part of post-operative adjuvant chemotherapy such as "DAV-IFN-β therapy", a combination of dacarbazie, nimustine, vincristine, and local subcutaneous injections of nIFN-β. After DAV-IFN-β therapy, nIFN-β alone can be administered for maintenance therapy. While the efficacy of nIFN-β when combined with DAV therapy has not yet been fully confirmed in clinical investigations, a recent study examining single-agent maintenance therapy with sequential, local injections of nIFN-β demonstrated significant improvement of the prognosis of stage II melanoma patients. Although further randomized studies are needed, adjuvant therapy using local injections of nIFN-β may be a viable option for post-operative melanoma patients.

---

* Correspondence: Dr. Yuta Kurashige, Department of Dermatology, Hachioji Medical Center, Tokyo Medical University, 1163 Tatemachi, Hachioji-shi, Tokyo 193-0998, Japan, E-Mail: kurasige@tokyo-med.ac.jp, Phone: +81.42.665.5611, Fax: +81.42.665.1796.

INTRODUCTION

The type I interferon (IFN) family consists of IFN-α, IFN-β, IFN-ε, IFN-κ, and IFN-ω [1]. As is well known, IFNs in general have anti-tumor activity, while individual types exhibit different biological behaviors. As a therapeutic agent for melanoma patients, adjuvant therapy with IFN-α has been tested clinically. As a result, "high-dose" IFN-α-2b and "pegylated" IFN-α-2b have been approved by the FDA for the treatment of stage II and III melanoma. In particular, pegylated IFN-α-2b can significantly improve recurrence-free survival (RFS) although no significant benefits were shown in overall survival (OS) [1]. In Japan the use of IFN-β has been approved and is covered by National Health Insurance for the treatment of melanoma patients. In this section, we review the previous literature regarding the effect of IFN-β on melanoma, and examine its molecular characteristics, the mechanism of its anti-tumor activity in both *in vitro* and *in vivo* studies, its clinical performance, and its practical clinical application in Japan.

MOLECUTLAR CHARACTERISTICS OF INTERFERON BETA

IFN-β is a naturally occurring secretary glycoprotein comprised of 166 amino acid residues and sugar chain structures. It has 30% amino acid homology with IFN-α but only 1% homology with IFN-γ [2]. IFN-α and IFN-β can bind to the same high-affinity receptor known as the type 1 receptor [3]. At present, two subtypes of IFN-β, namely, "natural" IFN-β (nIFN-β) and "recombinant" IFN-β (rIFN-β), which has structural variants, 1a and 1b, are used being clinically.

nIFN-β derives from human fibroblasts while rIFN-β has been produced using recombinant DNA techniques in host cells, specifically, rIFN-β-1a in Chinese hamster ovary (CHO) cells and rIFN-β-1b in *Escherichia coli*. rIFN-β-1a has an amino acid sequence identical to that of nIFN-β and like nIFN-β, has glycosylation as well. In contrast, rIFN-β-1b has a mutation of the amino acid sequence at position 17 involving a serine-cystine substitution and lacks glycosylation.

MECHANISMS THOUGHT TO UNDERLIE ANTI-TUMOR ACTIVITY OF INTERFERONS

Although the mechanisms underlying the anti-tumor activity of IFNs are not understood fully, previous experimental results suggest that this activity might be linked to several different processes that produce antiproliferative, antiangiogenic, and immunomodulating effects [4]. The anti-proliferative effects depend on the influence of IFN-β on the S phase of the cell cycle, namely, a delay from the G_1 to the S phase of the cell cycle was reportedly induced by IFNs [5]. The anti-angiogenic property of IFNs was seen in the results of *in vitro* or *in vivo* studies using cultured or transplanted tumor cells [6]. In their capacity as immuno-modulators, IFNs reportedly increased natural killer cell and lymphomononuclear cell activity and major histocompatibility complex class I and class II antigen expression [7].

In Vitro Studies of the Effect of Interferon Beta on the Growth of Human Melanoma Cells

A large number of studies have examined the anti-tumor activity of IFN-β on human melanoma cell lines. Most of these studies used nIFN-β as a representative form of IFN. In one of our own studies using cultured melanoma cell lines, we demonstrated the dose-dependent, anti-proliferative effect of nIFN-β. Specifically, at a dose of 300 IU/ml, nIFN-β almost completely inhibited the growth of melanoma cells [8]. Incorporation of [^{3}H] thymidine and [^{3}H] uridine was also inhibited by nIFN-β. With the exception of a few cases [9,10], most research on this aspect of nIFN-β activity demonstrated similar dose-dependent anti-proliferative effects on melanoma cells [3,5,11-14]. In addition, both rIFN-β 1a [15,16] and 1b [17] demonstrated an anti-proliferative effect on melanoma cells. On the whole, it must be noted that the anti-proliferative effect of IFN-β tends to be superior to that of IFN-α and IFN-γ [3,12,13,16,17]. It is also worth noting that nIFN-β was found to be capable of inducing apoptosis in melanoma cells. In some studies using the TUNEL method, for instance, apoptosis was demonstrated in melanoma cells cultured with nIFN-β [8,14]. Other studies have reported that nIFN-β inhibited the invasive potential of melanoma cells [3,10].

In Vivo Studies of the Effect of Interferon Beta on the Human Melanoma Cells Using Animal Models

In addition to *in vitro* experiments, a number of *in vivo* studies have also examined the effect of interferon beta on human melanoma cells. Most of the animal melanoma models used in such studies involved the transplantation of xenograftic human melanoma cell lines into genetically modified mice [18]. The results of these studies seem to indicate that the efficacy of IFN-β depends on the administration routes. Notably, local administration, including intratumoral or peritumoral injection, of each sub-type of IFN-β inhibited the growth, and induced apoptosis, of the transplanted melanoma cells [11,19,20,21]. In one comparative study, rIFN-β-1a showed a stronger anti-proliferative effect than IFN-α-2b. On the other hand, systemic administration of IFN-β, including intraperitonial and subcutaneous injections, failed to inhibit the growth of the transplanted melanoma cells sufficiently [9,11,22]. Only one study was able to demonstrate the anti-proliferative effect of the intravenous injection of nIFN-β and rIFN-β-1b [19]. These results suggest that local administration of IFN-β is more effective than systemic administration [11,19].

Clinical Trials of Interferon Beta in Advanced Melanoma Patients

Based on the anti-proliferative properties of IFN-β against various human tumor cell lines, some phase I clinical trials using nIFN-β [23-25], rIFN-β-1a [26], or rIFN-β-1b [27-31] were performed on various malignant tumors. Most of the trials confirmed the safety and tolerability of IFN-β, regardless of the route of administration and the variety of IFN-β used.

While fever, rigor, and fatigue were described as the most common side effects of IFN-β, its toxicity was mild and reversible. [25]. Single-agent phase II clinical trials using different subtypes of IFN-β and different administration routes were also conducted in order to analyze the clinical efficacy of IFN-β in advanced metastatic melanoma patients [7,32-35]. Of these trials, those that involved the systemic administration of IFN-β, including the subcutaneous injection of rIFN-β-1a [32], the intravenous administration of rIFN-β-1b [33, 34], and the intravenous low-dose administration of nIFN-β (0.6 x 10^6 IU/m^2) [7] showed no clinical benefit for advanced melanoma patients. Only the intravenous administration of high-dose nIFN-β (60 x 10^6 IU/m^2/day) demonstrated anti-tumor activity [35]. In contrast, a number of studies demonstrated the efficacy of the local administration of nIFN-β in cases of cutaneous metastatic melanoma [9,14,36,37]. For instance, one clinical trial conducted in Japan using daily intratumoral injections of nIFN-β at a dose of 3 x 10^6 IU/day showed an efficacy rate of 50% against cutaneous metastatic melanoma [36]. According to another clinical study of nIFN-β [38], 24 hours after a local subcutaneous injection a high concentration of nIFN-β was detected locally as well as in the lesional lymph nodes, while little nIFN-β was detected in the blood. These facts might corroborate the results from the above-mentioned *in vivo* studies.

Local Injection of Interferon Beta As Adjuvant Therapy for Melanoma Patients: Practical Clinical Application in Japan

On the basis of the findings mentioned above [36], local injections of nIFN-β were approved for treatment of melanoma patients in 1985 and have been frequently used since then, especially as post-operative adjuvant therapy. After surgical resection of the primary lesion, nIFN-β is routinely administrated as part of "DAV-IFN-β therapy", that is, a combination chemotherapy consisting of dacarbazie (on days 1-5), nimustine (on day 1), vincristine (on day 1) and local injections of nIFN-β (on days 1-10). This treatment is administered every 4 weeks in several cycles [39-41]. After DAV-IFN-β therapy, some hospitals administer nIFN-β alone once a month as maintenance therapy [42]. In such cases, nIFN-β should be administered by subcutaneous injection in the periphery of the surgical scar of the primary lesion. However, it should be noted that in addition to systemic adverse events such as neutropenia, fatigue, anemia and liver dysfunction, nIFN-β is known sometimes to induce adverse reactions locally, including redness, pain, swelling, and skin ulceration, at the injection sites [43,44].

Evaluation of the Efficacy of Adjuvant Therapy Using Local Injections of Interferon Beta

Despite its wide use in Japan, the efficacy of nIFN-β as part of post-operative "DAV-IFN-β therapy" has not yet been fully established. Although early nonrandomized retrospective studies have demonstrated that DAV-IFN-β therapy improved the 5-year survival rate for stage III melanoma patients than DAV therapy alone or DAV plus other agents [38, 40], recent propensity-score-matched analysis concluded that DAV-IFN-β therapy, compared with non-use, brought no significant improvement in either disease-free survival rates or melanoma-specific survival rates among stage II and III melanoma patients [39]. The efficacy of maintenance therapy using nIFN-β, however, was demonstrated in a single-institution matched case-controlled study; single-agent maintenance therapy with sequential local injections of nIFN-β significantly improved the OS and RFS in stage II melanoma patients [42]. Nonetheless, it should be noted that thus far there have been no randomized controlled studies investigating efficacy of nIFN-β for melanoma patients.

Summary and Conclusion

According to previous *in vitro* and *in vivo* studies, IFN-β showed stronger anti-proliferative effects than IFN-α on the growth of melanoma cells [28]. Nevertheless, in the majority of the phase II clinical trials, the systemic administration of IFN-β demonstrated no clinical benefit for advanced melanoma patients. On the other hand, adjuvant therapy consisting of local administration of nIFN-β, especially in sequential maintenance therapy, appeared to improve the prognosis of stage II melanoma patients.

In recent years, the two novel agents have shown a significant survival benefit for advanced melanoma patients: the immune system-stimulating human anti-CTLA-4 antibody ipilimumab, and the selective BRAF inhibitor, vemurafenib [45]. While these new agents may eventually supersede existing treatments for advanced melanoma, adjuvant therapy using local injections of nIFN-β will remain a viable option for the post-operative melanoma patients.

References

[1] Tarhini AA, Gogas H, Kirkwood JM. IFN-α in the treatment of melanoma. *J. Immunol.* 2012 Oct 15; 189: 3789-3793.

[2] Buchwalder PA, Buclin T, Trinchard I, Munafo A, Biollaz J. Pharmacokinetics and pharmacodynamics of IFN-beta 1a in healthy volunteers. *J. Interferon Cytokine Res.* 2000 Oct; 20: 857-866.

[3] Horikoshi T, Fukuzawa K, Hanada N, Ezoe K, Eguchi H, Hamaoka S, Tsujiya H, Tsukamoto T. In vitro comparative study of the antitumor effects of human interferon-alpha, beta and gamma on the growth and invasive potential of human melanoma cells. *J. Dermatol.* 1995 Sep; 22: 631-636.

[4] Borden EC. Interferons: pleiotropic cellular modulators. *Clin. Immunol. Immunopathol.* 1992 Jan; 62: S18-24.

[5] Nagao S, Tohgo A, Kohno M, Ogawa H. Cytostatic action of human fibroblast interferon in direct growth inhibition: effect on human malignant melanoma. *Gann.* 1983 Jun; 74: 452-458.

[6] Sidky YA, Borden EC. Inhibition of angiogenesis by interferons: effects on tumor- and lymphocyte-induced vascular responses. *Cancer Res.* 1987 Oct 1; 47: 5155-5161.

[7] Voelter-Mahlknecht S, Mahlknecht U, Letzel S, Fierlbeck G. Phase 2 trial of the continuous IV administration of interferon-beta in patients with disseminated malignant melanoma. *Skinmed.* 2006 Nov-Dec; 5: 271-276.
[8] Nagatani T, Okazawa H, Kambara T, Satoh K, Nishiyama T, Tokura H, Yamada R, Nakajima H. Effect of natural interferon-beta on the growth of melanoma cell lines. *Melanoma Res.* 1998 Aug; 8: 295-299.
[9] Horoszewicz JS, Leong SS, Ito M, Buffett RF, Karakousis C, Holyoke E, Job L, Dölen JG, Carter WA. Human fibroblast interferon in human neoplasia: clinical and laboratory study. *Cancer Treat Rep.* 1978 Nov; 62: 1899-1906.
[10] Fukuzawa K, Horikoshi T. Inhibitory effect of human fibroblast interferon (HuIFN-beta) on the growth and invasive potential of cultured human melanoma cells in vitro. *Br. J. Dermatol.* 1992 Apr; 126: 324-330.
[11] Ida N, Uenishi N, Kajita A, Satoh Y. Antitumor effect of human fibroblast interferon on the growth of human melanoma cells implanted in nude mice. *Gann.* 1982 Dec; 73: 952-960.
[12] Johns TG, Mackay IR, Callister KA, Hertzog PJ, Devenish RJ, Linnane AW. Antiproliferative potencies of interferons on melanoma cell lines and xenografts: higher efficacy of interferon beta. *J. Natl. Cancer Inst.* 1992 Aug 5; 84: 1185-1190.
[13] Krasagakis K, Garbe C, Krüger S, Orfanos CE. Effects of interferons on cultured human melanocytes in vitro: interferon-beta but not-alpha or -gamma inhibit proliferation and all interferons significantly modulate the cell phenotype. *J. Invest. Dermatol.* 1991 Aug; 97: 364-372.
[14] Kubo H, Ashida A, Matsumoto K, Kageshita T, Yamamoto A, Saida T. Interferon-beta therapy for malignant melanoma: the dose is crucial for inhibition of proliferation and induction of apoptosis of melanoma cells. *Arch. Dermatol. Res.* 2008 Jul; 300: 297-301.
[15] Chawla-Sarkar M, Leaman DW, Jacobs BS, Borden EC. IFN-beta pretreatment sensitizes human melanoma cells to TRAIL/Apo2 ligand-induced apoptosis. *J. Immunol.* 2002 Jul 15; 169: 847-855.
[16] Chawla-Sarkar M, Leaman DW, Borden EC. Preferential induction of apoptosis by interferon (IFN)-beta compared with IFN-alpha2: correlation with TRAIL/Apo2L induction in melanoma cell lines. *Clin. Cancer Res.* 2001 Jun; 7: 1821-1831.
[17] Köpf J, Hanson C, Delle U, Weimarck A, Stierner U. Action of interferon alpha and beta on four human melanoma cell lines in vitro. *Anticancer Res.* 1996 Mar-Apr; 16: 791-798.
[18] Becker JC, Houben R, Schrama D, Voigt H, Ugurel S, Reisfeld RA. Mouse models for melanoma: a personal perspective. *Exp. Dermatol.* 2010 Feb; 19: 157-164.
[19] Gomi K, Morimoto M, Nakamizo N. Antitumor effect of human recombinant interferon-beta against human melanomas transplanted into nude mice. *J. Pharmacobiodyn.* 1984 Dec; 7: 951-961.
[20] Kohno M, Ida N, Nagao S, Tanaka N, Sekiguchi F, Uenishi N, Kajita A, Ogawa H. Effects of human fibroblast interferon on human tumors transplanted into nude mice: sensitivity of human tumors to interferon. *Gann.* 1982 Dec; 73: 945-951.
[21] Roh MR, Zheng Z, Kim HS, Jeung HC, Rha SY, Chung KY. Difference of interferon-α and interferon-β on melanoma growth and lymph node metastasis in mice. *Melanoma Res.* 2013 Apr; 23: 114-124.

[22] de Clercq E, Georgiades J, Edy VG, Sobis H. Effect of human and mouse interferon and of polyriboinosinic acid.polyribocytidylic acid on the growth of human fibrosarcoma and melanoma tumors in nude mice. *Eur. J. Cancer.* 1978 Nov; 14: 1273-1282.

[23] Bukowski RM, Sergi JS, Sharfman WJ, Budd GT, Murthy S, Barna B, Medendorp SV, Yen-Lieberman B, Gibson V, Bauer L, Valenzuela R. Phase I trial of natural human interferon beta in metastatic malignancy. *Cancer Res.* 1991 Feb 1; 51: 836-840.

[24] Abdi EA, Kamitomo VJ, McPherson TA, Konrad MW, Inoue M, Tan YH. Extended phase I study of human beta-interferon in human cancer. *Clin. Invest. Med.* 1986; 9: 33-40.

[25] Hawkins MJ, Krown SE, Borden EC, Krim M, Real FX, Edwards BS, Anderson SA, Cunningham-Rundles S, Oettgen HF. American cancer society Phase I trial of naturally produced beta-interferon. *Cancer Res.* 1984 Dec; 44: 5934-5938.

[26] Ravandi F, Estrov Z, Kurzrock R, Breitmeyer JB, Maschek BJ, Talpaz M. A phase I study of recombinant interferon-beta in patients with advanced malignant disease. *Clin Cancer Res.* 1999 Dec; 5: 3990-3998.

[27] Grunberg SM, Kempf RA, Venturi CL, Mitchell MS. Phase I study of recombinant beta-interferon given by four-hour infusion. *Cancer Res.* 1987 Feb 15; 47: 1174-1178.

[28] Hawkins M, Horning S, Konrad M, Anderson S, Sielaff K, Rosno S, Schiesel J, Davis T, DeMets D, Merigan T, Borden E. Phase I evaluation of a synthetic mutant of beta-interferon. *Cancer Res.* 1985 Nov; 45: 5914-5920.

[29] Borden EC, Hawkins MJ, Sielaff KM, Storer BM, Schiesel JD, Smalley RV. Clinical and biological effects of recombinant interferon-beta administered intravenously daily in phase I trial. *J. Interferon Res.* 1988 Jun; 8: 357-366.

[30] Sarna G, Pertcheck M, Figlin R, Ardalan B. Phase I study of recombinant beta ser 17 interferon in the treatment of cancer. *Cancer Treat Rep.* 1986 Dec; 70: 1365-1372.

[31] Hu E, Horning SJ. Phase I study of recombinant human interferon beta in patients with advanced cancer. *J. Biol. Response Mod.* 1987 Apr; 6: 121-129.

[32] Borden EC, Jacobs B, Hollovary E, Rybicki L, Elson P, Olencki T, Triozzi P. Gene regulatory and clinical effects of interferon β in patients with metastatic melanoma: a phase II trial. *J. Interferon Cytokine Res.* 2011 May; 31: 433-440.

[33] Sarna GP, Figlin RA, Pertcheck M. Phase II study of betaseron (beta ser17-interferon) as treatment of advanced malignant melanoma. *J. Biol. Response Mod.* 1987 Aug; 6: 375-378.

[34] Schiller JH, Storer B, Bittner G, Willson JK, Borden EC. Phase II trial of a combination of interferon-beta ser and interferon-gamma in patients with advanced malignant melanoma. *J. Interferon Res.* 1988 Oct; 8: 581-589.

[35] Abdi EA, Tan YH, McPherson TA. Natural human interferon-beta in metastatic malignant melanoma. A phase II study. *Acta Oncol.* 1988; 27: 815-817.

[36] Ishihara K. Clinical studies of human fibroblast interferon in malignant tumors of the skinâ€"with special reference to local administration. *J. Jpn. Soc. Cancer Ther.* 1983; 18: 41-53. (in Japanese).

[37] Paul E, Müller I, Renner H, Bödeker RH, Cochran AJ. Treatment of locoregional metastases of malignant melanomas with radiotherapy and intralesional beta-interferon injection. *Melanoma Res.* 2003 Dec; 13: 611-617.

[38] Yamamoto A, Ishihara K. Clinical study of DAV+IFN - beta therapy (combination adjuvant therapy with DTIC, ACNU and VCR and local injection of IFN - beta) for malignant melanoma. *Int. J. Immunotherapy.* 1996; 12: 73-78.

[39] Matsumoto T, Yokota K, Sawada M, Sakakibara A, Shibata S, Yasue S, Tomita Y, Yatsuya H, Akiyama M. Postoperative DAV-IFN-β therapy does not improve survival rates of stage II and stage III melanoma patients significantly. *J. Eur. Acad. Dermatol. Venereol.* 2012 Dec 1. doi: 10.1111/jdv.12040. [Epub ahead of print]

[40] Nagatani T, Ichiyama S, Onuma R, Miyazawa M, Matsuzaki T, Miyagawa K, Baba N, Uchiyama M, Nakajima H. The use of DAV (DTIC, ACNU and VCR) and natural interferon-beta combination therapy in malignant melanoma. *Acta Derm. Venereol.* 1995 Nov; 75: 494.

[41] Nagatani T, Ichiyama S, Miyakawa K, Uchiyama M. Malignant melanoma treated with natural interferons alfa and beta and DAV. *Eur. J. Cancer.* 1992; 28A: 1774.

[42] Aoyagi S, Hata H, Homma E, Shimizu H. Sequential local injection of low-dose interferon-beta for maintenance therapy in stage II and III melanoma: a single-institution matched case-control study. *Oncology.* 2012; 82: 139-146.

[43] Ishihara K. The treatment of skin cancer and malignant melanoma using interferons. *Sogo Rinsho.* 2003; 52: 2593-2598 (in Japanese).

[44] Kurashige Y, Irisawa R, Abe N, Saito M, Tsuboi R. Two cases of malignant melanoma of the toe developed skin ulcers following local injection of natural beta-interferon. *J. Dermatol.* 2012 Dec; 39: 1037-1038.

[45] Wilmott JS, Scolyer RA, Long GV, Hersey P. Combined targeted therapy and immunotherapy in the treatment of advanced melanoma. *Oncoimmunology.* 2012 Sep 1; 1:997-999.

In: Melanoma
Editor: Alexander C. Jones

ISBN: 978-1-62808-608-9

Chapter 11

MOLECULAR TARGETED THERAPY AND DRUG RESISTANCE

Shigeo Masuda*
Gene Expression Laboratory,
The Salk Institute for Biological Studies, CA, US

ABSTRACT

Recent evidence suggests that molecular targeted therapy using BRAF or MEK inhibitors on melanoma (with BRAF V600E mutation) is promising. In addition, combined BRAF and MEK inhibition is proved to be superior, because MEK inhibitors are able to prevent BRAF-inhibitor-induced side effects; that is, cutaneous squamous cell carcinoma, which is associated with paradoxical activation of MAPK pathway by BRAF inhibitors.

Although molecular targeted therapy on melanoma seems to be successful, there remains an unsolved problem; drug resistance. Increasing volumes of evidence indicate that mechanisms of drug resistance are not only cell-intrinsic but also cell-extrinsic. One of cell-intrinsic mechanisms is BRAF gene amplification, and novel driver mutations reported recently may also contribute to drug resistance. On the other hand, regarding cell-extrinsic mechanisms, tumor-microenvironment-mediated drug resistance has been demonstrated; that is, HGF-high stroma is attributable to drug resistance, and HGF-cMet axis inhibitors are useful to resolve drug resistance.

Collectively, further understanding of drug resistance mechanisms will improve outcomes of molecular targeted therapy on melanoma.

Keywords: Molecular targeted therapy, BRAF, MEK, Paradoxical activation, Drug resistance, HGF

* Corresponding author: Shigeo Masuda. Address: 10010 North Torrey Pines Road, La Jolla, CA 92037, U.S.A. Tel: +1-858-453-4100 (ext. 1324). Fax: +1-858-453-2573. E-mail: smasuda@salk.edu, smasuda-tky@umin.ac.jp.

Molecular Targeted Therapy on Melanoma

Previously, it was revealed that mutations in the gene encoding BRAF kinase occurred in approximately 50% of melanomas. Melanomas harboring a BRAF V600E mutation constitutively activate the mitogen-activated protein kinase (MAPK) pathway, thus promoting cell proliferation and inhibiting apoptosis. Vemurafenib (also known as PLX4032) was developed as a selective kinase inhibitor for the BRAF V600E mutation. In the study by Sosman et al. [1], vemurafenib has clinical responses in 53% of patients with previously treated BRAF V600–mutant metastatic melanoma. Although patients with metastatic melanoma have a median survival of 6 to 10 months under conventional therapies, Sosman et al. demonstrated that the median overall survival was approximately 16 months by vemurafenib [1].

Activated BRAF phosphorylates MEK proteins (MEK1 and MEK2), which subsequently activate downstream MAPK pathway. The MAPK pathway is known to regulate proliferation and survival of tumor cells. Trametinib (also knonwn as GSK1120212, GlaxoSmithKline Pharmaceuticals) is an orally available, selective inhibitor of MEK1 and MEK2. In the study by Flaherty et al. [2], trametinib, as compared with chemotherapy, improved rates of progression-free and overall survival among patients with metastatic melanoma harboring a BRAF V600E or V600K mutation.

However, non-melanoma skin cancers (i.e. well-differentiated cutaneous squamous-cell carcinomas and keratoacanthomas) have developed in approximately 15 to 30% of patients treated with BRAF inhibitors such as vemurafenib or dabrafenib [3]. BRAF inhibitors are known to induce the opposite effect; i.e. increasing pERK in cell lines with wild-type BRAF that have upstream pathway activation such as oncogenic RAS. This RAF inhibitor–dependent activation of MAPK pathway in BRAF wild-type cells is referred to as "paradoxical MAPK-pathway activation", and is driven by the formation of RAF dimers that lead to signaling through CRAF and consequently MAPK-pathway hyperactivation [4-7].

Resistance to therapy with BRAF inhibitors is closely related to reactivation of MAPK pathway. Flaherty et al. [8] conducted a phase 1 and 2 trial of combined treatment with dabrafenib (a selective BRAF inhibitor) and trametinib (a selective MEK inhibitor). In this study, dose-limiting toxic effects were not frequently observed in patients under combination therapy with dabrafenib and trametinib. Interestingly, cutaneous squamous-cell carcinoma was seen in 7% of patients with combination therapy and in 19% with monotherapy (dabrafenib alone). Median progression-free survival in the combination therapy was 9.4 months, as compared with 5.8 months in monotherapy. The rate of (complete or partial) response with combination therapy was 76%, as compared with 54% with monotherapy. Collectively, dabrafenib and trametinib could be safely combined at full monotherapy doses; the rate of proliferative skin lesions was (non-significantly) reduced; progression-free survival was significantly improved.

DRUG RESISTANCE TO MELANOMA DURING MOLECULAR TARGETED THERAPY

Although molecular targeted therapy on melanoma has been proven to be promising, the problem is that melanoma would soon acquire resistance to molecular targeted drugs. Recent findings shed light on cell-extrinsic mechanisms, as well as cell-intrinsic mechanisms of drug resistance [9].

(1) Cell-intrinsic Mechanisms of Drug Resistance

One of the cell-intrinsic mechanisms is BRAF gene amplification [10-12]. Shi et al. [10] identified BRAF V600E copy-number gain as a mechanism of acquired BRAF inhibitor resistance in 20% of patients treated with BRAF inhibitor. BRAF V600E overexpression and knockdown in cell lines resulted in BRAF inhibitor resistance and sensitivity, respectively. In BRAF inhibitor-resistance driven by BRAF V600E amplification, ERK reactivation is saturable, with higher doses of vemurafenib downregulating pERK and re-sensitizing melanoma cells to BRAF inhibitor. The mechanism of ERK reactivation is sensitive to the MEK1/2 inhibitor or its combination with the BRAF inhibitor (vemurafenib).

Next, Novel driver mutations have been identified in melanoma [13, 14]. Hodis et al. [13] discovered six novel melanoma genes (PPP6C, RAC1, SNX31, TACC1, STK19, and ARID2), three of which (i.e. RAC1, PPP6C, and STK19) harbored recurrent and potentially targetable mutations. Krauthammer et al. [14] also found an activating mutation in RAC1 in melanoma. In clinical trials on melanoma using molecular targeted drugs, if these driver mutations are present in samples of patients, examination of whether they correlate with reduced responses to therapy with molecular targeted drugs would be interesting, because such examination would not only contribute to drug response predictions but also might help select other treatment options, including combination therapies [15].

(2) Cell-extrinsic Mechanisms of Drug Resistance

Many studies have focused on cell-intrinsic mechanisms of drug resistance. On the other hand, it has been proposed that the tumor microenvironment confers innate resistance to therapy. Strausman et al. [16] found that stroma-mediated resistance is common, particularly to targeted agents. They characterized the stroma-mediated resistance of BRAF-mutant melanoma to RAF inhibitors. By proteomic analysis, it was demonstrated that stromal cells secreted hepatocyte growth factor (HGF), which resulted in activation of the HGF receptor MET, reactivation of the MAPK, and immediate resistance to RAF inhibition. Immunohistochemistry experiments demonstrated stromal cell expression of HGF in patients with BRAF-mutant melanoma and revealed a significant correlation between HGF expression by stromal cells and innate resistance to RAF inhibitor treatment. Interestingly, HGF is not simply a prognostic biomarker because the combined inhibition of BRAF and the HGF–cMET axis (for example, using HGF-neutralizing antibodies or the MET-inhibitory small molecule crizotinib) can reverse drug resistance in BRAF-mutant melanoma. Wilson et al.

[17] also identified HGF as a factor that makes BRAF-mutant melanoma resistant to BRAF inhibitor. Using a panel of kinase-'addicted' human cancer cell lines, they found that most cells can be rescued from drug sensitivity by simply exposing them to one or more cytokines. They reported that the plasma HGF concentration was inversely related to the response to BRAF inhibition in patients with BRAF-mutant melanoma.

Another example of tumor microenvironment-mediated therapy resistance is that treatment-induced damage to tumor microenvironment promotes cancer therapy resistance through WNT16B [18]. Using a genome-wide analysis of transcriptional responses to genotoxic stress induced by cancer therapeutics, Sun et al. [18] identified a spectrum of secreted proteins derived from tumor microenvironment that includes WNT16B. They determined that WNT16B expression is regulated by NF-kB after DNA damage and subsequently signals in a paracrine manner to activate the canonical Wnt program in tumor cells. Although they used prostate cancer models, the expression of WNT16B in the tumor microenvironment attenuated the effects of cytotoxic chemotherapy *in vivo*, promoting tumor cell survival and disease progression.

(3) Other Demonstrations of Drug Resistance

Callahan et al. [19] report a case with progression of RAS-mutant leukemia during RAF inhibitor treatment for melanoma, which is alert for noncutaneous neoplasia after RAF inhibition. This leukemia was previously unsuspected. As mentioned above, paradoxical activation of ERK signaling is the mechanistic basis for the development of RAS mutant squamous-cell skin cancers in patients treated with RAF inhibitors. The authors showed that exposure to vemurafenib induced hyperactivation of ERK signaling and proliferation of the leukemic cell population, an effect that was reversed on drug withdrawal. Although proliferation of squamous-cell carcinomas and keratoacanthomas after paradoxical ERK activation by RAF inhibitors are known to be irreversible on drug withdrawal, it is curious that proliferation of the leukemic cell population in this report was reversible on drug withdrawal. As the authors speculate, the addition of a MEK inhibitor to this patient's treatment regimen would suppress the vemurafenib-induced leukemic proliferation in vivo (though the authors were unable to obtain a MEK inhibitor at that time).

Although it is a mechanism of resistance in colon cancer, Prahallad et al. [20] revealed unresponsiveness to BRAF V600E inhibition through feedback activation of EGFR. In general, colon cancer patients with BRAF V600E oncogenic lesion have poor prognosis and show only a very limited response. To explore the cause of the limited therapeutic effect of PLX4032 on BRAF V600E mutant colon tumors, they performed an RNA-interference based genetic screen in human cells. They report that blockade of EGFR shows strong synergy with BRAF V600E inhibition. Mechanistically, they find that BRAF V600E inhibition causes a rapid feedback activation of EGFR, which supports continued proliferation in the presence of BRAF V600E inhibition. Usually, melanoma cells express low levels of EGFR and are therefore not subject to this feedback activation, but if EGFR expression is high in a melanoma patient, combination therapy consisting of BRAF and EGFR inhibitors might have some efficacy.

Prevention of Drug Resistance

Although the following reports are based on mouse models in which human melanoma cells are used, if the results are reconfirmed in human clinical trials, the initial treatment strategy for patients with BRAF-mutant melanoma could be changed by the evidence of resistance to melanoma treatment.

Das Thakur et al. [21] demonstrated that intermittent dosing of vemurafenib can successfully prevent drug resistance; paradoxically, since drug-resistant cells have been shown to acquire drug dependency, drug withdrawal thereafter would induce a "fitness deficit" in the cells and result in tumor regression. Thus, "on–off treatment" with vemurafenib has shown efficacy in BRAF-mutant melanoma. Whether this strategy is also effective against other cancers treated with other inhibitors is of interest, and the underlying mechanisms should be fully elucidated. From a clinical point of view, both (i) stratification of patients according to prediction of drug responsiveness to on–off treatment and (ii) optimization of the treatment protocol are necessary [22]. For patient stratification, we should assess which people would be suitable for on–off treatment and establish a method to predict eligibility, which would enable us to stratify patients as putative responders or nonresponders. To optimize treatment protocols, we should decide on the appropriate timing for both drug initiation (restart) and cessation (which should be personalized for every patient); other parameters, including target rate of tumor regression for drug cessation (i.e., when to stop treatment) and target rate of tumor regrowth for drug restart (i.e., when to start treatment), should be established to find the appropriate schedule. Further clinical trials are necessary for evaluating efficacy of this strategy.

Landsberg et al. [23] demonstrated that inflammation in tumor microenvironment induces loss of melanocytic antigens in melanoma, which results in immune escape in mouse models. They showed that TNFα is a crucial factor and causes phenotypic plasticity (i.e., reversible loss of melanocytic antigens) in melanoma, which is referred to as dedifferentiation of melanoma. Whether anti-TNFα treatment is effective against this immunoediting would be of interest. Although combination treatment (e.g., BRAF inhibitor and immunotherapy) may be proposed, elucidation of whether TNFα (as an inhibitory factor for immunotherapy) is secreted during treatment with BRAF inhibitors is essential, to ensure that combination treatment is given synergistically rather than antagonistically [22].

References

[1] Sosman JA, Kim KB, Schuchter L, Gonzalez R, Pavlick AC, Weber JS, McArthur GA, Hutson TE, Moschos SJ, Flaherty KT, Hersey P, Kefford R, Lawrence D, Puzanov I, Lewis KD, Amaravadi RK, Chmielowski B, Lawrence HJ, Shyr Y, Ye F, Li J, Nolop KB, Lee RJ, Joe AK, Ribas A. Survival in BRAF V600-mutant advanced melanoma treated with vemurafenib. *N. Engl. J. Med.* 2012;366:707-714.

[2] Flaherty KT, Robert C, Hersey P, Nathan P, Garbe C, Milhem M, Demidov LV, Hassel JC, Rutkowski P, Mohr P, Dummer R, Trefzer U, Larkin JM, Utikal J, Dreno B, Nyakas M, Middleton MR, Becker JC, Casey M, Sherman LJ, Wu FS, Ouellet D,

Martin AM, Patel K, Schadendorf D; METRIC Study Group. Improved survival with MEK inhibition in BRAF-mutated melanoma. *N. Engl. J. Med.* 2012;367:107-114.

[3] Flaherty KT, Puzanov I, Kim KB, Ribas A, McArthur GA, Sosman JA, O'Dwyer PJ, Lee RJ, Grippo JF, Nolop K, Chapman PB. Inhibition of mutated, activated BRAF in metastatic melanoma. *N. Engl. J. Med.* 2010;363:809-819.

[4] Poulikakos PI, Zhang C, Bollag G, Shokat KM, Rosen N. RAF inhibitors transactivate RAF dimers and ERK signalling in cells with wild-type BRAF. *Nature*. 2010;464:427-430.

[5] Hatzivassiliou G, Song K, Yen I, Brandhuber BJ, Anderson DJ, Alvarado R, Ludlam MJ, Stokoe D, Gloor SL, Vigers G, Morales T, Aliagas I, Liu B, Sideris S, Hoeflich KP, Jaiswal BS, Seshagiri S, Koeppen H, Belvin M, Friedman LS, Malek S. RAF inhibitors prime wild-type RAF to activate the MAPK pathway and enhance growth. *Nature*. 2010;464:431-435.

[6] Heidorn SJ, Milagre C, Whittaker S, Nourry A, Niculescu-Duvas I, Dhomen N, Hussain J, Reis-Filho JS, Springer CJ, Pritchard C, Marais R. Kinase-dead BRAF and oncogenic RAS cooperate to drive tumor progression through CRAF. *Cell.* 2010; 140:209-221.

[7] Su F, Viros A, Milagre C, Trunzer K, Bollag G, Spleiss O, Reis-Filho JS, Kong X, Koya RC, Flaherty KT, Chapman PB, Kim MJ, Hayward R, Martin M, Yang H, Wang Q, Hilton H, Hang JS, Noe J, Lambros M, Geyer F, Dhomen N, Niculescu-Duvaz I, Zambon A, Niculescu-Duvaz D, Preece N, Robert L, Otte NJ, Mok S, Kee D, Ma Y, Zhang C, Habets G, Burton EA, Wong B, Nguyen H, Kockx M, Andries L, Lestini B, Nolop KB, Lee RJ, Joe AK, Troy JL, Gonzalez R, Hutson TE, Puzanov I, Chmielowski B, Springer CJ, McArthur GA, Sosman JA, Lo RS, Ribas A, Marais R. RAS mutations in cutaneous squamous-cell carcinomas in patients treated with BRAF inhibitors. *N. Engl. J. Med.* 2012;366:207-215.

[8] Flaherty KT, Infante JR, Daud A, Gonzalez R, Kefford RF, Sosman J, Hamid O, Schuchter L, Cebon J, Ibrahim N, Kudchadkar R, Burris HA 3rd, Falchook G, Algazi A, Lewis K, Long GV, Puzanov I, Lebowitz P, Singh A, Little S, Sun P, Allred A, Ouellet D, Kim KB, Patel K, Weber J. Combined BRAF and MEK inhibition in melanoma with BRAF V600 mutations. *N. Engl. J. Med.* 2012;367:1694-1703.

[9] Masuda S, Izpisua Belmonte JC. The microenvironment and resistance to personalized cancer therapy. *Nat. Rev. Clin. Oncol.* 2013 Feb;10(2). doi:10.1038/nrclinonc.2012.127-c1.

[10] Shi H, Moriceau G, Kong X, Lee MK, Lee H, Koya RC, Ng C, Chodon T, Scolyer RA, Dahlman KB, Sosman JA, Kefford RF, Long GV, Nelson SF, Ribas A, Lo RS. Melanoma whole-exome sequencing identifies (V600E)B-RAF amplification-mediated acquired B-RAF inhibitor resistance. *Nat. Commun.* 2012;3:724.

[11] Corcoran RB, Dias-Santagata D, Bergethon K, Iafrate AJ, Settleman J, Engelman JA. BRAF gene amplification can promote acquired resistance to MEK inhibitors in cancer cells harboring the BRAF V600E mutation. *Sci. Signal.* 2010;3:ra84.

[12] Little AS, Balmanno K, Sale MJ, Newman S, Dry JR, Hampson M, Edwards PA, Smith PD, Cook SJ. Amplification of the driving oncogene, KRAS or BRAF, underpins acquired resistance to MEK1/2 inhibitors in colorectal cancer cells. *Sci. Signal.* 2011;4:ra17.

[13] Hodis E, Watson IR, Kryukov GV, Arold ST, Imielinski M, Theurillat JP, Nickerson E, Auclair D, Li L, Place C, Dicara D, Ramos AH, Lawrence MS, Cibulskis K, Sivachenko A, Voet D, Saksena G, Stransky N, Onofrio RC, Winckler W, Ardlie K, Wagle N, Wargo J, Chong K, Morton DL, Stemke-Hale K, Chen G, Noble M, Meyerson M, Ladbury JE, Davies MA, Gershenwald JE, Wagner SN, Hoon DS, Schadendorf D, Lander ES, Gabriel SB, Getz G, Garraway LA, Chin L. A landscape of driver mutations in melanoma. *Cell*. 2012;150:251-263.

[14] Krauthammer M, Kong Y, Ha BH, Evans P, Bacchiocchi A, McCusker JP, Cheng E, Davis MJ, Goh G, Choi M, Ariyan S, Narayan D, Dutton-Regester K, Capatana A, Holman EC, Bosenberg M, Sznol M, Kluger HM, Brash DE, Stern DF, Materin MA, Lo RS, Mane S, Ma S, Kidd KK, Hayward NK, Lifton RP, Schlessinger J, Boggon TJ, Halaban R. Exome sequencing identifies recurrent somatic RAC1 mutations in melanoma. *Nat. Genet*. 2012;44:1006-1014.

[15] Masuda S, Izpisua Belmonte JC. Trametinib for patients with advanced melanoma. *Lancet Oncol*. 2012;13:e409.

[16] Straussman R, Morikawa T, Shee K, Barzily-Rokni M, Qian ZR, Du J, Davis A, Mongare MM, Gould J, Frederick DT, Cooper ZA, Chapman PB, Solit DB, Ribas A, Lo RS, Flaherty KT, Ogino S, Wargo JA, Golub TR. Tumour micro-environment elicits innate resistance to RAF inhibitors through HGF secretion. *Nature*. 2012;487:500-504.

[17] Wilson TR, Fridlyand J, Yan Y, Penuel E, Burton L, Chan E, Peng J, Lin E, Wang Y, Sosman J, Ribas A, Li J, Moffat J, Sutherlin DP, Koeppen H, Merchant M, Neve R, Settleman J. Widespread potential for growth-factor-driven resistance to anticancer kinase inhibitors. *Nature*. 2012;487:505-509.

[18] Sun Y, Campisi J, Higano C, Beer TM, Porter P, Coleman I, True L, Nelson PS. Treatment-induced damage to the tumor microenvironment promotes prostate cancer therapy resistance through WNT16B. *Nat. Med*. 2012;18:1359-1368.

[19] Callahan MK, Rampal R, Harding JJ, Klimek VM, Chung YR, Merghoub T, Wolchok JD, Solit DB, Rosen N, Abdel-Wahab O, Levine RL, Chapman PB. Progression of RAS-mutant leukemia during RAF inhibitor treatment. *N. Engl. J. Med.* 2012;367: 2316-2321.

[20] Prahallad A, Sun C, Huang S, Di Nicolantonio F, Salazar R, Zecchin D, Beijersbergen RL, Bardelli A, Bernards R. Unresponsiveness of colon cancer to BRAF(V600E) inhibition through feedback activation of EGFR. *Nature*. 2012;483:100-103.

[21] Das Thakur M, Salangsang F, Landman AS, Sellers WR, Pryer NK, Levesque MP, Dummer R, McMahon M, Stuart DD. Modelling vemurafenib resistance in melanoma reveals a strategy to forestall drug resistance. *Nature*. 2013;494:251-255.

[22] Masuda S, Izpisua Belmonte JC. At the crossroads of targeted treatment and resistance in melanoma. *Lancet Oncol*. 2013;14:e136-e137.

[23] Landsberg J, Kohlmeyer J, Renn M, Bald T, Rogava M, Cron M, Fatho M, Lennerz V, Wölfel T, Hölzel M, Tüting T. Melanomas resist T-cell therapy through inflammation-induced reversible dedifferentiation. *Nature*. 2012;490:412-416.

In: Melanoma
Editor: Alexander C. Jones

ISBN: 978-1-62808-608-9

Chapter 12

BORON NEUTRON CAPTURE THERAPY FOR MELANOMA TREATMENT

Fernanda Faião Flores*

School of Pharmaceutical Sciences, University of São Paulo, Brazil

ABSTRACT

Boron Neutron Capture Therapy (BNCT) is a therapeutic tool for treatment of many types of tumors. It is based on the administration of a compound containing the element boron - isotope 10 (^{10}B), followed by thermal neutron irradiation. This results in a nuclear reaction and consequent release of high linear energy transfer, by alpha particles and lithium production. The products created by this reaction have a short range (5-9 μm) and thus reaches only cells that incorporate ^{10}B. This therapy is therefore a cellular irradiation suited to treat tumors that have infiltrated into healthy tissues. Some compounds have been studied to increase the uptake selectivity by tumor cells. The most frequently compounds with 10B used clinically are BSH ($Na_2H_{11}{}^{10}B_{12}SH$, sulfhydryl borane) and an amino acid derivative known as BPA [$(HO)_2$ ^{10}B-C_6H_4-CH (NH_2) CO_2H, Boronophenylalanine]. These compounds are nontoxic and may be administered in high doses. BNCT has been used clinically to treat patients with cutaneous melanomas which have a high mortality. These patients were either not candidates for, or had declined, conventional therapy. Melanoma is the most aggressive skin cancer and frequently involves distant and locoregional spread, usually with no efficient treatment. Metastatic melanoma remains a highly lethal disease, with an incidence that continues to increase faster than any other cancer. Almost all adjuvant treatments fail to control this malignancy. This therapy can potentially target tumor tissue selectively, sparing normal cells damage due to radiation. BNCT induces cell cycle arrest by cyclin D1 decrease, antiproliferative effects by Ki67 decrease and apoptosis by mitochondrial electric potential decrease and cleaved caspase 3, 7, 8 and 9 protein levels increase only in melanoma cells. As a result, BNCT acts as a localized therapy with minimal side effects

* Corresponding author: Fernanda Faião Flores, 580 Professor Lineu Prestes Avenue, Zip code: 05508-900, São Paulo, Brazil, Phone: 55 11 3091 3632, Fax: 55 11 3813 2197, Email: fernandafaiao@usp.br; fernandafaiao@yahoo.com.br.

for the melanoma treatment. This way, BNCT can be used as an adjunctive treatment in combination with other modalities, including surgery and chemotherapy, may lead to an improvement in patient survival.

Keywords: Melanoma; boron neutron capture therapy; boronophenylalanine; apoptosis; cell cycle arrest

Boron neutron capture therapy (BNCT) of cancer relies on the administration of boron compounds, based on the harmless boron-10 isotope (^{10}B) combined with thermal or epithermal neutron radiation. The ^{10}B isotope is found in the ratio 1:4 in relation to ^{11}B isotope in nature and its use is due to the crash session 6 times higher. The neutron component has little effect on normal or tumor tissue because thermal neutrons have insufficient energy to damage tissue. In the absence of neutrons, the boron compound is a non-toxic and non-radioactive agent that accumulates into cancer cells. When the cells are irradiated with thermal neutrons a capture nuclear reaction is induced in ^{10}B converting it into ^{11}B, which decays by emission of highly ionizing alpha particles, quite toxic to cells, in other words, when the ^{10}B isotope is exposed to neutrons, the ^{10}B nucleus captures a neutron and promptly emits an alpha particle while the resulting lithium-7 nucleus recoils. Both the recoil lithium ion and the alpha particle are classified as high linear energy transfer radiation, and are highly destructive to cells within a short distance [1]. This therapy essentially combines a radiosensitizer, ^{10}B, with a nonionizing radiation, thermal neutrons, constituting a binary system. An advantage of a binary system would be that each component can be manipulated independently to maximize selectivity [2].

International efforts have been made by clinicians, physicists, chemists and biologists for over 60 years focused on the development and testing of BNCT in the cancer treatment [3-7]. The most clinical interest in BNCT has focused primarily on the treatment of gliomas, metastatic melanoma, head and neck and liver cancer [8-11]. Still, there are new studies in progress with other cell lines and patients' biopsies, including thyroid carcinoma, oral cancer, and prostate cancer, among others.

Research in the area of development of boron-containing delivery agents for BNCT started a few years ago with the investigation of a large number of low molecular weight boron compounds, from which the first generation agents emerged. The most important requirements for a BNCT delivery agent are: low toxicity and normal tissue uptake, with a tumor: normal tissue and tumor: blood (T:Bl) boron concentration ratios of 3; tumor boron concentration of 10-30 μg/g weight or 10^9 atoms/cell; relatively rapid clearance from blood and normal tissues, and persistence in tumor during neutron irradiations [12]. Furthermore, to have benefits, enough thermal neutrons must be absorbed to cause lethal damage from the ^{10}B (n,α) ^{7}Li capture reaction [3]. Neutron irradiations should be performed at the point in time after the boron compound is administered, when there is both a high absolute boron concentration in the tumor and high tumor/normal tissue and tumor/blood ratios. The destructive effects of these high energy particles are limited to boron containing cells and since they have short-range in tissues (5–9 μm). In-depth knowledge on the boron bioavailability in normal tissues may offer another starting point for treatment optimization, because it is an important parameter that influences normal tissue injury. Therefore, BNCT can potentially target neoplastic tissue selectively and provides a method to destroy malignant cells selectively with minimal effects on adjacent normal cells [12].

BNCT has two advantages. Firstly, the dose of radiation given in the neutron beam can be quite low; secondly, the local decay and action allow the surrounding healthy tissue to be spared damage due to radiation. This therapy can be used to eliminate tumor cells whose precise location may not be fully known to prevent residual cancer cells from causing tumors to recur [13]. This innovative therapy has been carried out in the USA, Japan, Netherlands, Argentina, Italy, Finland, German, Argentina, Sweden among others [14].

The success of BNCT depends on the preferential uptake of boron by the malignant cell. The two most common ^{10}B-carriers used in clinical BNCT trials designed for the treatment of melanomas, malignant gliomas, inoperable head and neck tumours and oral cancer are sodium mercaptoundecahydrododecaborate-^{10}B (sodium borocaptate-^{10}B, BSH, $Na_2{}^{10}B_{12}H_{11}SH$) and boronophenylalanine-^{10}B (BPA, C9H1210BNO4). The delivery of ^{10}B by BSH relies on passive diffusion from blood to brain tumor through a disrupted blood–brain barrier. Regularly, the BSH results in a high concentration of boron in blood and subsequent vascular damage during BNCT]. BPA is an analog of the essential amino acid phenylalanine and is actively taken up in cells not only as an amino acid analogue for protein synthesis, but also as a tyrosine analogue for melanogenesis [15]. Then, BPA is considered to be mostly taken up by active transport across the cancer cell membrane [16] and this transport mechanism happens even in normal cells leading to the accumulation of BPA in normal brain, although at a lower rate [17]. Furthermore, the system L-amino acid transporter-1 (LAT-1) can import BPA into cells and may play a major role in the effectiveness of BPA-based boron neutron capture therapy [18]. The availability of boron-containing compounds and new agents for selective delivery to the specimen with the help of boron nitride nanotubes, monoclonal antibodies, liposomal delivery, and immunoliposomal conjugation with endothelial growth factor and vascular endothelial growth factor receptors are being actively studied.

Although these two BNCT agents are being used in clinical trials in Europe and Japan focused on brain tumors, melanomas, head and neck tumors, and liver metastases, there is increasing emphasis on the need of better tumor-targeting BNCT agents [6, 19].

Boron compounds for BNCT do not themselves have any therapeutic effect, however, most boron biodistribution studies was carried out in cell lines or animals, because the methods used to measure the ^{10}B concentration in tissue are generally invasive. Thus, the number of patients who can be included in trials examining only the uptake of compounds in tissue is very limited [11]. Consequently, animal studies play a central role in characterizing the bioavailability of compounds for the rational design of future BNCT trials. Some articles have reported on the boron biodistribution in various models, for example, melanoma in hamsters [15] and in mice [20], undifferentiated thyroid carcinoma in mice [21] and Walker 256 tumors in rats [22].

In the application of BNCT to melanoma, good clinical outcome has been reported [23] because of the high uptake and accumulation of boron in melanoma cells due to elevated melanin synthesis process in these tumor cells [24].

The initial human clinical BNCT experience in patients with melanoma was performed by Mishima after extensive studies in vitro and in vivo. He incorporated ^{10}B into a precursor of melanina, BPA, to satisfy criteria for selective uptake [25]. The melanoma BNCT treatments in Japan by Mishima were followed by Fukuda (1999) [26] and by Busse (1997) [27] in the USA. All of them showed encouraging tumor control rates. BNCT project was started in Argentina during 1998 and thenceforth, the clinical trial phase I/II protocol on cutaneous melanoma have been done for toxicity evaluation [28].

For BNCT to afford selective treatment, it is essential that targeted delivery of boron is achieved; this has been realized using strategies that involve synthetic chemical approaches as well as biochemical and biophysical approaches [29]. Animal models have illustrated that BPA does indeed concentrate in melanoma tumors, however, accumulation is only temporary [30].

Studies in human and murine melanoma model confirm the cell proliferation inhibition by a decrease in cyclin D1 and mitochondrial electric potential, with apoptosis by DNA fragmentation and cell death mainly occurring in the tumor cells as a result of free radical production. BNCT also inhibited *in vivo* melanoma proliferation, extracellular matrix alteration and induced apoptosis by regulating Bcl-2/Bax expression, as well as increasing the levels of TNF receptor and cleaved caspases [31]. Moreover, normal melanocytes, used as normal cells control, did not present significant differences in cell density, metabolism, proliferation and cell death. There are few published results about the effects of BNCT on normal tissues compared to melanoma [32] and these data are extremely important in balancing the effectiveness of BNCT against its side effects on healthy tissues. Some mechanisms involved in damaging the tumor as a result of BNCT are still unknown.

There is still a need for studies that aim to BNCT radiobiology, as well as the development of new ^{10}B-carriers. The elucidation of the mechanisms involved in cell death and inhibition of tumor cell proliferation after BNCT treatment have been studied and will be the subject of further studies for the next years to include the BNCT as standard therapy for patients with melanoma.

References

[1] Petersen, MS; Petersen, CC; Agger, R; Sutmuller, M; Jensen, MR; Sørensen, PG; Mortensen, MW; Hansen, T; Bjørnholm, T; Gundersen, HJ; Huiskamp, R; Hokland, M. Boron nanoparticles inhibit tumour growth by boron neutron capture therapy in the murine B16-OVA model. *Anticancer Res*., 2008; 28(2A), 571-6.

[2] Byvaltsev, V; Kanygin, V; Belykh, E; Taskaev, S. Prospects in boron neutron capture therapy of brain tumors. *World Neurosurg*., 2012; 78(1-2), 8-9.

[3] Barth, RF; Coderre, JA; Vicente, MG; Blue, TE. Boron neutron capture therapy of cancer: current status and future prospects. *Clin Cancer Res*, 2005; 11:3987–4002.

[4] Coderre, JA; Turcotte, JC; Riley, KJ; Binns, PJ; Harling, OK; Kiger, WS 3rd. Boron neutron capture therapy, cellular targeting of high linear energy transfer radiation. *Technol Cancer Res Treat*, 2003; 2, 355–75.

[5] Hatanaka; H. *Boron neutron capture therapy for tumors*. Glioma, AB.; Karim, MF.; Lewis, ER., editors. Berlin: Springer; 1991. 233-249.

[6] Li, T; Hamdi, J; Hawthorne, MF. Unilamellar liposomes with enhanced boron content. *Bioconjugate Chem*, 2006; 17, 15–20.

[7] Pellettieri, L; H-Stenstam, B; Rezaei, A; Giusti, V; Skold, K. An investigation of boron neutron capture therapy for recurrent glioblastoma multiforme. *Acta Neurol. Scand*, 2008; 117, 191–197.

[8] Cordoso, JE; Trivillin, VA; Heber, EM; Nigg, DW; Calzetta, O; Blaumann, H; Longhino, J; Itoiz, ME; Bumaschny, E; Pozzi, E; Schwint, AE. Effect of boron neutron

capture therapy (BNCT) on normal liver regeneration: towards a novel therapy for liver metastases. *Int. J. Radiat. Biol*, 2007; 83, 699–706.

[9] Dagrosa, MA; Thomacz, L; Longhino, J; Perona, M; Calzetta, O; Blaumann, H; Rebagliati, RJ; Cabrini, R; Kahl, S; Juvenal, GJ; Pisarev, MA. Optimization of boron neutron capture therapy for the treatment of undifferentiated thyroid cancer. *Int. J. Radiat. Oncol. Biol. Phy*, 2007; 69, 1054–1066.

[10] Kankaaranta, L; Seppala, T; Kovinoro, H; Saarilhti, K; Atula, T; Collan, J; Salli, E; Kortensniemi, M; Uusi-Simola, J; Makitie, A; Seppanen, M; Minn, K; Kotilnoto, P; Anterinen, I; Savolainen, S; Kouri, M; Joensuu, H. Boron neutron capture therapy in the treatment of locally recurred head and neck cancer. *Int. J. Radiat. Oncol. Biol. Phy*, 2007; 69, 475–482.

[11] Wittig, A; Sauerwein, WA; Coderre, JA. Mechanisms of transport of p-boronophenylalanine through the cell membrane in vitro. *Radiat. Res*, 2000; 153, 173–180.

[12] Barth, RF; Vicente, MG; Harling, OK; Kiger, WS, 3rd; Riley, KJ; Binns, PJ; Wagner, FM; Suzuki, M; Aihara, T; Kato, I; Kawabata, S. Current status of boron neutron capture therapy of high grade gliomas and recurrent head and neck cancer. *Radiat Oncol.*, 2012; 7, 146.

[13] Chou, I; Chung, HP; Liu, HM; Chi, CW; Lui, WY. Suitability of boron carriers for BNCT: accumulation of boron in malignant and normal liver cells after treatment with BPA, BSH and BA. *Appl. Radiat. Isot.*, 2009; 67 (Suppl.7–8), S105–S108.

[14] Faião-Flores, F; Coelho, PR; Muniz, RO; Souza, GS; Arruda-Neto, J; Maria, DA. Antitumor potential induction and free radicals production in melanoma cells by Boron Neutron Capture Therapy. *Appl Radiat Isot.*, 2011; 69(12), 1748-51.

[15] Ichikawa, H; Taniguchi, E; Fujimoto, T; Fukumori, Y. Biodistribution of BPA and BSH after single, repeated and simultaneous administrations for neutron-capture therapy of cancer. *Appl Radiat Isot.*, 2009; 67(7-8 Suppl), S111-4.

[16] Wittig, A; Sauerwein, WA; Coderre, JA. Mechanisms of transport of p-boronophenylalanine through the cell membrane in vitro. *Radiat Res*, 2000; 153, 173–80.

[17] Masunaga, S; Sakurai, Y; Tanaka, H; Suzuki, M; Liu, Y; Kondo, N; Maruhashi, A; Kinashi, Y; Ono, K. Effects of employing a ^{10}B-carrier and manipulating intratumour hypoxia on local tumour response and lung metastatic potential in boron neutron capture therapy. *Br J Radiol.*, 2012; 85(1011), 249-58.

[18] Detta, A; Cruickshank, GS. L-amino acid transporter-1 and boronophenylalanine-based boron neutron capture therapy of human brain tumors. *Cancer Res.*, 2009; 69(5), 2126-32.

[19] Kabalka, GW; Yao, M-L. The synthesis and use of boronated amino acids for boron neutron capture therapy. *Anti-cancer Agents Med. Chem*, 2006; 6, 111–125.

[20] Faião-Flores, F; Coelho, PR; Arruda-Neto, JD; Camillo, MA; Maria-Engler, SS; Rici, RE; Sarkis, JE; Maria, DA. Boron uptake in normal melanocytes and melanoma cells and boron biodistribution study in mice bearing B16F10 melanoma for boron neutron capture therapy. Radiat Environ Biophys., 2012; 51(3), 319-29.

[21] Dagrosa, MA; Viaggi, M; Rebagliati, RJ; Batistoni, D; Kahl, SB; Juvenal, GJ; Pisarev, MA. Biodistribution of boron compounds in an animal model of human undifferentiated thyroid cancer for boron neutron capture therapy. *Mol Pharm.*, 2005; 2(2), 151-6.

[22] Suzuki, M; Nagata, K; Masunaga, S; Kinashi, Y; Sakurai, Y; Maruhashi, A; Ono, K. Biodistribution of 10B in a rat liver tumor model following intra-arterial administration of sodium borocaptate (BSH)/degradable starch microspheres (DSM) emulsion. *Appl Radiat Isot*., 2004; 61(5), 933-7.

[23] Mishima, Y. 1997. Melanoma and nonmelanoma neutron capture therapy using gene therapy: overview. In: Larsson, B., Crawford, J., Weinreich (Eds.), *Advances in Neutron Capture Therapy,* vol. 1. Elsevier, 10–25 Medicine and physics.

[24] Hiratsuka, J; Kondoh, H; Tsuboi, T; Yoshino, K; Imajo, Y; Mishima, Y. Selective uptake of para-boronophenylalanine increases in amelanotic elanoma cells transfected by the tyrosinase gene. *Melanoma Res*., 2000; 10(3), 297-302.

[25] Mishima, Y; Ichihashi, M; Hatta, S; Honda, C; Yamamura, K; Nakagawa, T. New thermal neutron capture therapy for malignant melanoma: melanogenesis seeking 10B molecule melanoma cell interaction from in vitro to first clinical trial. *Pigment Cell Res*. 1989; 2, 226–234.

[26] Fukuda, H; Honda, C; Wadabayashi, N; Kobayashi, T; Yoshino, K; Hiratsuka, J; Takahashi, J; Akaizawa, T; Abe, Y; Ichihashi, M; Mishima, Y. Pharmacokinetics of 10B-p-boronophenylalanine in tumors, skin and blood of melanoma patients: a study of boron neutron capture therapy for malignant melanoma. *Melanoma Res*. 1999; 9, 75–83.

[27] Busse, P; Zamenhof, R; MadocJones, H; Solares, G; Kiger, S; Riley, K; Chuang, C; Rogers, G; Harling, O. 1997. Clinical follow-up of patients with melanoma of extremity treated in phase I boron neutron capture therapy protocol. In: Larson, B., Crawford, J., Weinreich, R. (Eds.), *Advances in Neutron Capture Therapy*, vol.I. Elsevier, 60–64.

[28] Menéndez, PR; Roth, BM; Pereira, MD; Casal, MR; González, SJ; Feld, DB; Santa, Cruz, GA; Kessler, J; Longhino, J; Blaumann, H; Jiménez, Rebagliati, R; Calzetta, Larrieu, OA; Fernández, C; Nievas, SI; Liberman, SJ. BNCT for skin melanoma in extremities: updated Argentine clinical results. *Appl Radiat Isot*., 2009; 67(7-8 Suppl), S50-3.

[29] Mehta, SC; Lu, DR. Targeted drug delivery for boron neutron capture therapy. *Pharm Res*. 1996; 13(3), 344-51.

[30] Bonjoch, J; Drew, MG; González, A; Greco, F; Jawaid, S; Osborn, HM; Williams, NA; Yaqoob, P. Synthesis and evaluation of novel boron-containing complexes of potential use for the selective treatment of malignant melanoma. *J Med Chem*., 2008; 51(20), 6604-8.

[31] Faião-Flores, F; Coelho, PR; Toledo, Arruda-Neto, JD; Maria-Engler, SS; Tiago, M; Capelozzi, VL; Giorgi, RR; Maria, DA. Apoptosis through Bcl-2/Bax and cleaved caspase up-regulation in melanoma treated by boron neutron capture therapy. *PLoS One*., 2013; 8(3), e59639.

[32] Faião-Flores, F; Coelho, PR; Arruda-Neto, JD; Maria-Engler, SS; Maria, DA. Cell cycle arrest, extracellular matrix changes and intrinsic apoptosis in human melanoma cells are induced by Boron Neutron Capture Therapy. *Toxicol In Vitro*., 2013; 27(4), 1196-204.

INDEX

A

D

E

F

G

J

K

L

M

N

O

P

Q

R

S

T

U

V

W

X

Y